HEALING MEDICARE

HEALING MEDICARE

Managing Health System
Change the Canadian Way

Michael B. Decter

CANADIAN CATALOGUING IN PUBLICATION DATA

Decter, Michael B.

Healing medicare: managing health system change the Canadian way

Includes bibliographical references and index.

ISBN 0-9698064-1-8 (bound) ISBN 0-9698064-0-X (pbk.)

1. Medical care - Canada 2. Public health - Canada 3. Medical policy - Canada
4. Health planning - Canada I. Title

RA449.D43 1994   362.1'0971   C94-931685-7

Excerpts from the *Living Will* copyright Centre for Bioethics, University of
Toronto, used with permission.

Excerpts from the work of Brendan Kearney copyright Brendan Kearney, used
with permission.

Excerpts from the *KF News*, vol. 26, No. 2, copyright the King's Fund, U.K.

Excerpts from "The Economics of Self-Medication," *Social Policy and
Administration*, vol. 19, No. 3, copyright Professor Michael Cooper

Editor: Ann Decter
Copy editor: Angela Hryniuk
Cover design: Denise Maxwell
Layout: Heather Guylar
Printed and bound in Canada.

Dedication

For Una and Percy Decter, my parents, one a socialist politician and the other an orthopaedic surgeon, both of whom struggled for Medicare's creation during their lives.

And for my children, Geneviève and Riel, and my wife, Lucille, for whom I continue the struggle.

Contents

Preface

Medicare is among the most cherished of Canadian achievements. After twenty-five years, the elimination of finance as a barrier between individual citizens and health care services remains a true Canadian success story. Our pride in Medicare is vitally important. It is a national achievement that compares well with all other industrialized countries. It is as good or better than the others. It is home-grown, made the Canadian way, modelled on our values and not on the importation of a British or American system.

Yet, change is underway in Canadian Medicare; reform which alarms many and sparks emotional debate. Assumptions about what determines our health, and how we organize our health care delivery system, are undergoing profound, necessary rethinking and re-engineering. These changes are crucial to the future of health care in Canada, and on-going evaluation of this reform process is essential. We must monitor whether reforms are eroding or improving our health care system. Are we healing Medicare or harming it?

This book is about managing change. It is a journey, a search for the outlines of Canada's next health care system as it emerges from the struggles of healing professionals, managers, government leaders, researchers and teachers. No lofty utopian goal is intended and no precise description of the future shape of health care is offered. This is not a book about theory. Practical advice and advocacy for constructive and necessary reform are the objectives. Concrete examples of successful modifications illustrate the effectiveness of innovation and an open quest for a better way of doing things.

This book outlines two fundamental shifts — different but interwoven — happening in Canada. The first is a revolution in how we assess the real determinants of our health. Is it the formal health care delivery system or the broader way we live and organize our society that allows us to live longer, healthier lives? Do more doctors and hospitals make us healthier or just treat us more extensively when we are ill? The second revolution is in how we view health care services. There is a dramatic shift from an unquestioning provision of inputs, to a mounting and sustained questioning of outcomes. A debate rages about appropriateness of care, about what works, and how well it works. Consumers no longer take a backseat to providers in the struggle for resource allocation. Re-engineering the supply side of health services is underway. Managing the demand for health services is the next key challenge.

This is not a sterile book of policy concepts. It is a chronicle of the efforts of tens of thousands of Canadians — from Ministers of Health to ward nurses — to keep our health care system affordable and of high quality through constructive change. If I have one clear hope in writing these ideas and experiences it is that we may learn from each other how to succeed in saving our Medicare. We need to accelerate our learning. Providing health care to all Canadians on the basis of needs is a proud, national accomplishment, but sustaining it into the twenty-first century will be hard, hard work.

Complacency and self-congratulation will not serve us well in a difficult financial and policy environment. Resting on our laurels will not maintain public confidence. Openness to change and to learning is essential. The preservation of Medicare is not a task for museum curators who can capture a glorious past like a fossil in amber. Medicare was born out of a struggle for a better way. Healthy Medicare means waging a continuing struggle to serve the larger purpose of the nation. We need the advice and determination of all those who have invested their working lives in health care. We need the nurses as well as the doctors, the workers as well as the managers, the orderlies as well as the researchers. We need leaders in business and labour, as well as those in government and in our universities. We need to care and struggle to succeed. Leadership and vision, not curatorship and hindsight, will enable Medicare to continue.

Quality and Affordability

Many commentators — Canadians and non-Canadians — have fallen into the trap of believing that affordable cost and quality are mutually exclusive objectives. Quality is quite wrongly seen by some as something added on at extra cost. This is not my view. Quality flows from how well the system is organized, from how both consumers and providers are educated, and how individual decisions about care are implemented. The United States spends 35% more of its GNP on health care than Canada, yet this additional spending does not result in better quality medical care or improved health outcomes. Reforms across Canada provide clear evidence that others quality and affordability can be improved *simultaneously*. Day by day quality and affordability are joining the five statutory principles of the *Canada Health Act* as practical foundations of our approach to health care. The right question is not whether we can afford Medicare, it is how can we better allocate resources within health.

Health Economic Development

In Canada, we have a high standard of living. We are no longer able to sustain our living standard by selling wheat or nickel or other natural resources. Canada has developed valuable expertise in various aspects of health care, including health care products, expertise we can export. We can concurrently help the rest of the world to be healthier and boost our economy.

Health care systems are rooted in the culture and values of the society they serve. In 1969, my parents drove me to Boston to begin studies at Harvard College. As we crossed the border I saw a New Hampshire license plate with its very American motto "Live Free or Die," our's read "Friendly Manitoba." I knew I had arrived in another country. The American Declaration of Independence premise of "life, liberty and the pursuit of happiness" contrasts drastically with the Canadian constitutional tradition of "peace, order and good government." The values of Canadians are as deeply entrenched in our health care system as they are in our constitution. The transformation we are undergoing must continue to respect those values.

Healing Medicare is a hopeful book, because I am an optimist about the prospects for our health as individuals and for the health of a reformed Medicare. I draw my confidence from my encounters with the thousands of individual Canadians who work in health care, whether as part-time volunteer hospital trustees, Ministers of Health, ambulance attendants, nurses or doctors. Each contact has left me filled with respect and hope.

We are managing change in Canadian Medicare in our own very distinct classically Canadian fashion. Change is taking place at a different pace with a slightly different approach in each province. Quebec is unique in how it's implementing change in health care.

We invest vast energy debating these changes in each provincial legislatures and in the media. The Government of Canada is somewhat uncertain of its role. There is great, loud political debate. All of this is very Canadian and quite healthy.

There is much to be done. Canadians have the will and the talent to succeed in reforming, healing and sustaining Canadian Medicare. We also have an obligation and an opportunity to use our expertise in the larger world beyond our borders to improve the health of the other five billion people with whom we share this planet. There is urgency to both challenges.

Introduction:
Our Health as a Nation

Over the past forty years life expectancy has improved more than during the entire previous span of human history.... Small-pox which killed more than five million annually in the 1950's, has been eradicated entirely.... Vaccines have dramatically re-duced the occurrence of polio and measles.... Despite these improvements enormous health problems remain.... By 2000 the growing toll from (AIDS) in developing countries could easily rise to more than 1.8 million deaths annually.... Tobacco related deaths from heart disease and cancers alone are likely to double by the first decade of the next century, to two million a year, and, if present smoking patterns continue, they will grow to more than twelve million a year in developing countries in the second quarter of the next century.[1]

The story of the first era of Medicare belongs to Tommy Douglas in his role as Premier of Saskatchewan from 1944 to 1961. As a child, the charity of a doctor enabled Tommy Douglas to avoid permanent damage to his leg. Later in life, the political leader created Medicare amidst the relative poverty of Saskatchewan. Driven by the dream of saving others, not from the charity of physicians, but from the necessity of that charity, Premier Douglas introduced universal hos-pital insurance in Saskatchewan in 1948. The Government of Canada followed in 1957 with the *Hospital and Diagnostic Services Act*, which provided 50/50 cost-sharing to the provinces. By 1961, the entire country had this coverage. When the Co-operative Common-wealth Federation (CCF) — later the New Democratic Party (NDP) — Government of Saskatchewan endured a doctors' strike in 1962

---

1   *Investing In Health, The 16th Annual Development Report of The World Bank,* 1993, Overview, p.1.

to introduce government insurance of physician services, the federal government felt the pressure. The Royal Commission on Health Services, headed by Justice Emmett Hall, prepared the blueprint, and, by 1968, Canada had the Medical Care Act and 50/50 cost-sharing. By 1972, all provinces were in. Canadian Medicare, as we know it, was born.

But, there was a flaw in Medicare. The design, with government as the sole insurer, did not solve the leadership question. Nor did it ensure the dynamism to change and evolve. In 1982, Tommy Douglas reflected on Medicare's progress: "When we began to plan Medicare, we pointed out that it would be in two phases. The first phase would be to remove the financial barrier between those giving the service and those receiving it. The second phase would be to reorganize and revamp the delivery system — and of course, that's the big item. It's the big thing we haven't done yet." [2]

In 1994, Canada has already entered the second era of reorganizing and revamping Medicare. A rational starting point for this second phase of Canadian Medicare is to examine health goals as individuals, and as a nation. Once they are established, we can discuss how to behave and what to invest to achieve these goals. It is also instructive to look beyond the borders of Canada. Which of our goals are shared by other nations, and which are uniquely Canadian?

The key story of the second era may already have taken place in Saskatchewan. In that province, Health Minister Louise Simard converted fifty small, rural hospitals to health centres and transferred the budgets to regional boards, in order to invest in health services. Saskatchewan galvanized other provinces to question what promotes good health and whether health services need to be hospital-based.[3]

Some Canadians doubt that Medicare, stable as it has been, can be made to change fast enough to survive. Their sense of the impossibility of this task often derives from earlier, failed attempts to lead change before it was seen as absolutely necessary. They will

---

2 T.C. (Tommy) Douglas, Interview, 1982, as quoted in *Alberta Roundtable Report*, Government of Alberta, August, 1993, p. 17.

3 Saskatchewan's hospital situation, it should be noted, was more extreme than that of other provinces. For a population of under one million people, Saskatchewan was operating 137 separate hospitals prior to reform or about one hospital for every 7000 residents compared to Ontario with 10.8 million people and 223 hospitals for a ratio of one hospital for every 50,000 residents. Hospital consolidation is an active issue in Ontario, Saskatchewan and virtually every other province.

not be the last reformers to become casualties of the status quo in Canadian health care. My considered view is that necessary chan es are already underway in every Canadian jurisdiction and they are *essential. It is not reform that will bring about the demise of Medicare but the absence of it.*

This book follows four broad themes in the healing of Canadian Medicare and its evolution into a dynamic - and therefore sustainable — system for the next century:

- Re-engineering care delivery
- Restructuring health work, re-skilling and redeploying health workers
- Taking control of individual health and health care
- Health economic development

This agenda for action can achieve the affordability and quality improvements our nation needs from Medicare. The road ahead is not easy or smooth, but the map has been planned and charted by the ideas, advocacy and actions of thinkers and leaders at every level in Canadian health. We only need to look carefully at the evidence and learn from our experiences.

The road ahead cannot be travelled simply by health ministers and their officials. No one group has the legal, intellectual or moral authority to affect the needed reforms alone. We need a much broader base of understanding and popular acceptance. We need requisite political will, leadership and citizen support. Changes require local decisions about how health services are to be delivered, by whom, to whom and where, in the future. Upward delegation to the political level will, in most instances, delay change, making it more abrupt and painful when it finally occurs. Health ministers and premiers have an obligation to provide leadership. But leadership alone will not be enough. The tens of thousands of Canadians who serve as hospital trustees, members of health boards and directors of health organizations must understand and support change. So must the hundreds of thousands of workers who deliver health care services. Without their active support, our elected leaders will have no one to lead.

In a period of change, leaders are among the first casualties. The accelerated turnover of Canadian health ministers, both provincially and federally, reflects the anxiety and political turmoil which accompanies altering our view of health. New methods of leading and consulting are evolving as governments seek to share the difficult burden of public policy choices. We must understand our health care history and learn from it.

Health and health care are different concepts, requiring different goals. For health, a broader agenda is crucial. Our population needs positive action on the issues that pose the greatest threat to life expectancy and health status: unemployment, cigarette smoking, substance abuse, Aboriginal impoverishment and social disintegration, obesity, adolescent suicide and AIDS. As social issues, not illnesses, these cannot be cured by doctors in hospitals. They must, however, be the core of our approach to investing in our health as a nation. Through determined efforts in our communities and workplaces, redirected spending and new laws, we can *improve health where it is really decided.*

In Canada, we invest in health in a myriad of different ways. As individuals when we join a fitness club, buy a bicycle, our weekly groceries or a car, we invest in our health. Some of our investments are subtle. The purchase of a desk chair may have a long-term impact on our back, qualifying it as yet another health investment.

At the community level, housing bylaws, fire regulations and public health initiatives are all health investments. At the provincial government level, investing in health occurs not only when the health ministry budget is shaped but also when decisions are made about housing programmes, environmental regulations and road safety. How should we make these investments? Should we be guided by history and politics or by health evidence? Should we please the crowd by doing what is immediately popular or is there a better way? Governments not only expend financial capital raised by taxation or borrowing, they also expend their "political capital" or credibility, by leading change in society. Narrow interests, hostile to change, are always noisier and more disruptive than the broad public at large. Seat belt legislation was very unpopular with some segments of society when it was introduced. Toughening restrictions on smoking is a continuing challenge. For governments, these are investments, not of tax dollars, but of even scarcer political capital. They are also key investments in determining our future health.

We have success stories to learn from in this field. Automobiles, long a source of pollution, death and injury, have been redesigned and vastly improved. Product safety changes, forced by law and consumers, are only part of this story. Safer roads and greater success in regulating dangerous drivers are also important levers. Non-coercive sanctions, such as altered societal attitudes, are essential tools.

Much remains to be done in restoring the health of our environment, through combatting tobacco use and improving the health of our most impoverished citizens. Investing in health must rank as the most important of our societal goals.

For nearly forty years, our attention has been focused on building an excellent, modern care delivery system. In that period, about half the lifetime of the average person born in our country, life expectancy has grown more than in the previous 5,000 years. Are these two realities connected? Is it really the health care system which has given us greater health status and longer lives? Credit belongs mainly to improvements in income, diet, housing, sanitation and other public policy and social factors. The state of our health is a social issue. And the state of our health determines, to a significant degree, the demands placed upon our health care system.

Re-Engineering Care Delivery

Rapid progress in technology, strained public finances and shifting public expectations are all strong drivers of re-engineering in the care delivery system. Frustrated consumers want a health care system that meets their needs in a high quality, timely fashion. Weary taxpayers want an affordable, cost-efficient system. Technology can help with both tasks, but significant changes in how we do business will be necessary. Simply automating current practices is not evolution. We need to re-engineer care delivery, starting with the basic questions: what are we trying to achieve and how can we achieve it? It means starting over and rethinking the system, using technology as a powerful tool.

Re-structuring/Re-skilling/Re-deploying

How we make change is as important as the change we make. Our humanity demands we pay careful attention to Canadian health care workers, providing opportunities for them to gain the skills to flourish in the new Medicare. Forcing thousands of skilled health workers into unemployment will damage individuals and the nation. Yet any attempt to resist financial and technological pressures, in support of an employment status quo, is doomed to failure. There is a better way, which will require greater cooperation among workers, managers, bargaining agents and governments.

Mechanisms and solid workable approaches are emerging to

create a more skilled *and* flexible workforce in health care. We need to learn from the early successes emerging in hospitals and communities across Canada. We need to ensure that people who work in health care are able to gain the skills to cope with changes in where and how health care is delivered.

Taking Control

Assuming greater personal responsibility for our health and health care is a necessary ingredient in healing Medicare. By taking control of our own health we can live longer in good health. The simple steps are well-known. Stop smoking (or don't start), eat a healthy diet, exercise, and you are well along the road to maintaining health. We can also take more responsibility as consumers of care services by becoming informed decision-makers. We need to ask more questions of health care providers and insist on more and better answers. Effectiveness of treatment depends not only on the skill of the provider, but, also, on the fit between patient circumstance and outcome. Just as we have learned to conserve energy, we must now learn to access health care services, when needed and with full knowledge of consequences. We have an obligation to become *informed* consumers.

Health Economic Development

Health care is one of the major activities in every nation on earth. Although Canadian Medicare should not be slavishly copied from elsewhere, we can learn from experiences in the United States, in Europe and even in the less developed nations of the south.

We also need to heal the Canadian economy. Unemployed Canadians, particularly 1.5 million unemployed Canadians, are a large health problem. Developing a greater capacity to export our excellence in health, by making more health products in Canada and by expanding research, can be a strong contributor to enhanced Canadian economic renewal. Health economic development can improve our economic performance and create jobs in Canada. Jobs and wealth are major determinants of health.

Why Less of the Same Will Not Work

In *The Learning Organization*, Peter Senge points out that sawing a large elephant in two does not give you two smaller elephants.[4] I would add that starving a large elephant will not leave you with a smaller but healthy one, either.

We need to change *how* we do things in Canadian health care, not simply reduce what we do. Less of the same will not work. We need to focus on how we define health and pursue it and how we deliver care and measure its outcome. Simply doing a little less of everything would give us a very expensive and wholly unsatisfactory outcome.

Bad Ideas Which Will Do Harm

There are a few very dangerous ideas loose in the health debate, ideas with surface appeal that camouflage potentially damaging impact. The most seductive and dangerous is the thought that more money will solve the problem. If government can't afford to pay *all* the costs, the refrain runs, why not let consumers pay some of the cost? We already have the second most expensive health care system on the planet. We don't need more money, but better value for the existing spending. Adding more money works to postpone, however briefly, needed reforms.

User fees, often proposed as a funding mechanism, would cause a fundamental and negative shift in the basis of our health care system. There are two foundations on which nations have constructed health and health care delivery systems: ability-to-pay and ability-to-benefit. The American system, which the Clinton administration is trying to reform, is based on ability-to-pay. Our Canadian system is based on ability-to-benefit. In the United States, the care you receive — even the decision about whether you receive care or not — is based upon whether you, or someone else can pay for it. In Canada, the decision about care is based on need. There is no way to "co-mingle" these principles successfully. Once user fees are introduced, there is an inevitable shift towards a mixed or two-tier system. Ability-to-pay takes precedence. How ironic it would be for the Canadian health care system to mirror the American system at the very point when the Americans have decided to shift toward the Canadian ability-to-benefit or, in President Clinton's terms, health

---

4   Peter Senge, *The Fifth Discipline, The Art & Practice of the Learning Organization* (New York: Doubleday, 1990) p. 66.

security, model. Adam Smith's invisible hand works less well when it is wearing a surgical glove. It is neither invisible nor efficient.

Another idea given currency is the Oregon Plan.[5] While the Oregon Plan may constitute progress for Oregon, it offers an old direction for Canada. Concerned about citizens with no coverage, the State of Oregon decided to rank necessary medical procedures. Through a massive public consultation process it created a list of services for which all residents of Oregon would be insured. Oregon chose to draw the line on the list of procedures, rather than on the list of those eligible for coverage. This is accurately viewed as the introduction of the ability-to-benefit principle into the American health care system. Canada may have problems with providing each and every Canadian in our vast territory with access to the same quality of services, but we do not have any groups without coverage. Coverage for all medically necessary services is a basic principle of Medicare. That the definition of medically necessary is undergoing debate and examination in Canada should not cause us to confuse our situation with that of Oregon.

Oregon-style consultation has lessons for Canada, but our situation is fundamentally different. Adopting their approach would be a huge step backward. Canada can go backward and reinstate financial barriers to access or forward and reform the health care system. It is an easy choice.

Technology is often offered as a possible panacea. Like other tools, it depends on how it is applied. Technology without compassion is a bad idea; technology with compassion is a good one. For example, we need to examine whether the technology of respirators and heart pumps is being used to restore life or to prolong death in an intrusive and undesired way. What is the impact of a new information system? Does it assist better patient care? Technology itself, neither possesses or lacks compassion. How we use it determines its outcome. It's not wise to greet each new technology as a universal good and embrace it unquestioningly. A thorough assessment of new technology and thoughtful consideration of the ethics of applying it, is.

---

5 *Prioritization of Health Services*, A Report to the Governor and Legislature, Oregon. Health Services Commission 1993.

Health Goals

Focus on health goals is emerging as the new religion of international development on health. Among international development issues, health has gained prominence with the World Bank. It has agreed to lend money for health purposes and devoted its entire sixteenth annual *World Development Report* (1993) to considerations of health. Closer to home, health goals and visions of health have had prominence in the provinces pursuing health care reforms.

Advocacy for broader health goals and a wider view of health has been with us for two decades. The *Lalonde Report* in 1974 and the *Alma-Ato Conference on Health for All* in 1978 set a framework. The *Alma-Ato Conference* concluded with the goal of:

> The attainment of all of the peoples of the world by the year 2000 of a level of health that will permit them to lead a socially and economically productive life.

An array of Canadian royal commissions, task forces and advisory councils have each made a persuasive case for a vision of health based on broad population health, rather than a narrow treatment of illness. We are gradually embracing these views and acting upon them. Seat belt and tobacco control legislation have their roots in this fertile soil.

Population Health and Health Care Delivery

In Canada, debate about health is generally framed in the terms population health or determinants of health. Depending on provincial jurisdiction and analysis, the argument runs that, while the health delivery system is a contributor to the health status and life expectancy of a population, far larger contributions are made by socio-economic factors. Some of these are: income and its distribution, healthy public policy, the safety of the environment, quality of air, water, and lifestyle choices about consumption of alcohol, tobacco and other substances, as well as diet.

The determinants of health view points to the significant allocation — generally over 90% — of financial resources to the delivery system, and argues that Canada is over-invested in health care delivery at the expense of progress on the other determinants of health. We spend our health dollars treating illness, not developing health. However, Canadian governments do spend significant dollars in housing, education, transportation. Ministries of Health are not the sole players when it comes to investments in health. Advocates of a broad determinants of health approach cite significant differences in health outcomes based on socio-economic status.

At an historic 1992 meeting of all of Canada's Federal, Provincial and Territorial Health and Finance Ministers, a presentation made by the Government of Manitoba indicated that the poorest 20% of Canadians would gain thirteen years of disability-free life if their socio-economic status was the same as the top 40% of income earners in the population. This contrasted with gains of three to five years which could be achieved by the complete eradication of all forms of cancer or heart disease. Evidence of this sort has been available for a number of years. A focus on broader socio-economic factors is now gaining currency, as fiscal pressures force politicians to restrict investment in the health care delivery system.

Public health advocates have suggested that the population health view is simply a rediscovery of the basic principles of public health in Canada. A recent Government of Manitoba document,[6] sets out the argument in this fashion:

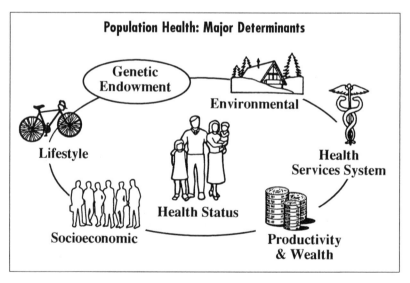

Population Health: Major Determinants

Genetic Endowment

Environmental

Lifestyle

Health Services System

Socioeconomic

Health Status

Productivity & Wealth

Ontario captured the same basic concepts in a vision statement and related health goals.

6 *Quality Health for Manitobans: The Action Plan*, published by the Government of Manitoba, May, 1992, p.9.

A Vision of Health

We see an Ontario in which people live longer in good health, and disease and disability are progressively reduced. We see people empowered to realize their full health potential through a safe non-violent environment, adequate income, housing, food and education, and a valued role to play in family, work, and the community. We see people having equitable access to affordable and appropriate health care regardless of geography, income, age, gender or cultural background. Finally, we see everyone working together to achieve better health for all.

Health Goals for Ontario

Goal 1   Shift the emphasis to health promotion and disease prevention.

Goal 2   Foster strong and supportive families and communities.

Goal 3   Ensure a safe, high-quality physical environment.

Goal 4   Increase the number of years of good health for the citizens of Ontario by reducing illness, disability and premature death.

Goal 5   Provide accessible, affordable, appropriate health services for all.[7]

In Canada, there has been an increased emphasis on *healthy* public policy, following previously explored roads such as compulsory seat belt laws and the much harsher penalties for drinking and driving. New initiatives likely to proceed in some provinces include compulsory use of bicycle helmets, further emphasis on reduction of access to tobacco for young people and diminishing second-hand smoke in various environments. Most Canadian public transportation modes — airplanes, buses, trains — are now largely smoke-free.

Generally, these intrusions by government are met with initial public resistance and become accepted social values. Most governments have newly-appointed senior officials responsible for healthy public policy or population health. In most Canadian jurisdictions, there is a strong emphasis on shifting from investment in the delivery system to a greater focus on population health. Investments in health

---

7   Health goals adopted by the Government of Ontario in 1992 on the advice of the Premier's Council on Health Well Being and Social Justice.

promotion, prevention and healthy public policy are being pursued at both the national and provincial level.

Over the past twenty years a series of commissions, task forces, studies and reports have concluded that:

- The formal health care system is only one factor that affects the health of the population. More important factors are our wealth as a society and how we distribute it, our physical environment, lifestyle choices, educational opportunities, housing, social supports and employment.
- The existing health system concentrates too much on treatment, and the necessary investments in population health are not being made.

What Health Goals Are Not — Eternal Life and Medical Myth-Making

We have been convinced by miracle technology dreams and endless television portrayals of valiant surgeons restoring life that immortality is a goal just beyond the grasp of modern medicine. It is not. Our expectations, and the burdens we place on health goals, must take reality into account. For our species, at this evolutionary point, a life span of seventy to eighty years in reasonable health is achievable. The factors which deprive billions of our fellow human beings of the reasonable expectation of a healthy life are rooted in economic disparities. Poverty is our most damaging global epidemic. Within Canada, our poor are disproportionately our sick.

Our health goals must focus our resources on the greatest good to the greatest number while respecting extraordinary cases. If we are true to our fundamental principle of directing health and health care resources on ability-to-benefit, then our goals must reflect that core value. We must rank comprehensive immunization, safer automobiles, a less violent society and other health goals that can benefit our children and their children, ahead of vastly expensive technologies that prolong dying without gains to quality of life. How to establish, and, more importantly, how to gain acceptance of such broad goals is a challenge faced by each health minister in Canada.

Goals in Health Care Delivery Reform

What should be our health *reform* goal in Canada? What will determine whether we are able to look back on this period, from the vantage point of the late 1990s, and say we made change that led us back to a stable, efficient health and health care? What will cause us to say we are proud of our work in managing change, that it reinforced our core values and principles? It really turns on being able to simultaneously improve both quality and affordability.

The turbulence you see in every provincial jurisdiction as governments, the medical profession and hospitals, try different approaches, is a process of change that will lead us to health care services that are affordable and of better quality. That statement clearly puts me in the category of optimists. I would probably have had trouble getting up in the morning and going to work as Ontario's Deputy Minister of Health if I were not an optimist, because the obstacles to change are formidable.

There are several themes to this shift, all of them essential. There has been a tendency to think we are going to find one answer. That total quality management or clinical epidemiology or determinants of health is *the* answer. We like to think some magic equation or formula is going to get us out of our difficulties. I am not optimistic about magic. We are going to have to work very hard to bring about transformation or improvements that will let us look back at this period as one of constructive reform. There is not likely to be an end to reform. Continuous improvements of quality and a continuous pressure for affordability are most probably permanent features.

Population health requires a revitalized public health system. One of the less-featured aspects of Canada is that we have had historically a very high quality public health system. That system is seen by many as a building block in an approach to healthy communities. Seeing health as an environmental issue, and environment as a health issue, we move forward. It is crucial for communities and individuals, to have a sense of responsibility. Health is not simply a repair business after the fact. Health has a lot to do with individual lifestyle choices: how safe our communities are; how well-designed our roads and cars are; and other aspects of our broader public policy. Within government, it means that the health ministry must advocate in other ministries for change in policies that go to the root causes.

Another theme is clinical epidemiology. Across Canada, in virtually every province, governments are finding ways of establishing, whether it is through commissions or institutes, benchmarking or quality processes, clinical guidelines (essentially applied clinical epidemiology) for the practice of medicine. This cannot be achieved through government dictates that have no credibility with the medical profession. It can be accomplished, rather, by having the best available talent that we have (and we have a good deal of it in this country) communicate with both providers and consumers. This will certainly impact on the knowledge and practice of medicine.

Our health goals underwent a great historic narrowing from the early broad goals of public health to a focus on health care. We are now in the second long wave, a return to comprehensive health goals.

Risk-Taking

Getting to a sustainable future will be neither easy nor smooth. Quality leadership is essential. Professional risks are real for those who lead change and those who support it. Improvements can stall, and those in favour will be discredited and hurt. Risks must not be taken carelessly or recklessly, but they must be taken. Without Tommy Douglas taking a risk, without Emmett Hall and Claude Castonguay possessing courage and vision, we could not have built Medicare.

Stop Blaming

There are no bad guys in the Canadian health care dilemma. We are here with the best of intentions. To quote the famous medical ethicist and philosopher, Pogo:

We have met the enemy
And he is us.

We need to reach beyond the search for villains and into the healing process.

Optimism in a Time of Transition

Change is stressful. One good definition of health is the ability of the organism — be it a person, an organization or a nation — to cope with change. Optimism is an important ingredient in dealing with change and a key ingredient in health. Thankfully, it is also somewhat contagious.

Confidence is part of the necessary optimism for this transition. Confidence to venture along the road of change, without a detailed map, without knowing every twist and turn in advance. Our leaders will be from among us, not delivered from on high. As Peter Senge notes:

> Most of the outstanding leaders I have worked with are neither tall, nor especially handsome; they are often mediocre public speakers; they do not stand out in a crowd; and they do not mesmerize an attending audience with their brilliance or eloquence. Rather, what distinguishes them is the clarity and persuasiveness of their ideas, the depth of their commitment and their openness to continually learning more. They do not have the answer. [8]

Confidence, optimism and openness to learning new ways of working are required attributes to heal Medicare. There are more intelligent questions to be asked than there are answers offered. We will learn by doing, by making mistakes and learning from them. And it is not beyond reason that we might enjoy the challenge of change, rather than facing it with grim determination to survive. Greater mastery over our work should be both a source of pride and joy to each of us.

We have started to build some of the necessary machinery, but it is far from finished. Change might bruise some of the people involved: elected officials and those who serve them; those that deliver care; and those that receive it. It will take some very broad support in our Canadian society to get the job done. I remain an optimist because I see the beginnings of the kind of change that we need.

Good Stuff To Read

World Development Report — 1993 Investing in Health-World Development Indicators published for the World Bank by Oxford University Press, New York, June 1993, is rich in data and analysis. Offering an overview of health and health systems on a worldwide base, it is required reading for those serious about understanding health and health care policy in both the developed and developing worlds. The decision as to which health investments to make is aided by the analytical tools provided. The report advocates sensible investments in public health and essential clinical services.

8   Op. cit., Senge p. 359.

The advocacy of a greater private sector role in clinical services is the sole bit of dubious advice which may reflect the World Bank's private enterprise roots and the current American fascination with managed competition. There is certainly no evidence to support this particular advocacy. The notion that a competitive health insurer model will produce more money for health care is debunked by every serious comparison of Canada and the United States whether conducted by the U.S. General Accounting Office or others. Single payer systems are efficient in administrative terms and should not be discarded as an option by the developing world simply because the United States has moved past the point where vested interests can be overcome in favour of a single payer approach.

Report of the Ontario Premier's Council on Health Strategy. This report and the related reports of the Premier's Council which have evolved to the Premier's Council on Health, Well-Being and Social Justice are solid approaches to broader population health goals. The advice of the Premier's Council was adopted as policy by the Government of Ontario.

Restructuring Canada's Health Services System — How Do We Get from Here to There? Proceedings of The Fourth Canadian Conference on Health Economics, edited by Raisa B. Deber and Gail G. Thompson, University of Toronto Press, 1992, is a rich, well-edited collection of interesting insights and powerful data. It captures valuable drivers of change and a variety of perspectives in a series of readable presentations. A solid, one-stop-shop on Canadian health care issues.

Part 1

Re-Engineering the Care Delivery System

Whatever the grand scheme of things, I hope many people in health services will recognize that small scale change, personal involvement and acceptance of responsibility, some creativity, imagination and friendliness are likely to make things better, and unlikely to make things worse. So far, a better idea eludes us. [1]

Fiona Hastings
Beyond Provider Dominance

Of our twin challenges — investing in health and re-engineering our current health care delivery systems — re-engineering is the more difficult task. Achieving affordability and quality at the same time requires significant change in the way we do business. We may like the results of reform but no one really likes the process. Change means uncertainty, unease and even fear. Exceptional leaders who enjoy change, often have the courage to accept its necessity and decide to have some fun along the way. We will meet a few of these remarkable people, Canadians who are leading reform in health care.

Conceptually, re-engineering the system requires more dramatic reconstruction than simple marginal improvements. As Michael Hammer and James Champy note in *Re-engineering the Corporation,* "When someone asks us for a quick definition of business re-engineering, we say that it means 'starting over.'" Re-engineering doesn't mean tinkering with what already exists or making incremental changes that leave basic structures intact.[2] Instead, Champy and Hammer define it as "the fundamental rethinking and radical redesign of business processes to achieve dramatic improvements in critical, contemporary measures of performance, such as cost, quality, service and speed."[3]

Let there be no doubt about the urgency of the re-engineering challenge in our health care delivery system. Without improvements it will drift rapidly into unaffordable crisis. Fortunately, the urgency of the situation is motivating boards, managers, providers and gov-

1   Fiona Hastings, *Beyond Provider Dominance*, King's Fund, 1993, p.169.
2   Michael Hammer and James Champy, *Re-engineering the Corporation* (New York: Harper Collins Publishers Inc., 1993), p.31.
3   Ibid., 32.

ernments from coast to coast to act quickly. What follows is an effort to capture the direction of constructive reform as well as many of the worthwhile stories about those leading it. Few successes are transportable holus-bolus from one province to another or from one hospital to another. Circumstances are always unique due to differing histories. Nevertheless, we can learn and successfully adapt experiences and ideas to our own situation.

We must keep in mind that we are not starting with a blank canvas. Re-engineering occurs while we continue to deliver care. We need to balance history and values against imperatives for change. The next health care system must arise in an evolutionary way from current realities and cannot be designed or implemented in a vacuum. There are few 'eurekas' in health reform.

Our objective in re-engineering must be to achieve the highest quality health care service possible, in the most appropriate setting, in response to patient needs. This has several implications. We must take a more consumer-centred view, shift to a continuum of care model and detach health care from the hospital bed to which it has been yoked in the past. As services and institutions are unlinked, the basis for previously-defined roles shifts. What was once done by a physician in a hospital might be accomplished, with equal effectiveness, by a nurse in a home. We are headed toward more holistic, integrated health systems planning. Parts of Canada have implemented these approaches, but the shift from a hospital-physician image of health care to a wider, broader view of services and providers is still difficult for many people. New Brunswick's Extramural Hospital[4] — literally, a hospital without walls — is a powerful example of where we must move.

From Insured Services to Managed Delivery Systems

Movement to greater management of the present system is concur-

---

4   The New Brunswick Extra-Mural Hospital was established by the New Brunswick
    Government in 1981. The role of the Extra-Mural Hospital is to provide health
    services in the home setting. With fourteen service delivery units the emphasis has
    been on long-term care. Caseloads in the range of 3400 patients and a spectrum of
    active, palliative and chronic care characterize the activities. In 1992, when New
    Brunswick announced the regionalization and consolidation of the hospital system
    it also announced an expansion of the Extra-Mural Hospital. The most striking
    aspect of the Extra-Mural Hospital is how long it has been a success without
    drawing many imitators across the country. A non-bricks and mortar hospital is
    still too distant a concept for most of us.

rent with the shift to population health. Restructuring, in many parts of Canada, means rapid consolidation. The era of the largely independent hospital, operated by a volunteer board of directors, with a loose relationship to an overall delivery system, is ending. Hospital mergers, regionalization and measurements of outcomes are all themes in recent reforms. Movement towards shared services, regional or district needs-based planning and regional systems is underway.

Five provinces — New Brunswick, British Columbia, Alberta, Nova Scotia and Saskatchewan — have introduced legislation to bring hospitals within regional systems. This follows Quebec. Other jurisdictions are proceeding on a more evolutionary, less legislative path, but are still consolidating hospitals, particularly in multi-hospital centres. Religious owners, largely Catholic, are also examining and undertaking movement towards systems.

In other provinces, major shifts in bed usage and bed allocation is underway. Manitoba has mandated a transfer in bed use of shift patients to community hospital and community care settings. This has been accomplished by significant bed reductions in the two teaching hospitals — the Health Sciences Centre and St. Boniface General Hospital — as well a movement of patients to community hospitals. The opening of additional beds in chronic care hospitals and increased home care are the necessary investments which have enabled the restructuring to proceed.

Restructuring the System to Achieve Effective Patient Care[5]

Re-engineering is not confined to the hospital sector. Major change is also occurring in long-term care, in public health and in how drugs are prescribed, dispensed and managed. In fact, there are few areas of health care which are not undergoing questioning and reworking. The pressures driving these changes are not limited to the financial problems of governments in Canada. Other impetuses, which may be more powerful over the medium term, are changing consumer expectations and the dramatic impact of technology, particularly information technology. It may be that the silicon chip, with its incredible capacity to make information an inexpensive commodity,

5 *Quality Health for Manitobans: The Action Plan*, Government of Manitoba, May, 1992, p.28.

Restructuring the System to Achieve Effective Patient Care: An Example

becomes one of our greatest allies in re-engineering health care services.

Where does the responsibility for re-engineering lie? Is it the job of ministries of health? Of hospital managers? Of trustees? Of all those who represent the public interest on District Health Councils in Ontario or on health services boards in Saskatchewan? *All of the above* is the best answer. The task is so large and diverse that all parties will need to be involved and share responsibility. There is no single right answer or pat, cookie-cutter solution.

Ministers and departments of health will need to show leadership through clear direction and policies. They may decide to restructure health governance in order to provide a broader investment in health and health services. This process has gone through several phases in Quebec. Government should not, however, try to micro-manage change and usurp the role of hospital and community health governances. Rather, the citizen governors who serve as board members of hospitals, health councils, community health centres and the like should shoulder the governance role in times of change, as well as in times of preserving services. It is not enough for a board to meekly accept the advice of management. Board members must ensure that the advice conforms to changing and evolving community expectations. It is no longer enough to know that physicians, nurses and other providers support new directions. Consumers must also have a voice. Boards must carefully balance the views of providers and management but they must *act* in the interests of those with health care needs. Service to the consumer hasn't often received the central role in health care delivery discussions. Boards have a vital role in shifting this aspect of decisionmaking. Archimedes once commented that with a long enough lever he could move the earth. The consumer is a lever long and powerful enough to move the health care system, but only with the active support of informed board members.

Hospital management teams need to lead change and ensure more active participation from staff at all levels. Advisory groups established at the community, district or regional level must balance their advice. The need for evolutionary, not revolutionary, reform of service delivery must be accompanied by tough-minded questioning of old solutions and conventional wisdom. As advisors on health as well as health care delivery, these groups must be open to new investments that assist health status. Each group playing its appropriate role will combine to create successful change.

New partnerships are being created to bring together the necessary participants in managing change. Partnerships evolving between providers of health services and payers (largely governments) is one essential element. However, broader partnerships must involve representatives of an array of community and institutional governances, the boards that direct managers in the system. In most provinces, reforms are consolidating governances and agencies. Consumers must occupy more seats at more decision-making tables. Partnerships need to share risks and rewards to succeed. They also require clarity as to roles, not a naive assumption of common interests.

Successful policy making is tough in health care delivery, implementation is far more difficult. Making change at the field level will be a major, continuing theme. Some parts of the medical profession have long since adopted clinical practice guidelines, and others are contemplating them. Clinical guidelines will only work if they are seen to be developed independent of government, scientifically credible and based on the evidence. If we apply more of what we know about outcomes and evidence to the practice, we will simultaneously improve both quality and affordability in the system. Physicians will change their behaviour when confronted with evidence, not exhortation.

Better Management

Better management at all levels, improved application of technology and more feedback loops for information, are some areas of significant success. Better management will require new tools and new incentives. Managers are rewarded for maintaining the status quo, not for administrating change. In fact, the stability of Canadian Medicare supports the skill of managers in resisting change. There must be a shift in the incentive structure to reward managers for implementing change.

In comparison with the Americans, we are often complimented for our leanness on the management side. In fact, recent studies published by both the *New England Journal of Medicine*[6] and the General Accounting Office in the United States,[7] concluded that if the Americans could reduce their administrative costs to the Canadian level they could provide coverage for those thirty-five million Americans currently without it. Though this may be heresy, I would suggest that we may be a little too lean on the management side. I know many readers will say that "My hospital management doesn't feel very lean. It has been adding layers of management for as long as I can remember," and that may well be true. However, at the central or government level we have largely been an insurance agency, a collection of bill payers, rather than having analytical capacity to ask real outcome questions. We have not been asking tough enough questions about results as we pay for the inputs. We have lacked management in managing the outcomes rather than inputs. This additional management should not be translated as more managers' jobs but rather as more managerial responsibility for everyone who works in health care delivery.

This situation is changing. In Canada, there has been a dramatic movement in the last few years to more day and outpatient surgery

---

6 Redelmeier et al., "Hospital Expenditures in the United States and Canada," *New England Journal of Medicine*, March 18, 1993.
7 General Accounting Office, *Canadian Health Insurance Lessons for the United States: Report to the Chairman, Committee on Government Operations, House of Representatives*. GAO Publication No. GAO/HRD-91-90, B-244081. U.S. Government Printing Office, Washington, 1991.

resulting in profound impact on the system of enhanced affordability and quality. Rethinking how hospitals look at themselves — from essentially a collection of beds that are managed, to being a collection of services that may or may not be linked to a bed — has begun.

In Windsor, Calgary, Edmonton and Vancouver and in many other communities, the more difficult task of the inter-hospital rationalization is underway. Across the country, governments are putting significant funding into information systems. In the Ontario Drug Benefit Program, as a result of automation, the government will be able to not pay for the dispensing of the same prescription multiple times to a senior who has visited multiple doctors. Ontario, like Saskatchewan, will have a real time, on-line drug information system and will catch fraudulent transactions. The pharmacist filling the prescription will know whether that prescription has been filled recently and whether the prescription they are filling will interact in a negative way with other medication the patient is on. Eventually, all hospital emergency rooms will be linked into the system. Patients presenting for treatment will have their drugs identified rapidly whether they are conscious or unconscious. Physicians offices will eventually be linked up, but that is a longer term proposition.

These are a few examples. The point is that there are real gains in better management at all levels. This is not advocacy for more managers, rather, for acquiring the tools to really manage. Information systems and outcomes research are part of getting management information to providers to make decisions about health care. We must not add layers of management, instead we should be removing layers. We should increase accountability — whether with physicians or nurses — at the front line, for managers and workers. The purpose is not to put anyone in conflict with their professional responsibilities to the patient by imposing additional work, but to enlist the help of those who know what actually goes on. The possibility of improvement depends on the active support and participation of all health workers in change.

Technology Assessment

Finding the right place for technology, and harnessing it to care and compassion, is a priority in many areas of health care reform. Technology includes not only medical devices and equipment, but also drugs, techniques and procedures, plus the systems that support the delivery of care. Decision-making through technology assessment is about balancing cost containment and the desire to provide the latest technology.

The image of new technology as always driving up costs is simplistic and inaccurate. For example, laparoscopic surgery has been receiving coverage in the journals as a minimally-invasive alternative to traditional surgery. Laparoscopic or "keyhole" surgery involves small incisions rather than large ones and use of new techniques like fibre-optics. Laparascopic cholecystectomy or "lap-choly" is the removal of the gall bladder utilizing the techniques of laparoscopic surgery. Patients can expect a one-night stay in hospital and a return to work within seven to ten days, rather than five to seven days in hospital and six weeks recovering at home from conventional gall bladder removal surgery.[8] In fact, in the U.S. today 30% of patients undergo the operation on a day-surgery basis.

From the patient's point of view, this surgical option also means less pain and probably lower risk of complications. For the hospital, the significant reduction in length of stay produces major savings in acute service costs. The capital costs of setting up the service can be quickly recovered, after which the hospital is ahead financially. Laparoscopic surgery is a technology that has potential to cut costs and improve quality. However recent evidence suggests that cholecystectomy rates are rising due to the convenience and speed of the laparoscopic procedure.[9]

To continue to afford the latest technology, we need better assessment and better planning. Technology assessment is the basis for information-based decision-making and it is an integral part of the move toward more accountable, quality-assured, outcome-oriented health care.

Through more rigorous analysis the bane of medical technology, the fact that in health care the new rarely drives out the old, might be overcome. Every new development tends to become an add-on, creating new demands rather than replacing existing services. Better comparisons between technologies can tell us exactly which old

---

8   Dr. John V. White, "Laparoscopic Cholecystectomy: The Evolution of General Surgery," Dr. John V. White, *Annals of Internal Medicine*, October 15, 1991, Volume 115, Number 8, p. 651-653.

9   Private correspondence June 2, 1994 with Dr. David Naylor in which he references work by the Epstein Group at Harvard as published in the *New England Journal of Medicine*, 1994 and unpublished work by Marsha Cohen of Institute for Clinical Evaluative Sciences (ICES). Rising number of procedures with lower rates of death and complication per procedure. This underscores the complexity of any technology change in health care.

devices and services should be replaced when new options come on stream.

The essential first step in assessing a technology is randomised clinical trials to demonstrate clinical effectiveness. Such trials are routinely performed on drug therapies but, are used much less for other therapeutic and diagnostic technologies. It is clear from the literature that uncontrolled studies often produce wrong answers. There is no substitute for rigorous scientific controls. More and more, those who pay for new technologies are going to insist on proof that they work. This will challenge medical device manufacturers to conduct clinical trials and produce credible research results.

But clinical effectiveness is not the end of the issue. We also need to weigh cost effectiveness. We need to ask how a new technology compares to existing alternatives in terms of costs and benefits. Cost-benefit analysis is based on quantitative measurements, such as the cost in dollars per life-year gained. Work is also being done on ratios that reflect quality of life factors. The techniques of economic evaluation will continue to become more refined and helpful to decision-makers. There is still a great distance to be travelled to make this analysis of practical value in day-to-day decisions.

A recent article in the *New England Journal of Medicine*[10] compared hospital expenditures in Canada and the United States. After adjusting for case mix and other variables, the authors estimated that resources used for inpatient care per admission were 24% higher in the U.S. than in Canada. One of the main reasons appeared to be greater centralization of specialized equipment and personnel in Canada, leading to higher efficiency.

MRI — Magnetic Resonance Imaging — the most effective replacement to old X-Ray technology, is an example. In the U.S. there are about 3,000 MRI machines, whereas in Canada there are twenty-eight, eleven units per million population in the U.S. and one per million in this country. In Ontario, there are ten MRI units operating and one more approved, all in health science centres. We must proceed with caution in relaxing our controls on the proliferation of technology. Nevertheless, ministries of health in every Canadian jurisdiction are under some pressure to revise policies regarding MRI, and a range of other technologies.

The stakes are high. If we misallocate financial and human

10 Redelmeier, Donald and Victor Fuchs, "Hospital Expenditures in the United States and Canada," *New England Journal of Medicine*, March 18, 1993, p. 772-778.

resources to an inappropriate technology, we are diverting resources from cost-effective technologies. And that means patients who would have benefited will not. On the other hand, if we invest wisely in technology, population health will improve.

We can also take cost-benefit analysis the next logical step and compare new medical technologies, not with other medical technologies, but with alternative investments in the broader determinants of health. Perhaps instead of buying the latest medical equipment we should insist on better driver training, add fibre to foods or invest more in job training. These questions on the determinants of health are ultimately political ones for government to decide on behalf of and in consultation with the public.

The key to getting the maximum value from technology — to meeting patient needs within affordable budgets — is co-operation among hospitals and physicians. We are beginning to see a determined effort at various levels in health care to assess technology more rigorously and distribute it more rationally. Assessments are occurring within the larger context of the managed re-engineering of the health care delivery system to bring costs under control and emphasize the larger determinants of health. Through partnership we can succeed in creating a sustainable and affordable health care system in which continuous quality improvement is a reasonable expectation.

Chapter 1
Hospital Services

Boards should meddle. To begin with, there is no way to stop them, and if you can't lick them, you had better join them! Board members of a non-profit organization should be committed to the cause. They should be deeply interested and involved in it, they should know the programmes and the people who work on them, and they should *care*. But also, non-profit boards are usually organized in such a way that 'meddling' is part of their job.[1]

Managing For The Future
Peter F. Drucker

In attempting to arrive at the truth I have applied everywhere for information, but in scarcely an instance have I been able to obtain hospital records fit for any purposes of comparison. If they could be obtained they would enable us to decide many other questions besides the one alluded to. They would show subscribers how their money was being spent, what amount of good was really being done with it, or whether the money was not doing mischief rather than good.[2]

Florence Nightingale, 1863

The re-engineering of health services delivery in Canada is changing

---

1 Peter Drucker, *Managing For the Future* (Butterworth and Heinemann: London, U.K. 1993), p. 176-177.
2 Florence Nightingale, as quoted by Mr. Frank Maynard, Deputy Minister of Health for Manitoba in presentation to meeting of Deputy Ministers of Health, Fall 1993, Hull, Quebec.

the nature of our nine hundred hospitals in many ways. Fifty-two small hospitals in rural Saskatchewan are being closed or converted to community health services. Large hospitals across Canada are closing, in total, thousands of beds. In many mid-sized Canadian cities, the existing four or five hospitals will be reorganized in the next few years into one or two facilities. In a number of two-hospital towns or small cities one hospital is to remain for acute care while the other becomes a long-term care facility. Why is this happening? Is this re-engineering or simply shutdown?

The forces driving hospital change are powerful and continuing. The changes which we are witnessing need to be accelerated, not slowed down, if our hospitals are to keep pace with the combined forces of technology and changing medical practice, and cope with reduced funding from governments. Historically, our hospitals were like hotels, where doctors and nurses provided care to patients. Hospitals were measured by how many beds they had and the task of the hospital administrator was very focussed on managing the 'inn'. Our vocabulary has lagged behind the dramatic change in the role and management of the hospital. Ask the president of a hospital to describe his or her facility and, in most cases, you will still get the bed count early in the reply. But beds are no longer the right measure. Hospitals have become a key delivery point for a vast array of services, which have been unbundled from the bed or hospital stay. Rapid movement of many services from inpatient to outpatient, the explosion in growth of day surgery and impressive technological advances to much less intrusive ways of treating patients, have altered hospitals. The new role of a hospital is as physical structure where a range of treatment services is managed, some of which may involve a hospital stay, but many of which do not.

For health services which still require a hospital stay, the length of that stay is being dramatically shortened and the quality in the outcome improved. Techniques for better management of bed utilisation have gained importance. Many hospitals are working out the consequences of these changes and finding ways of reshaping their operations. The smart ones are asking their workers for ideas. The Woodstock General Hospital in Ontario is one of the smart ones. Some comments on the Woodstock re-generation:

We decided to reduce our days, cycle days from a fourteen-day menu cycle to an eight-day cycle menu. That depresses our food inventories in the department. So that helps our cost and we don't have food just sitting in inventories waiting to be used.

Kris Lavoie,
food services manager

For years, the menus changed every two weeks. Then, one of the kitchen workers pointed out that patients don't stay in hospital for two weeks anymore, so they changed the cycle and that saves money. They changed the way they scheduled Operating Rooms and that saves $100,000 a year. They consolidated two critical care units and saved $300,000.

Bob Johnston,
CBC News

Just a few years ago, we used to bring them in for a couple of days to do tests on them. Before we made this change, you'd have two more days; now, we do all that testing on an out-patient basis. Just bring you in, in many cases, on the day of your surgery. And with the changes in techniques, more and more folks are going home that same day.[3]

William Pobe,
hospital administrator

The Woodstock General Hospital changed its employee suggestion programme two years ago. The new rule was that employees would be told where their idea had gone and why. The number of suggestions increased from twelve the year before the new rule, to 366 the following year.

When St. Boniface Hospital in Manitoba undertook a major restructuring project[4] in 1993, it gathered ideas from all staff at all levels. Of the 2,300 ideas submitted, a steering committee, with representation from all levels including the bargaining agent, approved 129 recommendations to proceed to implementation. These ideas will save the hospital $13.5 million over three years or nearly 10% of the hospital's budget.

These examples suggest a dangerously radical three-step plan for

3   C.B.C. Radio News Broadcast, Toronto 7:30 a.m. EDT, October 18, 1993.
4   Presentation by Mr. Jack Litvack, CEO, St. Boniface General Hospital, to the Canadian Institute Conference, Re-engineering Hospitals, Toronto, April 11-12, 1994.

achieving efficiencies through changing the way activities are carried out in hospitals:

Step 1. **Ask the people who work there, all of them.**

Step 2. **Take the ideas seriously — implement the good ones.**

Step 3. **Have enough respect to tell them what happened to their ideas, both the good and the not-so-good ones.**

The Japanese quality revolution in the automobile industry was accomplished by re-engineering the car and how it was made. Employee suggestions played a key role in Japan's automotive success, as did continuous quality improvement processes. Eventually, as their market share eroded, North American car makers had to follow suit.

Consider the dramatic changes in the automobile over thirty years. Consider also that you would have been regarded as a dangerous radical to predict in 1963 that today's cars would be lighter, more fuel efficient, safer and less polluting. In developments which have saved hundreds of thousands of lives, the automobile has advanced dramatically. The one thousand dollar plus per car of safety equipment includes seat belts, side impact bracing in doors, airbags, anti-lock brakes, and crash crumple zones, front and back. All this and cars are still about one thousand pounds lighter due to advanced materials. On the pollution side the progress is even more dramatic. The 1963 model emitted 96% more hydrocarbons, 96% more carbon monoxide, and 76% more nitrous oxide.[5] Lead fumes have been totally eliminated by taking lead out of the fuel. Can we re-engineer the hospital in as total a fashion as the automobile? Are hospitals so different from our automakers? The scale of hospital enterprise dwarfs the automobile industry. The nine hundred hospitals in Canada employ three hundred and fifty-thousand workers, the auto industry barely one hundred thousand.

Canada's nine hundred hospitals are overseen by volunteer boards of trustees. This aspect of health care governance is a significant strength, if the trustees take their governance responsibilities

---

5   Al Haas, ''Today's cars are leaps ahead of yesterday's guzzlers,'' *Toronto Star*, March 28, 1992, p. K23.

seriously and if they have the tools to do their job. High quality information is the most important of these tools, without it, effective governance is thwarted and the board of trustees can be quietly reduced to fundraisers and boosters for the hospital's cause. These are both legitimate and necessary roles, but fall short of full, responsible governance. Trustees must demand sufficient information to do their jobs, and hold hospital management accountable for achieving the goals and mission of the hospital.

Advocating that hospital boards fulfil their entire role is not an argument for their intrusion into the role of hospital management. A proper balance of roles clearly separates the task of *governing* — setting direction, priorities, establishing policy, approving a strategic plan and approving the budget — from the task of *managing* — hiring and managing staff, monitoring progress towards goals, implementing policy and administering the spending of the approved budget.

What follows are my best twenty ideas for saving money and improving quality in the hospital system, gleaned from three decades of visiting hospitals, consulting in hospitals and serving in government. Where possible, I have given examples, named names and told stories. I apologize to my colleagues and many friends in the health consulting business for giving away trade secrets at a low price. However, my apology is limited by the limited time we have to keep Medicare accessible and affordable. There is also no shortage of work for health care consultants. Every single idea on the list has already been successfully implemented somewhere in Canada. By sharing, we can all climb the necessary learning curve at a faster pace.

If you are a health care manager you have a ready source of hundreds of additional ideas available from your employees, and from the physicians and other professionals, who are part of your institution. If you are willing to listen and to let them know which ideas worked and which did not, this is a well that will not run dry. If you are a trustee or board member, here are a few meddlesome questions to ask yourself, your fellow trustees and your management team. I don't completely subscribe to management guru Peter Drucker's meddlesome views of boards noted earlier. A gently managed conspiracy between the board chair and the chief executive officer should focus the meddling board on a constructive set of tasks.

Here is the hospital-money-saving-quality-improving question and idea list. A word of warning: while some of these questions should only be attempted by trained professionals, most are just organized common sense!

Informed and Dangerous
— A Few Questions Trustees
To Ask Themselves and Hospital Management

Big Questions About Hospitals

1 **Does your hospital really need to exist at all?**

We might as well deal with the toughest question first. Is there another nearly identical hospital across the street or down the road? Are you both needed or would one hospital be enough? Could the elimination of all the non-patient care costs in one hospital provide both savings and more dollars for patient care in your community? Who are the major beneficiaries of the continued existence of the hospital? Providers? Consumers? The community? Is the benefit primarily a health benefit or an economic benefit? This is one for the chair of the board to consider with a handful of key and trusted board members.

A gut-wrenching, but good litmus test for chairs of small hospitals is whether they would themselves use the services of the hospital in an urgent care situation. If the answer is no, that may be the beginning of the answer to the basic question.

In many communities, consumers are voting with their feet by seeking care in the nearest regional centre. In communities such as Sault Ste. Marie, Ontario, two hospitals across the street from each other have merged into one hospital. The bottom line needs to be resources for health care not preservation of bricks and mortar.

2 **Could your hospital dramatically alter its role with a benefit to the overall system?**

The future of Doctor's Hospital in Toronto has brought down health ministers and sparked enormous political controversies over the past fifteen years. Yet, recently the board of the hospital, the Ontario Government and the Metro Toronto District Health Council unanimously agreed to rebuild the aging facility as an innovative ambulatory care centre. Downtown Toronto is knee-deep in closed, never to be re-opened hospital beds. The Doctor's Hospital decision is to transform into a sensible accommodation with a new and important role, which builds on the strengths of the organization without adding to a growing problem of excess hospital bed capacity.

Does it still need to be an acute care hospital? Across Saskatchewan a number of small, under utilized community hospitals are being converted to better serve chronic care needs or to become community health centres.

 Should your hospital's role be a smaller subset of its current activities? Should you specialize or become a long-term care facility? Do more of what you're really good at and less or none of the rest?

In Guelph, Ontario, twenty-five years of discussion and a report by a Committee chaired by Bill Blundell culminated in the decision by the Sisters of St. Joseph where their hospital would become a long-term care facility and the Guelph General Hospital would focus on acute care.

When the Toronto Hospital, Canada's largest hospital, declared two years ago that it would no longer be all things to all patients, the world moved in Canadian hospital thinking. If even the biggest cannot do everything well, should other hospitals consider a narrower, more collaborative role? In June, 1994, the Toronto Hospital and the Princess Margaret Hospital have formed a Joint Venture Council to lead comprehensive cancer care services.

 How are you restructuring services and roles with other hospitals and health service providers?

Planning for restructuring of hospital services has become a central activity in Windsor, Ontario,[6] in Victoria, B.C. and in dozens of other cities and regions across Canada. Has your hospital joined as an active participant in planning for future services or are you waiting for someone else to take the lead?

As governments continue to pressure for a broader continuum of care extending from home to community to hospital and back, your linkages with community services will become extremely important. How strong are those linkages? Do patients remain longer in hospital because relationships with home care are not well developed? Does your emergency ward fill with social admissions who might be better

6   *An Evolving Plan For Total Health System Reconfiguration* — The Essex County
    Win-Win Model — The Final Report of the Steering Committee on
    Reconfiguration, Essex County, District Health Council, Windsor, February, 1994.

served by a community shelter or drop-in centre? Have you considered an advisory board or board committee link to other service providers in the community? Have you ever considered using your hospital's ability to raise capital dollars as an asset in a partnership with community agencies who may need new facilities?

In Edmonton, a report by Dr. John Atkinson recommends extensive consolidation of hospital services.[7] In Calgary, Mr. Lou Hyndman has chaired a similar review.[8] In Winnipeg, the Bell-Wade Report[9] recommends a reordering of teaching hospital programme responsibilities. Will your hospital undertake a constructive, leadership role in the realignment heading your way? Are you preparing your board, management team and staff for change?

Some Questions on Patient Care Servies

What patient care services does your hospital provide? Where and how? Before we get to all the standard and important questions of effectiveness and efficiency, we need to consider what services are delivered and in what setting. The unbundling of services from the bed extends the full spectrum.

5 **Inpatient, Outpatient or Somewhere Else?**

Changing the setting for delivering health care services has been the major shift in the hospital sector over the past five years. In 1989, Ontario's hospitals had 48,989 beds. By 1994, we had reduced the number of beds by 7,889. How? Did people in Ontario become miraculously healthier in this period? No. The answer lies in a real shift in hospital activity from inpatient to outpatient and day surgery. Services increased during this period. With nearly 8,000 fewer beds, Ontario hospitals increased acute cases by 1.3 million or 8.8% (1989-90 to 1993-94) and outpatient services by 10.4%. Overall productivity increased by 18.5% due to a 20% decline in length of stay from 8.2. days to 6.5. days.[10]

---

7   Dr. John Atkinson, Tannis Chefurka, "Principles and Programs for Edmonton Regional Health," a.k.a. the *PAPER* Report, for the Edmonton Region Health Faculties Planning Council, Edmonton, March 1994.

8   *Report of the Calgary Facilitation Group on Health Services in Calgary, Alberta*, Chair Mr. Lou Hyndman, Members, Dr. C. Wright, Mr. Ken Fyke, April 11, 1994 Report to the Calgary Regional Acute Care Planning Group.

9   Dr. John Wade, Mr. Bob Bell, *Bell-Wade Report*, Government of Manitoba, 1993.

10 "Managing Health Care Resources 1994-95 Meeting Priorities," Ministry of Health Ontario, Queen's Printer, 1994, p. 5.

The Alberta Government has established targets for bed use in that province. From 1,083 patient days per 1,000 population and 4.3 hospital beds per 1,000 population in 1991/92, Alberta intends to reduce to 745 patient days per 1000 and only 2.4 acute care beds per 1,000 by 1996/97.[11] Data from elsewhere in Canada reveals the same trends.

The Saskatchewan Health Services Utilization and Research Commission (HSURC) published a study in August of 1993[12] showing that hospitals in that province could save $16 million per year by increasing day surgeries and reducing pre-surgical admissions. Dr. Stewart McMillan, who heads HSURC, noted these changes could cut costs and improve quality of care to patients. There have been dramatic increases in the use of day surgery in Canada in the past five years but we still lag well behind the American hospital system in this area. There are many free-standing ambulatory care centres in the U.S. which do nothing but day surgery and outpatient work. In Canada, day surgery is undertaken largely in converted operating rooms within hospitals. There is considerable merit in facilities which are purpose built and managed for day surgery. Staffing patterns and other major cost factors in a twenty-four hour a day hospital setting can be dramatically reduced in a centre that operates from seven a.m. to six p.m.

Reviewing the facilities and location in which day surgery is carried out, coupled with a review of inpatient stays for procedures which need not require inpatient stay, are both worthwhile efforts. Lists of procedures approved for day surgery are available from U.S. health authorities and might form the basis for a review by your hospital's medical and management staff.

Good integration and communication with home care services are required to ensure follow-up care for day surgery patients. These linkages have been discussed in general above and will require attention as you expand day surgery to more complex procedures. As well, patient education and education of patient's families will be necessary to provide an understanding and peace of mind to post-surgery patients recuperating at home.

The Mulcahy Outpatient Centre at Loyola University Medical Centre in Chicago is an excellent example of a free-standing outpa-

---

11 "Healthy Albertans Living In A Healthy Alberta; A Three Year Business Plan," *Alberta Health*, February, 1994.
12 Deana Driver, "Hospital days acutely overused in Sask," Deana Driver, *The Medical Post*, Vol. 29, No. 24, June 15, 1993, p. 2.

tient centre with a significant volume of day surgery. An extensive library of videos for viewing by patients in advance of their day surgery is a valuable tool in Mulcahy's patient education approach, as is the use of nursing visits for patient education purposes.

6 How are you managing utilization? How *well* are you managing service utilization?

Utilization, that is, what services and how many are used by patients is extremely important to improved management. Most Canadian hospitals have some form of utilization management review in place but there has been little formal evaluation of the effectiveness of these efforts. In the U.S., where market forces and government incentives have forced more intensive efforts, the trend is towards explicit criteria for review of bed utilisation. In a June, 1993 review of the recent Canadian experience, an Institute for Clinical Evaluative Sciences — ICES — study team found a number of techniques that demonstrated effectiveness in improving management. These included:

- screening emergency departments and using quick response teams to prevent unwarranted admissions
- pre-admission testing to reduce cancellations of surgery
- guidelines are useful in reducing lengths of stay but their development process impacts significantly on their success
- short stay units
- a range of other techniques including co-operative care and self-care units, expected date of discharge programmes

Decisions about approach to utilization of beds are best taken in a collaborative fashion by hospital management, physicians and nurses. Formal bed utilization review tools such as SWITCH, ISD-A, MCAP establish criteria for admission and days of stay. These tools are in use in Canada: SWITCH at several Ontario hospitals, ISD-A in Victoria, B.C. and Saskatchewan and MCAP at the Hospital for Sick Children in Toronto. The ICES evaluation concluded that MCAP and ISD-A were the highest scoring against the criteria used.[13]

---

13 Paula Blackstein-Hirsh et. al., "Management of Hospital Bed Utilization in Canada," Institute for Clinical Evaluative Sciences, Working Paper #10, Toronto, June 1993. A6 SWITCH, ISD-A, MCAP are all acronyms for computerized tools to assess hospital performance. ISD-A — Intensity of service, severity of illness and discharge screens. MCAP — Managed Care Appropriateness Protocol. AEP — appropriateness evaluation protocol. SMI — standardized Medereview Instrument.

We are at a very early stage in applying the rigour necessary to develop a fully effective set of tools and properly evaluate their impacts in random trials. Nevertheless, the direction is clear. Much more management of admissions, discharges and lengths of stay, based on explicit criteria, are the new tool kit.

A good example of learning across Canada is the quick response team idea made prominent by the Victoria Health project in B.C. and later adopted by the Greater Niagara and Windsor Hotel Dieu in Ontario. The simple idea of screening patients prior to admission and determining whether the patient could be safely returned home without a hospital admission is a powerful and successful approach. Getting beyond "bed" management to services management is essential.

7 Benchmarking and Performance Measurement

Benchmarking is a powerful technique for comparing your performance to the performance of other similar peer organizations in comparable circumstances. In other instances, you may wish to benchmark your hospital with perceived leaders in the field. How do you compare with the best? Common measures are length of stay for patients of a particular type, percentage of surgery undertaken on a day basis, bed use and resource use, for various conditions or procedures.

For Ontario Hospitals the recently published ICES — Practice Atlas is a superb source of comparative data for benchmarking purposes.[14]

In 1992, Arthur Anderson & Co., a leading consulting firm, published a study based on a review of best practices in 120 ambulatory surgery facilities in the United States.[15] Their results showed an average time from arrival to surgery of forty minutes for the best performer, fifty-six minutes for the top twenty group of performers and ninety-eight minutes for all other facilities surveyed. The leader was saving nearly one hour per case! The study identified forty-three best practices or benchmarks in eleven areas such as patient registration, recovery, physician relations and diagnostic testing.

A leading American in the benchmarking field, James Heidbreder of the James Group Ltd., identifies four key qualities of true process benchmarking. These are:

14 *ICES Practice Atlas*, Institute for Clinical Evaluative Sciences, Toronto, 1994.
15 Arthur Andersen, ''Ambulatory Surgery Best Practices,'' Dallas, Texas, 1992.

1. "It deals with the "how's" as well as the "what's."[16] Benchmarking is not simply about performance measurement but it is also about how superior performance is achieved.
2. "It stimulates breakthrough thinking that results in quantum improvements."[17] Not incremental improvements but real breakthroughs with process improvement of 20% or more.
3. "It is grounded in a customer orientation."[18] What should be benchmarked should be determined by the customer. This quality is a shared foundation with Total Quality Management which is discussed below.
4. "It is a carefully structured analytical process."[19] This is a back of the envelope approach. Organized data, analysis and an intelligent plan, executed in a systematic fashion is necessary for success.

Mr. Heidbreder concludes on the following note:

As health care organizations come to test — and then to institutionalize — benchmarking, we will learn from the best and adapt that learning to our critical processes. The result will be the ability to do more with less and do it faster. We will be working smarter. And, above all, we will have a predictable ability to bring substantial improvement to our critical processes that produce both patient customer delight and superior financial performance.[20]

The Ontario Ministry of Health began sharing benchmarking software and peer hospital comparative data with Ontario hospitals in 1993. Data is available for Canadian hospitals from — MIS — or Hospital Management Records Institute — HMRI — which are merging to form the National Health Information Institute in 1994. The *ICES Practice Atlas* provides some useful advice on how to make this data of relevance to clinical practice and hospital management.

16 James E. Heidbreder, "Looking for the Light — Not the Heat," *Healthcare Forum Journal*, January-February 1993, p. 26.
17 Ibid., p. 26.
18 Ibid., p. 27.
19 Ibid., p. 27.
20 Ibid., p. 29.

8 Hospital Pharmacy: Managing Your Drug Costs

One of the fastest rising cost aspects of the hospital system is the drug bill. As new drugs have been developed, often with important advantages over the ones they replace, drug pricing has resulted in significant cost increase.

A lesson from down under: at an international meeting in Adelaide, Australia I had an opportunity to meet the talented CEO of the Royal Adelaide Hospital, a one thousand bed adult general teaching hospital in that city. He shared an interesting approach to drug decisions and allocation of scarce resources.

The Royal Adelaide on Drugs!

... The Hospital Drug Committee remained concerned at the continuing pressure on the drug budget and the growing request to use new drugs in the Hospital. By mid 1992, nineteen new drugs that had been assessed as clinically effective were waiting to be released for use within the Hospital. The Drug Committee devised the following methodology to address this problem.

With the increasing number of applications for drugs falling into the category of being approved on clinical/scientific grounds but unable to be available because of financial restrictions, the Drug Committee decided to develop a priority list for outstanding drug requests.

In developing a method for prioritisation, it was important that the method be:
   a. simple to use (i.e., use data that are readily available through the published literature)
   b. objective where possible
   c. reproducible and reliable
   d. discriminative

After many meetings, considerable discussion and several draft models, the RAH Drug Committee developed the following model.

The principles used were:
   1. Specific guidelines for each drug are developed by the relevant experts to establish the protocol for drug use at the RAH.
   2. Only those requests which have received approval from the Drug Committee on clinical/scientific grounds are considered for priority ranking.
   3. A ranking system based on supply and cost is utilised to minimise subjectivity and enhance consistency in the decision making process.

The goal was to provide a ranking of drug requests on the basis of obtaining the greatest benefit for the most patients for each dollar spent. For each drug request, scores are allocated for each of the subsections under —

1. **Quality score**
2. **Cost score**

Scores are obtained from the information provided with the submission. The guidelines established by the relevant experts and a further review of the scientific literature is necessary. A final ratio of total quality score over total cost score is used to rank requests (i.e., the higher the ratio the greater the priority).

1. QUALITY SCORE

1.1 Outcome

    a. Individual patient benefit

cure/prevention	(30)
prolongation of life	(15)
palliation/symptom control	(7)
placebo	(0)

    b. Mortality/Morbidity of Disease

mortality:	- high risk	(9)
	- moderate risk	(6)
	- low risk	(3)
morbidity :	- severe	(5)
	- moderate	(3)
	- mild	(1)

    c. Response
expected response fraction
(e.g. 80% of patients respond = 0.8 response fraction)

Outcome = (a + b) x c

1.2 Therapy Type (Based on Literature Support)

a.	established indication/effectiveness	(5)
b.	new therapy	(3)
c.	trial/investigational studies	(1)

1.3 Clinical Comparison with Available Alternative Therapy
(considering efficacy, side effects, administration, etc.)

a.	no alternative	(15)
b.	new treatment better than existing	(10)
c.	new treatment equals existing	(5)
d.	existing treatment better than new	(0)

2. COST SCORE

   2.1 Cost Comparison with Alternative Therapy

      a.   new treatment less expensive than existing (0)
      b.   no alternative (2)
      c.   new treatment equals existing (5)
      d.   new treatment more expensive (10)

   2.2 Total Cost per Year

      a.   less than $7,500 (1)
      b. $7,500 — $15,000 (2)
      c. $15,000 — $22,000 (3)
      d. $22,000 — $30,000 (4)
      e. $30,000 — $37,500 (5)
      f. $37,500 — $45,000 (6)
      g.   greater than $45,000 (7)

   2.3 Cost per Patient

      a.   less than $750 (1)
      b. $750 — $1,500 (2)
      c. $1,500 — $2,250 (3)
      d. $2,250 — $3,000 (4)
      e. $3,000 — $3,750 (5)
      f. $3,750 — $4,500 (6)
      g.   greater than $4,500 (7)

Final Cost Score =

Cost Comparison	+ Total Cost per Year	+ Cost Per Patient
(2.1)	+ (2.2)	+ (2.3)

By using this method, the Drug Committee was able to deal with fourteen new drug requests for nineteen indications during the 1991/92 financial year. If all of these drugs were approved for use then the total cost would be $750,000 per annum and the drug budget for this year was not able to accommodate it. The chart indicating the summary data for each of the newly marketed drugs and the final rankings is attached.

The Hospital decided that it only had $300,000 to apply to new drug use in this period. As a result of the nineteen drugs forwarded for funding, the first eleven only were released for use in patient care. This process was described in full not only at the Drug Committee but at several clinical staff meetings and gained acceptance by those staff as a fair and appropriate method to rank drugs in priority for use of patient care.[21]

21 Dr. Brendan Kearney, ''The RHA Drug Priority Scheme,'' *Physician's Executive*, Vol. 19, No. 5, p. 63

The Ottawa General Hospital achieved a $500,000 saving on their drug budget in a twelve month period through collaboration of doctors, pharmacists and administrators. The Ottawa General Hospital leaders believe 5 – 10 % reduction in hospital drug budgets are possible, without compromising the quality of patient care.[22]

9 Hospital Laboratories

Do you know how much each test costs in your hospital lab? Have you invested in lab systems and telecommunications systems to reduce costs and improve quality? What tests do you send elsewhere that you could do? Should your lab testing be a shared service with some other facility?

Dr. John Atkinson has recommended in his recent report[23] that Edmonton hospitals integrate their labs. Among the specific recommendations are a single lab manager for Edmonton, one integrated computer system and a lead site. Overall, an integrated single service, rather than each hospital's lab as an independent entity. Savings from the Edmonton Caritas Group, which has already integrated three hospital sites, are estimated to be in the millions. Atkinson suggests further savings may be possible in the $8 million range on a total budget of $42 million.[24] An ambitious target. Has your hospital considered lab integration?

10 Emergency Services

Does your hospital have an Emergency Department? How long are waiting times? How many of the people visiting your Emergency Department really need to be there? Is there another Emergency Department across the street or down the block?

In most Canadian communities fundamental questions about emergency services have not been asked. Some alternatives to visiting emergency departments such as urgent care clinics exist across Canada but there coverage is uneven at best. Only Quebec, through

---

22 "One Hospital's Success with Medication Budget Control," *Leadership in Health Services*, March/April, 1994. Published by the Canadian Hospital Association, p. 16.

23 Dr. John Atkinson, and Tannis Chefurka, "Principles and Programs for Edmonton Regional Health," a.k.a. the *PAPER* Report, for the Edmonton Region Health Faculties Planning Council, Edmonton, March 1994.

24 Ibid., p. 21.

its CLSC's,[26] offers a widely available clinic alternative. Quebec has been struggling to convince its citizens to use CLSC care clinics rather than hospitals. A telephone help number, as an alternative to a visit, is not commonly available in Canada although the Hospital for Sick Children in Toronto has a service and Nova Scotia has promised one.

Our American cousins have a good idea in this regard.

Ask-A-Nurse

Access Health's signature product, Ask-A-Nurse, is the country's leading telephone-based health care information and referral service. It responded to more than 5.5 million calls in 1992.

Created in 1986, Ask-A-Nurse offers health care consumers 24-hour access to specially trained registered nurse counsellors. Based on the caller's symptoms or concerns, the counsellors offer personalized, confidential information. This enables callers to make an informed decision about when, how, or whether to seek medical care, and assists them in selecting appropriate sources of care.

Sponsored by hospitals and other providers within their service areas, Ask-A-Nurse helps hospitals to increase their market share by assisting consumers with their health care needs. When appropriate, Ask-A-Nurse also helps them locate care from the hospital's network of services and affiliated physicians.

Ask-A-Nurse is currently used by 195 hospitals throughout the U.S., and has become the nation's most widely recognized health care information and referral service. Hospitals sponsoring Ask-A-Nurse offer it as a free service to their local communities to build goodwill and assist individuals in finding appropriate health care services within the hospital's network.[27]

The company that developed Ask-A-Nurse has gone on to develop a newer product — Personal Health Advisor — which combines access to an audio-library on health topics with a nursing information service. In recent trials with Blue Cross of Oregon and

26 C.L.S.C. (Centre locale de services communautataires) Quebec has a full network of integrated health and social service centres unlike any other province. These centres include physician, nursing and social services.
27 Access Health Marketing Inc., Annual Reports 1992, 1993 and supplementary material available from Access Health: Access Health 11020 White Rock Road, Rancho Cordova, CA, 95670.

California, Personal Health Advisor has dramatically reduced inappropriate emergency room visits and increased consumer satisfaction.[27]

Dr. Ron Stewart, an expert in emergency medicine and the Minister of Health for Nova Scotia, has recently announced that his department will reform emergency health services. One of the improvements will be the addition of health information by telephone. Why not uncouple the information from the visit?

Your Hospital As A "Factory"

Devote significant attention to the sizeable slice of your hospital budget that goes to heat, light, food, supplies and all of the other non-direct health care activities. Certainly fewer beds and shorter stays will mean fewer, sicker guests at the inn, but no matter how numerous or how acute those guests, you still have lots of room to improve purchasing and non-patient care.

11 Linking to Other Management Resources

There are many lessons to be learned about re-engineering from outside the hospital sector. Is there someone on your board who manages a manufacturing operation? An information technology-driven services company? A bank?

Perhaps the senior management team of the hospital could visit the relevant manufacturing plant or bank and meet their counterparts. Is there learning that could be shared? Are there experts who could be "borrowed" to help with a problem or issue?

This will work best as a partnership or two-way street. What expertise does the hospital have that could be of value to firms? Is a partnership with mutual learning possible? In Ontario, the Ontario Hospital Association has become active in promoting the export of hospital expertise to other countries.

The strength of this type of collaboration is that it can draw managers out of their conventional wisdom ruts causing new questions to be asked and answered.

---

27 Evaluation material on Oregon and California Blue Cross studies, unpublished material, 1993-1994.

12   Management and Purchasing

Materials management! I hear you sigh. How dull! How boring!

A recent Ontario study[28] estimated that Ontario hospitals could save $250 million per year through improvements to materials management including purchase, distribution and storage of products. Not sexy, but you sure could use the money saved to improve your performance and be a hero or heroine to your hard-pressed finance committee and board of directors. Beginning to sound less dull?

There are two joint buying groups among the Ontario hospitals, Carecor and the Ontario Hospital Association. With personnel and support from the Ministry of Health, the buying groups formed a Health Care Materials Management Task Force. What did the Task Force and its expert consultants discover? First, that Ontario hospitals lagged behind other Canadian and worldwide industry leaders in this field. Second, and more important, they identified five activities which will lead to significant cost reductions:

- more extensive use of information technology
- improvements in, and greater use of, hospital buying groups
- buying from fewer vendors
- use of just-in-time delivery (stockless supply systems)
- use of shared off-site warehousing

The Ontario situation in materials management may be a little better or a little worse than that in other parts of Canada. There is significant savings potential in every hospital in Canada in the better management of materials. Has your hospital Board ever heard a presentation from the management team on materials management? A full consideration of the potential for shared services among hospitals and others is highly recommended. What are the potential savings of shared services and a systems approach? In 1992, I met Scott Parker, the calm, thoughtful Chief Executive Officer of Inter-Mountain Health Care (IHC). This charitable, non-profit health care system serves communities in the states of Utah, Idaho and Wyoming. Scott Parker had commissioned Ernst & Young Management Consultants to examine IHC. In particular, they studied nine services

---

28   Report of the Ontario Healthcare Materials Management Taskforce, by Carecor Health Services Inc., Ontario Ministry of Health, Ontario Hospital Association, October 1993.

provided by the corporate office to IHC hospitals.[29] The savings attributable to the system were \$36.7 million for the year 1990, allocated as follows:

Purchasing	**\$9.3 m**
General liability, Malpractice and WCB	**7.7 m**
Data processing	**6.2 m**
Financing	**5.2 m**
Cash management	**1.1 m**
Collection agency	**3.5 m**
Clinical engineering	**2.8 m**
Equipment rental	**.8 m**
Central laundry	**.1 m**
	\$ 36.7 m[30]

Although each and every hospital cost is not comparable between the U.S. and Canada, enough similarities exist to make Scott Parker's IHC a system worth investigating. Canadian hospitals are less likely to need a collection agency but just as likely to benefit from rethinking purchasing decisions.

13 Food Services

We have already considered the menu cycle cost-saving idea from our leaders in Woodstock. What about the bigger question? Catering management firms have streamlined food service production across the country. Does a hospital in the 1990's need to prepare all its own meals from scratch? Airlines don't. In many cases hotels don't. Even many restaurants don't! Has your hospital considered buying meals, prepared foods, becoming part of a commissary group? The Ottawa hospitals own the Ottawa Commissariat and are saving significant costs through shared food services. The Commissariat serves hospitals and other institutional customers, such as the homes for the aged. The result is smaller kitchens, less expense and more attention to patient care.

Seven Oaks Hospital in Winnipeg is in the process of working out a new menu option approach jointly with Nestle Canada which could lead to a total re-engineering of food services in that hospital. The Toronto Hospital and Bitove are teaming up on a venture which

---

29 "Ernst & Young Report Savings from Corporate Office Activities to Intermountain Health Care," Salt Lake City, 1991. Further material can be found in the Intermountain Health Annual Report, 1992.
30 Ibid., p. 4.

could signal the beginning of mini-commissariats serving several hospitals.

Are you in the health care business or the food services business?

14 Energy Management

Energy conservation sounds almost passé but what about co-generation? Have you devoted a senior management meeting or a finance committee meeting to hearing from experts in the energy conservation and energy management fields?

Energy Costs

- How much energy does your hospital use each year?
- Have energy conservation actions been undertaken?
- Has your management team explored energy co-generation options?
- Is a regular energy audit part of your management plan?

15 Management of Labour Relations Matters

Hospitals are people-intensive organizations, 75% + of the budget is the payroll, with potential for very difficult labour relations if serious effort is not devoted to managing this area. Early warning signals are the numbers and types of grievances being filed. An abundance of grievances may reflect a lack of skills on the part of front-line managers, or it may reflect an insufficient delegation of authority by senior management to settle grievances at early stages. Front-line supervisors need to be able to problem-solve with the bargaining agent. If the bargaining agent is willing, joint training of union and management staff, in dispute resolution, can lead to dramatic improvement. Left to fester, bad labour relations only get worse with expensive and disruptive results. With proper attention, good labour relations can save dollars, aggravation and contribute sound ideas to the savings process.

16 Employee Benefits, Workers Compensation,
Workplace Health and Safety: Hospital Heal Thy Self

In recent years hospitals have eclipsed the construction industry as a growing site of workplace injuries. As older, heavier patients are cared for by older, more easily injured workers, the result unsurprisingly, has been a steady growth of at-work injuries.

To heal themselves, hospitals are going to need a greater focus on workplace health and safety. This is cost-avoiding. Today's injury is a workers compensation claim for tomorrow and tomorrow and tomorrow. Hospitals can also play a key role in early rehabilitation services which prevent a short-term injury from becoming a chronic condition. Needless to say, this is part of being a decent employer and human being, not just a cost-saving measure.

The results can be startling. In Whitby Psychiatric Hospital in Ontario total Workers Compensation Board costs were reduced by 20% in a three-month intensive effort with full labour-management cooperation.[31]

What about employee benefit plans? Have you moved your drug benefit plan to a mail-order pharmacy with much lower dispensing fees? Have you insisted on less expensive but equally effective generic drugs in your employee benefit plan?

17 Insurance and Financial Management

When I met with the London Teaching Hospital Council and the Thames Valley District Health Council in 1992 they told me about the substantial savings the London, Ontario hospitals had achieved by purchasing their insurance as a group. Does your provincial hospital association offer a plan? Would you benefit from joining it?

Do you have an ATM (automated teller machine) in your hospital? Is your bank paying for the privilege of using your facility to shelter their machine? How about cash management? Have you undertaken a thorough review of factors that could improve your financial efficiency and lower costs?

A few constructive thoughts would include better terms from major suppliers and direct deposit of payroll cheques for employees. Have you examined the merits of a payroll service? How much does it cost you to issue a single paycheque?

18 Selecting and Managing Consultants and Other Advisors

If they are well-selected and well-managed, external advisors can provide a worthwhile addition to a hospital. The external "team" is

31 Whitby Psychiatric Hospital, Ministry of Health-OPSEU project team, 1993.

typically composed of the accounting firm represented by a partner, the legal firm represented by a partner, and one or many consulting firms advising on strategy and managing projects. Under-managed or completely unmanaged external advisors can be a very expensive and redundant proposition. Getting the most out of your external team is important. Often the experience of the external advisors is vast, and they can help identify major versus minor problems or issues to be tackled.

A good first rule is not to ask external advisors to do work which properly belongs to the management team. If your vice president of finance is not up to the challenge, then you should recruit a new vice president of finance, not expect your external audit partner to cover inadequacies. If your strategic planning is a once-in-four-year affair, then a consultant is probably a good person to lead the way. If you are a large hospital and the change effort is permanent perhaps you need a fully dedicated member of the management team for planning.

If you require the expertise of an external team of consultants, insist on a partnership. Insist that the consultants train staff at the hospital and that data used for the restructuring remain connected to your decision-making process. Consultants earn their fees if you have both an immediate result and a value-added process left after their departure.

Recruit a high quality team and use their talents well.

Total Quality Management (TQM)

19 How to Benefit From TQM

What is TQM or Total Quality Management? It is an approach to customer-centred quality management focused on doing the task right the first time. A Total Quality Management approach can yield important benefits, but requires leadership from a very committed CEO and management team. A purely externally-led TQM effort will fail due to lack of understanding within the decision-making structure of your hospital.

To encourage the application of Total Quality Management approaches to health care, in 1992 the Conference of Deputy Ministers of Health hired Ernst & Young Management Consultants to undertake a study. They reviewed seven case studies of excellence in quality management in Canada with companies as diverse as Inco and Bombardier. The consultants identified the major thrusts and captured their implications for health care in Canada. The following chart indicates their findings.[33]

Quality Champions

ORGANIZATION (sector)	RESULTS OF TQM APPROACH
Whistler Mountain Ski Corporation (Tourism)	- premier customer services - development of measurement systems to evaluate impacts of customer service initiative
Nodak Associates Inc. processes (Information Technology Consulting)	- quality embedded in management - has not lost a customer in 7 years of operation
Inco Ltd. Manitoba Division (Mining)	- involvement of union from the start - redefinition of customers to include both internal and external
Bombardier Inc. (Manufacturing)	- value system linked to teamwork - shared vision of customers and shareholders as important
Maritime Telegraph and Telephone (Utility telecommunications)	- measuring results on a continuous basis (customer satisfaction surveys, etc.) - quality as integral to jobs, not an add-on
Standard Aero (Aircraft engine servicing)	- targets to be 50% better than the world's best in every business activity - focus on value-added activities with others dropped
MDS Laboratories	- cost reduction and improved (Medical labs) service levels - MDS transformed from a collection of labs into specimen-collection centres - consolidation of information - consolidation of existing 150 indicators of performance into Quality Improvement Binder

---

33 Adapted from Ernst & Young Report to Deputy Ministers of Health, Steering Committee on Quality and Effectiveness, *Quality Champions: Case Studies and Implications for Health Care in Canada*, June, 1993, p. 5-42.

20 Applied Clinical Epidemiology: Tapping the Best and Brightest

Applied clinical epidemiology — gasp! But it's not as obscurely technical as it sounds. Epidemiology looks at patterns of disease and their occurrence in the population. Clinical epidemiology looks at patterns of outcome from various medical interventions. "Applied" is my own addition to underscore the practical bent of it.

Across Canada there has been a wave of "best and brightest" approaches to increasing the effectiveness of the health care system. These are new ways to make public policy choices. In each the focus is outcomes. This shift from examining inputs — how much we spend — to examining outcomes — what works and how well it works — is a major shift.

In Manitoba, Dr. Nora Lou Roos heads the Centre for Health Policy; in Saskatchewan, Dr. Stewart McMillan is Chair of the Saskatchewan Health Services Utilization and Research Commission (HSURC), and in Ontario, Dr. David Naylor heads The Institute for Clinical Evaluative Sciences (ICES). Whatever the name on the door, these institutes are research tanks filled with very bright researchers focused on how to judge outcome: what works and how well it works. Their goals are not simply to do good research driven by intellectual curiosity and publish the results in technical journals. Governments have funded these initiatives to focus on improving both quality and affordability through *applying* knowledge and intelligence to the measurement of outcomes. Governments also believe that practitioners are more likely to accept the results and findings of independent think tanks. The results are available in user friendly formats.

Let us examine a few examples of a non-technical sort. ICES published a study in October of 1993 which calculated that if all vasectomies were done in doctor's offices, rather than in hospitals, the saving would be about $4.26 million per year in Ontario alone.[33] The cost for a vasectomy in an outpatient department of a hospital was found to be $324 versus a fee paid in a doctor's office of $10.30. How many vasectomies per year does your hospital perform? How

33 Wendy Young and Vivek Goel, *The Impact of Relocating Vasectomies from Hospital Outpatient Departments to Non-Hospital Sites*, Institute for Clinical Evaluative Sciences, Working and Research Paper Series #19, October 1993.

many other procedures are better performed in other settings? How could you create incentives to shift work to the most appropriate setting?

The bottom line for hospital managers is clear. Each study released by ICES, or the Manitoba Centre or the Saskatchewan Commission is a source of good, well-researched ideas. Why not ask your vice president medical and the president of your medical staff to co-chair a group to review these ideas and findings as they apply to YOUR hospital. Successfully managing change in health care is probably 80% implementation and 20% bright ideas. The work of the health service researchers needs to affect behaviour changes in hospitals and in the delivery of health care. It must be a key driver of intelligent change. The tough, essential job is to build bridges between what we *know* and what we *do* in health care.

Managing Non-Government Revenues

21 Meals, Parking and All of That (extra-bonus special idea No.21!)

In difficult economic times it is easy and tempting to devote too much effort to schemes to attract additional revenues. This can have a negative effect on organizational performance, if it diverts management and board attention away from pressing challenges in the expenditure management side. Here are a few initiatives worth taking. Be careful — do not divert your attention from the real management challenge of doing more with less. The revenue side can be seductive and treacherous.

The sad story of the financial crisis[34] which engulfed St. Michael's Hospital in Toronto flowed from a wholesale shift of management effort to a revenue project, contributing to both large losses and a rapid growth in deficit and debt in the late 1980's and early 1990's. The current hospital president described the situation at St. Michael's Hospital during their troubled period as follows:

Management team — out of control

Board — asleep at the switch

---

34 Lone et al. *Report of the Investigation of St. Michael's Hospital,* August 30, 1991, Details the difficulties of St. Michael's presented by Jeff Lozon, Canadian Hospital Association Conference, Halifax, June 7, 1994.

Medical Staff appetite for new technology — insatiable

Owners — trusted the wrong people[35]

The happy news is that the dynamic team of Sister Mary Beth Montcalm, Board Chair Patrick Keenan and President Jeff Lozon, who replaced the previous revenue-fixated folk, achieved a remarkable turnaround by putting their focus back on the expenditure side of the ledger. They have reduced St. Michael's Hospital spending by 15% without damaging care services. This was accomplished with a 25% reduction in overall management, a 55% reduction in senior management and the closure of 126 beds. Total staff reductions were 500 positions with 300 actual layoffs.

There is reason to ask your financial team to review all revenue possibilities, including options such as the sale of surplus land assets. Revenues from parking and other non-health care services should be at market rates and effectively managed. "Are we in the health business or the parking lot management business?" and other such questions are worth asking. What hidden subsidies do you have in place for direct employees or doctors? Are these still justified, if they ever were? But, don't let the great revenue search become a dangerous diversion from managing.

Advocating Change Is Easy, Doing It Is Hard

These ideas focus much more on re-engineering hospital activities than on the human consequences for the hospital workforce. This is not a pointless or thoughtless omission. The people aspects are dealt with in Part 2. Hospital boards, managers and other key players have the challenging task of pursuing change rapidly enough to get the necessary job done but taking sufficient time to bring along their health care people. Without their support little lasting and constructive change can be accomplished. With their active support and participation, this process can be interesting and very productive.

Our wins in health care in the next while will require a daily "grinding it out on the ground" in re-engineering care delivery. We need a lot of help from trustees. It is worthwhile to note that the British are scrambling to create what they call trust hospitals, i.e. hospitals with boards from the community. We have that. It is a tremendous asset. If the trustees can be persuaded to ask the difficult

35 Presentation by Jeffrey Lozon, Canadian Hospital Association Conference, Halifax, Nova Scotia, June 7, 1994.

questions, we can see a rationalization of the system that will maintain affordability and quality.

Look West — Look Way West

Canadian hospital trustees and managers looking for inspiration should look to the Greater Victoria Hospital Society (GVHS) and to Ken Fyke, its remarkable CEO. In the past decade, since the three hospitals on four sites in Victoria have been brought under one governance and management, a virtual transformation has occurred. All of the progress has been achieved despite the high portion of Victoria's population over the age of sixty-five. Fully 20% have reached this age in Canada's retirement capital. Far from overwhelming the hospital system, as some have predicted, the GVHS is using fewer hospital beds than nearly anywhere else in Canada.

With a reduction from 25% to 2.3% in the number of beds utilized by people best served elsewhere, and with an emphasis on home nursing care, including pain control and palliation, the GVHS has returned dying to the home. The benefits include both the creation of a more compassionate end-of-life setting and the availability of resources for other needs. Significant progress has also been made in the quest to improve community care. Through patient education, the number of nursing home visits associated with cataract surgery had been reduced from twelve to one per patient.

So, learn about Ken Fyke and the Greater Victoria Hospital Society — they are 80% of the way to the future of hospital services.

Good Stuff To Read

Re-engineering the Corporation by Michael Hammer and James Champy. Published by Harper, New York, 1993. This is a powerful book of insight and advocacy for starting from scratch in the redesign of how we do business. The authors argue persuasively for an abandonment of orthodoxy and a thoughtful, participatory reworking of the processes and organization of the enterprise. Their case studies have application to customer service in the health care sector.

Rx for Hospitals New Hope for Medicare in the Nineties by Philip Hassen. Published by Stoddart, Toronto 1993. Phil Hassen is the president of St. Joseph's Health Centre in London, Ontario. He is also a leading Canadian advocate and practitioner of Total Quality

Management (TQM). A first rate book which brings together the practical and the theoretical, it is a must-read for hospital board members, hospital managers, hospital based nurses, physicians and those who sit on various health planning bodies. It offers sound practical ideas on how to make continuous improvement through TQM in a hospital setting.

The Challenge of Organization Change or *When Giants Learn to Dance*, London, Simon & Schuster, 1989 or *The Change Masters, Corporate Entrepreneurs at Work*, London, Unwin, 1985 both by Rosabeth Kantor. Any of these books by this Harvard professor are a wonderful read with strong ideas on how organizations can manage change.

Quality Champions: Case Studies and Implications for Health Care in Canada. "A Profile of Findings" for the Conference of Deputy Ministers of Health, Ernst & Young, September, 1993. An excellent review of the experience of seven major Canadian corporations. Implications for health care management are clearly outlined.

Report of the Investigation of St. Michael's Hospital by Edward Lane, Ralph Coombs, Donald Holmes, August 30, 1991. Available from St. Michael's Hospital. A guidebook on how not to manage the affairs of a hospital. A gripping read.

Get on the Mailing List

Institute for Clinical Evaluative Sciences
G-2, 2075 Bayview Avenue
North York, Ontario
M4N 3M5
The ICES Working Paper series is an excellent source of ideas. A variety of key topics from surgical rates to drug utilization to surveys of key medical literature are included in the series. The ICES monograph, *Patterns of Health Care in Ontario — ICES Practice Atlas, First Edition*, 1994 published by the Canadian Medical Association is available from the CMA at 1867 Alta Vista Drive, Ottawa, Ontario K1G 3Y6. It is an insightful and data rich source for all concerned with health policy and managing the delivery of health services. Issues covered include patterns of drug use, variations in surgical procedures by region, variations in lengths of stay and day

surgery use. This is the most thorough work in Canada on these issues. It is a must read for health policy makers and health care managers. It is also a powerful tool for consumers and consumer groups.

Saskatchewan Health Services Utilization Commission
Box 46
GMO 41
Saskatoon, Saskatchewan
S7N 8W8
(306) 966-1500

The Manitoba Centre for Health Policy and Evaluation
St. Boniface Hospital Research Centre
409 Tache Avenue, Room 2008
St. Boniface, Manitoba
R2H 2A6
(204) 233-8563

Council for the Evaluation of Health Care Technology
522 Pine Avenue West
Montreal, Quebec
H2W 1S6

Hospital Annual Reports — Another excellent source of ideas and advice is to obtain annual reports from individual hospitals which are leaders and learn from their experiences. My own list of hospital annual reports always includes Foothills Hospital in Calgary, University of Alberta Hospital in Edmonton, St. Boniface Hospital in St.Boniface, Manitoba and a range of Ontario hospitals including The Hospital for Sick Children, Mt. Sinai, Wellesley, Sunnybrook, Toronto, Kingston General, St. Joseph's in London, Chedoke — McMaster in Hamilton and CHEO (Children's Hospital of Eastern Ontario).

International Benchmarking Clearinghouse — Part of the American Productivity & Quality Centre, the Clearinghouse is an excellent source of books and other publications on benchmarking and can be reached at 1-800-366-9606.

Chapter 2
Long Term Care Services

The elderly benefit as much as other age groups from good nutrition, regular exercise and other health promoting activities.[1]

Long-term care is likely to be the 'sleeper' health issue in Canada. As a baby-boomer, I realize that re-engineering for the aging of my generation will create major change, as it did in the school system, universities and labour markets. Soon, in planning terms, the long-term care system will feel aging boomers' demands. Countries with older populations, such as Germany and the United Kingdom, are already experiencing these enormous pressures. Occasionally, in stories about the inability of current levels of contribution to sustain the Canada Pension Plan, we get a glimpse of a much tougher future ahead. The good news is that we are living longer in good health. The bad news is that a small percentage of a larger group of us needing long-term care can devastate current funding arrangements. Our need to better balance health care approaches to mental illness between institutions and communities is directly linked to the long-term care issue.

Mental and physical health are both part of long-term care. As we live longer and become more frail a variety of health issues arise. Many of these correspond to issues addressed later in the book having to do with advance directives for our care. Much of the dilemma of treating the elderly in need of care, stems from disorders

---

1 June Engel, ed., "Keep up the quality of life with advancing years," Chapter 15, *The Complete Canadian Health Guide* (Toronto: Key Porter, 1993), p. 392.

such as Alzheimer's disease, which rob people of their ability to decide for themselves about care. A vast majority of seniors experience greater needs for company, companionship and a social context than for intensive medical care.

In the long-term care sector we are seeing the same shift to community and broadening of continuum of services as in the acute care sector. The unlinking of services from institutions, and the desire of most elderly persons to remain in their own homes and live independently, is providing opportunities for rapid growth in non-institutionally-based services. For example, in the United States, there are estimated to be three thousand day care centres for the elderly, a growth rate of 50% in the last three years and forecast to soon reach ten thousand centres. The benefits of these centres and other efforts of a non-institutional nature are supported by a range of studies. One such study conducted by California's Department of Aging in the early 1980s concluded that between 87% and 96% of people who attended senior citizens' day centres either improved or maintained their functional abilities in such daily activities as bathing, dressing, problem solving, and so on. There is both a humanity and a cost-effectiveness embodied in this approach. In some cases these types of services will delay institutionalization by a period of months or years; in other cases they will prevent its necessity all together.

Of the myriad issues in the long term care field this chapter focuses on three key challenges:

- the need to integrate health and social services in a comprehensive and manageable fashion
- the need to examine the financial issues sooner rather than later at a national level
- the role technologies can play in long term care services.

Integrating Services

Across Canada changes are going on in how long-term care services are organized. In Ontario, after two successive governments engaged in lengthy policy analysis and extensive consultation, a movement toward a reformed system is underway. The key elements of the Ontario reform can be summarized as a more needs-based funding approach on the institutional care side and significant new investment to build a high quality, comprehensive, set of services in the home and community setting. One of the most interesting aspects of the Ontario long-term care policy process was the surprisingly strong impact of advocacy organizations for seniors in the policy process.

Consultation changed the government's programme design in a fairly dramatic way. The government's original intention had been to establish placement coordination agencies to perform the gate-keeper function, replacing individual physicians and institutions. Advocacy by seniors' organizations pushed the government a step further, into the more radical reorganization of the system just beginning. At its core is the principle of one-stop shopping. Seniors, as consumers, indicated their very strong preference for a more accessible and centralized service provision network. At present, thousands of small agencies deliver services ranging from meals on wheels to home care to visiting nursing services. The clear message from seniors was to pull these together and put the access to them under one roof. The policy response, called multi-service agencies, offers the prospect of both administrative efficiency in a system which suffers from fragmentation, as well as the much sought after one-stop shopping. The process of moving the thousands of small agencies into perhaps one hundred to two hundred larger multi-services agencies will be an enormous political and managerial struggle.

Evelyn Shapiro, the founder of Manitoba's innovative home care programme and a sound thinker on health policy and delivery captured the need to integrate in a very practical fashion:

> ...the problem is that most provinces have not included representation from their community care program in their overall planning for health care. In some provinces, this occurs because community care reports to the Minister of Community Services or to the Ministry of Social Services, whereas other health care sectors report to the Ministry of Health. In provinces that do not have this division of responsibility, community care, probably because it is not a major spender, is regarded as nice and maybe even necessary, but peripheral. Each province, in my view, should have some conjoint vehicle for:
>
> 1) reviewing what changes in treatment modalities require changes in the kind or amount of home care services delivered,
> 2) anticipating what effect changes in one sector will have on another

3) deciding whether a new type of service should be delivered, and

4) ensuring that serving a new sub-population does not jeopardize serving vulnerable elders.[2]

Financing For Future Needs

Other nations are also examining their long-term care system. One of the most intriguing policy processes is underway in Germany. The European countries, including Germany, have much older populations than Canada. They provide a window on the future which Canadians would be well advised to look through. With a larger proportion of the population in the seventy plus and particularly in the eight-five plus age group, the German system is experiencing rapidly increasing costs for long-term care. The conclusion the Germans are reaching is that they need a separate form of insurance for long-term care. They delineated insurances for health services, for unemployment, for injury, in short, for the major risks in life. The purpose of an organized national societal approach is to share these risks on a broader basis rather than having them fall on individuals. The options are to create a marketplace in which individuals can insure themselves privately against such future risks, or take the risks on as a collective responsibility as a society. In Canada we have taken health insurance as a societal risk. Through Unemployment Insurance we have shared the burden of insuring the risk of unemployment among employees, employers and governments.

With regard to long-term care, Canada has not set an overall approach in a comprehensive way. We do not have a long-term care system yet. At present, there are a range of approaches in the different provinces. In general, individuals are expected to contribute some or all of their room and board charge while governments pay the health care component. In the home or community setting, there is a mix, with governments paying for a number of services, and individuals being charged cost-sharing in the form of co-payments for some other services. As well, there is an enormous voluntary sector active in the care of the elderly and the provision of services to the elderly. In some ways, the long-term care system shows the mix of funding sources and approaches evident in health care,

2   Evelyn Shapiro in Deber and Thompson, *Restructuring Canada's Health Services System* (Toronto: University of Toronto Press, 1992), p. 103.

generally prior to the introduction of Medicare. Some aspects of long-term care are, of course, covered under the Canada Health Act and the health insurance acts of the provinces. Medical care and hospital services are insured, drug costs are insured in institutional settings. There is an array of different approaches to drug coverage among the provinces in the home and community sector.

The institutional side of the long-term care system supports a range of institutions including guest homes with minimal care; nursing homes with a moderate amount of care; homes for the aged, both municipal and charitable; and, at the more intensive end of the spectrum, chronic care hospitals. These different institutions have evolved historically on a very fragmented basis. They have become part of the system largely through the development of government funding and therefore standards. Until recently, when several provinces moved toward needs-based or levels of care funding, there was no particular connection between the needs of any individual and the funding received by the institution. The general tendency to have dollars follow patient needs in the system is a good one. If sufficiently sound methodologies can continue to evolve, it will provide a way of increasing both the fairness and the effectiveness of care services within the institutional system.

We have also come to realize that not institutionalizing elderly people who aren't in need of institutionalization, and who could cope in their home on an independent basis with a range of support services, is a far better option. The growth of home care in various provinces is illustrated by a dramatic increase in spending through the past two decades. This mirrors the acceptance by government of care in the home as an alternative to institutionalization in acute care hospitals or long-term care facilities.

We need to have a hard national look at the trends and the numbers. Do we need an additional insurance approach for long term care? Should it be modeled on Germany or the Canada Pension Plan or the Registered Retirement Savings Plan approach? There is a lot to be gained by answering the design questions early.

The Chip Meets Seniors - Welcome to The Caring Network

For a fascinating example of a product which utilizes modern information and telecommunications technology to improve both quality and affordability, a visit with a British company, Tunstall PLC, is worthwhile. Tunstall started out in the alarm business and thirty years later has evolved into a high-technology manufacturer. One of their leading-edge products is called The Caring Network. In their own description:

> A British technology company - Tunstall PLC - has developed a very interesting product by combining software, hardware and a lot of common sense. The Caring Network is a clever use of telecommunications technology and people to provide the elderly with security in their homes while assisting the management of in-home services.[3]

The elements of the system are straightforward: a special, modified telephone for your home, a control switchboard staffed by trained personnel and a computer capable of tracking and storing an accessible record of all care provided.

The Caring Network system allows elderly persons to remain in their home with the security of immediate access to care and a friendly, familiar voice by telephone. By including the record keeping function for all home visits the system begins to reduce dramatically the paperwork burden on providers. Paperwork is not just a hospital phenomena!

Good Stuff to Read

The Eldercare Sourcebook, by Ann Rhodes, Key Porter, Toronto, 1993 ($18.95). Until one-stop shopping is achieved this is a good guidebook of services for seniors. Very readable and current. There is an intention to update annually which will keep it current.

Anything written by Evelyn Shapiro on home care and long term care is highly recommended.

When Older is Wiser: A guide to health care decisions for older adults and their families, by Patricia Parsons and Arthur Parsons, Doubleday Canada, Toronto 1994. A very user friendly guide to rights issues and to various seniors organizations. Accessible and practical in its tone.

---

3   ''The Caring Network,'' Tunstall PLC Corporate brochure, 1993.

Chapter 3
Drugs and Pharmacy Services

Statistics Canada estimates that in 1989, four thousand Canadian seniors died as a result of inappropriate medication use.

- Up to 20 % of seniors entering hospitals are there because of a "drug problem" — too many drugs, the wrong dosage, drug interactions, or the failure to take drugs properly.
- Inappropriate medication use is "one of the five most important quality of care problems among the elderly in terms of morbidity."[1]
- Seniors are being "drugged silly," given medications they don't need or given new expensive drugs that don't work any better than the older, cheaper ones.

Doctors need drugs, but do drugs need doctors? Could the pharmacological revolution ultimately cast aside the physicians? Many patients regulate their own medicines rather skilfully after an initial diagnosis and medical advice. Many simple remedies are available over the counter in pharmacies and their numbers will grow as patents expire on relatively safe medicines like ibuprofen. Large research-intensive pharmaceutical houses are buying up generic manufacturers and suppliers of inexpensive drugs directly to patients.

The challenge is for physicians to develop greater skill and understanding in the use of therapeutic drugs. If they do not,

---

1 *Consumer Response*: Prepared by the Senior Citizens Consumer Alliance for Long-Term Care Reform, Ontario, 1993.

their role in the treatment of many common conditions may become marginal.[2]

Drugs and their use is an area of miraculous breakthroughs, rapid cost growth and horrendous misuse. We have been able to eliminate whole classes of disease and the pain and suffering they cause through drug therapies. But our ability to manage drug therapies has not kept pace with advances in the products or with the market power of the pharmaceutical industry. Technological change is rapidly overtaking our traditional drug distribution systems and replacing them with new, information-rich approaches. Pharmaceutical companies quest for an extended monopoly on new products is giving way to purchase of generic companies and a drive for greater, non-prescription, over-the-counter-sales.

Four ideas are presented which will greatly improve the Canadian situation in the drug policy area. They go to the heart of the needed re-engineering in how we evaluate drugs, how we distribute them and pay for them. By adopting a cost-effectiveness approach to assessing new drugs, re-engineering the drug distribution system and re-skilling the pharmacist, we can create significant efficiencies. By adopting a new national approach, Canada can improve the fairness of the access to necessary drugs.

Drug Use and Abuse

All recent studies of the problems of drug misuse reach two key conclusions. The first is adverse drug reactions are common due to mis-prescribing, inappropriate consumption and lack of conformity to the optimum use of drugs. The second conclusion is that adverse reactions are a high cost to the total health care system, measured in unnecessary human suffering and in millions, perhaps billions, of dollars. Available studies reach roughly the same conclusions on the need for better management of drugs and greater efficiency in the distribution system. As Dr. Barry Sherman, president of generic drug manufacturer, Apotex Inc., argues: "Drugs cost Canada $6 billion to $7 billion per year. With rational prescribing and competition that could come down to $2 billion."[3]

A somewhat remarkable statement for someone in the drug

2   Sir Colin Dollery, "The Harveian Oration," Royal College of Physicians, London, U.K. October 19, 1993.
3   "Profile of Dr. Berry Sherman," *Profit Magazine*, Sept., 1992, p. 37.

manufacturing business! It underscores the huge potential for improvement in the drug use field.

A Changing Marketplace

The day Merck decided to pay $6 billion for Medco Cost Containment the pharmaceutical industry was forever transformed. Merck paid sixty times the earnings for a company that, far from manufacturing drugs, makes its living by managing the cost and distribution of drugs. Medco has its original roots in finding a better way to deliver drug benefits to organizations like the International Ladies Garment Workers Union. Through rapid growth, it has expanded to cover nearly one in every eight Americans for drug benefits. Merck is the largest global pharmaceutical manufacturing firm with sales greater than the GNP of many small nations.

A new drug costs some $300 million to bring to market. Merck have decided that Medco is a better investment than 20 new drugs — a remarkable shift.

WalMart is coming to Canada. The giant U.S. retailer has purchased the Woolco stores and is preparing their conversion to WalMarts. Among the areas in which WalMart is known as aggressive price competitors is pharmacy. Large advertisements in the national *Globe and Mail* are recruiting pharmacists to staff these new Wal-Mart pharmacy operations.

What will a changing marketplace mean for Canadians? Certainly more price competition and a wider array of ways of obtaining drugs. But, also, the fundamental reordering of the pharmaceutical and pharmacy industries.

The Chip Meets Norman Paul — Result: Meditrust

Norman Paul is a pharmacist. When he was in his twenties he was part of the Shopper's Drug Mart revolution in Canada. In this first wave, a large chain of pharmacies was assembled by Murray Koffler and significant results achieved. Many more products were added and Shoppers became the drug supermarket. The corner drugstore gave way to the mall superstore as the franchise overwhelmed small businesses owned by the pharmacist. Shopper's Drug Mart used the leverage of a customer flow to sell all sorts of other merchandise. The pharmacy is always at the back of the store and few of us can resist the other products enroute to our prescription. Now, thirty years later, Norman Paul is leading the second revolution in pharmacy distribution in Canada. His company, Meditrust, is often labelled as Canada's first mail order pharmacy, an inadequate description. A better way of looking at Meditrust is as a fundamental re-engineering of the pharmacy business. From the computerized data base record on each client, to the arrival of prescriptions by fax, to the automated assembly line for filling orders and courier delivery, the entire operation is the application of information technology to re-engineering. Without the information and telecommunications technology made possible by the silicon chip, this revolution would not be possible.

Norman Paul is also providing a higher quality service for his customers. Into each dispensed prescription, an information sheet on the drug is included. The patient receives much more than the traditional tiny label with "take before each meal." As well, patient profiles maintained by Meditrust allow them to identify and prevent potential, harmful drug interactions before dispensing. In New Brunswick, Meditrust is piloting interactive telephone booths connected to its national operation along a state of the art information highway.

Meditrust will face competition and resistance in this revolution. Already traditional pharmacies in Ontario have resisted. The largest U.S. mail order pharmacy, Medco Cost Containment, with thirty-three million Americans enrolled, will look to Canada for new markets. Aggressive expansion in Canada by Medco is likely. As well, the advent of WalMart competition in the pharmacy market will bring extremely low prices. WalMart assisted by its massive purchasing clout will push other pharmacies out of business. If this competition follows the course of reducing prices charged to both patients and insurers, including governments, as well as increasing information to patients, then it will assist our Medicare challenge. This second pharmacy revolution has significant potential to simultaneously improve affordability and quality.

A Good Idea: Re-skilling the Pharmacist

Another piece of the pharmacy reform puzzle are pharmacists, their training and their model of practice. Dean Perrier of the University of Toronto, Faculty of Pharmacy, sees a major shift in the role of pharmacists. In a February, 1993, paper he noted that historically, pharmacists were very product-focused but, by the middle of this century this role had been largely taken over by pharmaceutical companies. This narrowed the pharmacist's role to drug distribution. Gradually, many of these tasks passed to the pharmacy technician or dispensing assistant.

Are pharmacists to become more and more, de-skilled assistants to the pharmaceutical industry? Dean Perrier sees a new and evolving role, which is patient-focused rather than product-focused. He calls this expanded role the "pharmaceutical care" model. Perrier describes it as "the responsible provision of drug therapy for the purpose of achieving definite outcomes which improve a patient's quality of life."[4]

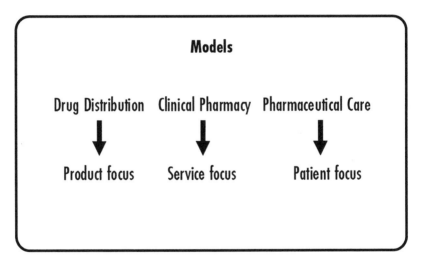

Models

Drug Distribution   Clinical Pharmacy   Pharmaceutical Care

↓   ↓   ↓

Product focus   Service focus   Patient focus

4   Dean Perrier, "The Pharmaceutical Care Model," (Toronto: University of Toronto, 1992).

Pharmaceutical Care Model

In the following pharmaceutical care model three distinct functions can be detailed for the pharmacist. These are:
- Identifying a patient's actual or potential drug related problem (DRP)
- Resolving a patient's actual DRP
- Preventing a patient's potential DRP

Eight categories of problems pharmacists can solve:
1. The patient is taking/receiving a drug for no medically valid indication
2. The patient is requiring drug therapy (a drug indication) but not receiving/taking a drug for that indication
3. The patient is being treated with the wrong drug or drug product
4. The patient is being treated with too little of the correct drug (subtherapeutic dose)
5. The patient is being treated with too much of the correct drug (toxicity)
6. The patient is not receiving/taking the prescribed drug appropriately
7. The patient is experiencing an adverse drug reaction (any undesirable effect from the drug which is not dose related)
8. The patient is experiencing a drug-drug, drug-disease, drug-food, drug-laboratory interaction

There are several prerequisites for a pharmacist to successfully undertake Dean Perrier's vision of an expanded and very desirable role. The first is a diversification in pharmacy training programmes to properly prepare pharmacists. This is underway.

The second necessary reform is the application of information technology to pharmaceutical care activity. Only with full patient information at the point of service can the pharmacist successfully treat the range of problems identified above. Computerized information systems which provide point of service information have been created in Saskatchewan, and started in several other provinces, including Ontario. These information networks will allow a pharmacist to know all the drugs a patient is already taking and how those drugs might interact with the prescription to be filled.

The third necessity is for a fundamental shift in the method of payment for pharmacists. As long as the only two sources of income for community pharmacy are prescription dispensing fees and product mark-ups, it will be difficult to move from a transaction or product-focus to a patient-focus.

With these three improvements, two of which are substantially underway, pharmacists can perform an expanded and needed role in tackling our very serious over-medication and inappropriate medication problems.

Good Ideas: A National Drug Benefit Plan for Canada

As more and more health care services are delivered in a home or community setting, one of the weaknesses of the Canada Health Act has become evident. Because drugs administered in the community setting are not insured medical services under the Canada Health Act, each province has devised its own drug plan, without the benefit of a national standard or framework. The consequences are unfair and expensive. This state of affairs is the major unfinished piece of phase one — the removal of the financial barrier between the individual and appropriate care — of Medicare.

The drug cost issue is very real for Canadians. Their access to appropriate medication is determined by their province of residence. Access to medical and hospital services are reasonably comparable across the country. Variations in access exist, but they are minor and predictable, for example, bigger cities have more sophisticated hospitals than smaller centres. There are, however, major and as yet unexplained variations in use of services. This is not true of how drug costs and benefits are organized. Here access and financial barriers vary dramatically, depending on which province you reside. In Ontario, those over sixty-five years of age or on welfare do not pay for their drugs. If you are working at a low wage you are likely to receive no help from government with your drug bills. Your employer may or may not cover you. Next door in Manitoba, everyone has some coverage under the government Pharmacare plan. A senior citizen would pay the first $117.25 per year of their drug costs and 30% of the balance. Others would pay the first $206.90

per annum and then 30%. In Alberta, seniors pay 20% per prescription but no deductible. Others, under sixty-five pay $50 annually plus 20%. In P.E.I. only seniors and social assistance recipients are covered. Seniors pay $7.85 for the dispensing fee and $4 towards the drug cost. In Ontario, if you are over 65 and wealthy you can send your chauffeur to the pharmacy and the taxpayer will pay the whole cost for your drugs. But if you are without coverage and trying to pay your own drug costs while working, you get no help.

This patchwork of provincial programmes illustrates the problem of unfair coverage across the country. The inequity of this situation is getting worse as the smaller, poorer provinces have been forced to raise deductibles and co-payments. And the very real issue of misuse of drugs through inappropriate prescribing and dispensing require national efforts to tackle. This work need not be undertaken by the federal government, although federal leadership has historically been key to achieving interprovincial cooperation in the health field.

A national plan with provincial discretion over both the scale of their formulary (what drugs are covered) and the level of premiums collected, would better serve our country than the current inequitable and inefficient hodgepodge of programmes. There are two major advantages of a national drug plan approach. The first is that it would allow far better management of drug use. Canada has a limited number of experts in the drug evaluation field (also known as pharmacological epidemiology). By having the relative merit and cost-effectiveness of each existing and new drug assessed once and the results shared among the provinces, better decisions could be made. The second major benefit is increased bargaining power to obtain lower prices.

A national plan would also benefit Canada's drug manufacturers. Many complaints have been voiced by manufacturers about the fragmented nature of Canada's drug market. Because each province operates a separate plan with different rules for listing products and paying for them, the companies incur considerable additional costs conforming to variant prices and policies in the different provinces. A national plan could reduce company costs in this regard. A good case could be made that some of these savings should flow through to taxpayers and consumers in the form of lower prices. Recently the industry, through the Pharmaceutical Manufacturers Association of Canada, has undertaken to promote better use of drugs. As noted earlier, this area requires significant attention in Canada.

The Australians have a national approach to drugs. The Pharmaceutical Benefits Scheme PBS is a monopoly purchaser of drugs in Australia, accounting for approximately 80% of the market and directly influencing the prices of drugs in the hospital market (12%). Expenditure in 1989/90 was approximately $1 billion, accounting for 8% of Australian Federal Government health expenditure.

The PBS has a long history. It was originally developed in 1950 to pay for 'lifesaving and disease preventing drugs' to the community at no cost. The list was originally quite small but has grown to about 1300 items, including different strengths and dosage forms.

Co-payment, that is payments by patients, for general users was introduced in 1960, and is now $15 per script. Co-payments for pensions were introduced for the first time in 1991 and are set at $2.50 per script (prescription), the same as for other subsidized users, with a safety net.

The Australian PBS

The goals of the PBS balance health care, economic development and fiscal objectives of the government. They are designed to:

- provide access to safe, efficacious and high quality pharmaceuticals to the Australian population, irrespective of income
- limit the budgetary cost to Government
- encourage the development of an Australian pharmaceutical industry

The PBS prices are determined taking into account eight pricing factors:

i   the prices of alternative brands of the same drug
ii comparative prices of the drugs in the same therapeutic group
iii cost information supplied by the manufacturer
iv prescription volumes, economies of scale and other factors such as expiry date, storage requirements, product stability and special manufacturing requirements
v   prices of the drug in reasonably comparable overseas countries

vi the level of activity being undertaken by the company in Australia including new investment, production and research development

vii other relevant factors which the applicant company wishes the Authority to consider

viii other directions as advised by the Minister

Drug companies can launch a drug onto the market after it receives general marketing approval from the Australian Drug Evaluation Committee. In reality true market access is only provided through a drug attaining PBS listing. Companies lodge applications for listing on the PBS to the Pharmaceutical Benefits Advisory Committee (PBAC) after marketing approval is received. PBAC considers applications and advises the Pharmaceutical Benefits Pricing Authority (PBPA) of its recommendation for listing. PBPA is then responsible for negotiating the price with the company. The PBPA determines prices taking into account factors such as the advice of PBAC on the therapeutic benefits of the drugs in comparison with other drugs and the cost of manufacture, or import, plus an amount meant to cover indirect costs such as research and development, administration and profit. A gross margin of 30% over direct costs is used as a guide although this varies with the level of usage of the product and other factors.

More recently a number of companies have indicated an increased willingness to de-list products, or not to seek listing not being prepared to accept the price determined by the PBPA. The private prescription market may eventually provide a greater share of the total market, but under existing arrangements it will probably always be small.

In addition, an increasing number of drugs listed on the PBS have restrictions on use. This is done by an authority system where drugs are rationed by making it difficult for patients to fill prescriptions and by building in delays between scripts. Restricted listings include products for which prescribing is permitted only after the doctor attests that all cheaper alternatives have been tried. These include cancer drugs and human growth hormone.

The list of restricted access drugs is likely to grow
because of the increasing numbers of effective but very
expensive drugs.[5]

How Would We Pay For This Programme?

The major obstacle to a national drug plan — the perilous state of
public finance in our nation — will be readily and rapidly identified.
This dictates a careful approach, without new public dollars, but it
is not an excuse for inaction. The savings inherent in a national
approach, plus a revenue stream from fair, monthly premiums, plus
existing provincial spending would be a good start. The necessary
federal investment may well be political will, leadership and a small
amount of funds. The gains to a strengthened Canadian Medicare
and a true adherence to the principles of comprehension and port-
ability in the Canada Health Act are well worth the effort.

Major savings would be realized from improved utilization and
tougher price bargaining. The cost of the plan could be born by the
Government of Canada through price rebates negotiated nationally,
the governments of the provinces, and individual Canadians through
payment of modest monthly premiums. This would spread the burden more fairly. It would also put drug costs on the same footing as
medical or hospital costs, rather than continuing a patchwork quilt
coverage that resembles the current, and discredited, approach of
Americans to health care in general. Where employers are now
paying for drug coverage they would continue by paying premiums
for their employees.

It would be a fitting twenty-fifth anniversary of Medicare to
replace the inequity inherent in our fragmented approach to drugs by
a fair national plan, administered by each province.

Good Stuff to Read

Reflections on a Month in the Life of the Ontario Drug Plan, by
Warren McIsaac. C. David Naylor, Geoffrey M. Anderson, Bernie J.
O'Brien, published a ICES Paper #004, April, 1993.

The Real Pushers — A Critical Analysis of the Canadian Drug

---

5   Adapted from Brendan Kearney paper. Presented to the King's Fund International
     Seminar, October, 1992, Adelaide, Australia.

Industry, by Joel Lexchin, New Star Books, 1984. Although nearly a decade old, Joel Lexchin's book asks all the tough and necessary questions in a critical and readable fashion. Dr. Lexchin's criticism caused more questioning of the industry's role by policy makers in Canada and lead to some improvements.

Controlling Drug Expenditure in Canada, the Ontario Experience, by Paul Gorecki, 1992, published by the Economic Council of Canada. A data-rich analysis of the Ontario Drug Benefit Program.

Part 2

The 3 R's of Human Resource Management: Restructuring Re-skilling Redeployment

Health care services are a labour-intensive, person to person endeavour. Of the over $64 billion expended on the health care delivery system in Canada in 1994, about 80% will be taken home as a paycheque by a nurse, doctor or other health care worker. Health care creates jobs for nearly 750,000 Canadians.

Within Canadian health care the trend has been toward increasing expenditures on the wage component. In 1961, 68.6% of total hospital spending was wage costs. By 1988, wage costs had climbed to 76.3%. Managing change in how we deliver services is about managing the human issues, about managing transformation in careers and lives. The human side of the equation must be central to achieve success, as work is restructured to coincide with a re-engineered health care delivery system. Restructuring will require us to shape our training and our retraining systems on the assumption that once-in-a-lifetime training is not the route to success in a world with significant technology advances.

There are 3R's on the human side of the re-engineering challenge in our health care delivery system:

- restructuring of work;
- re-skilling of workers;
- redeployment of workers.

With serious attention to these 3R's and a new infrastructure for the people side, a humane transition from our current health care system is possible. How do we manage our most important health care resource — our health care providers/workers — through this re-engineering period? First, we must recognize the need to alter the work itself. Second, we must recognize the need for all health workers, whether physicians or orderlies, cooks or nurses, to gain the new skills to undertake restructured work. And, thirdly, we must implement redeployment mechanisms. Redeployment is a fancy term for moving health workers to the new work from the old. Redeployment mechanisms will allow continuity and permit workers to follow health care work as it moves from inpatient to outpatient, from the hospital to the community and the home. Where an overall reduction in the workforce of a hospital or other health sector employer is required, effort must be made to maximize voluntary exits through measures such as enhanced early retirements or leaves of absence. Involuntary exits, i.e. layoffs should be a last, not a first, resort.

We have badly undermanaged human resources in Canadian health care. Unfortunately this situation is not unique to the health care sector of our economy. Generally, we focus on training young people, rather than retraining our existing workforce. Health care has been no better or worse than the steel industry or retail trade. We are now turning the demographic corner into a country of middle-aged workers. The only rationale response is to shift from a pure focus on initial training to ongoing workforce training for new skills.

The second major force driving change in human resources is technology. As it alters how and where we work, our skills are being surpassed. It goes without saying, revolutions in information and telecommunication technologies have created powerful new tools which we must learn to use effectively. We need skills to manage these new tools and to adapt to restructured work. These skills will not appear by magic. Training is essential.

Human resource management, training and redeployment apply to *all* health care workers, physicians, orderlies, nurses and managers. The Canadian policy effort to tackle the physician resource issue provides important lessons.

Job security for individual health workers will not come from opposing all change. The necessity of change is too great, the timing too urgent. Instead, we require careful attention to minimize the adverse consequences for individuals. Continuity of employment will depend upon ability to cope with modifications and evolution.

Bargaining agents in the health care sector are gradually acknowledging these realities, without much enthusiasm. They seek mechanisms to protect their members by equipping them for change in the work environment. We need new infrastructure to ensure re-skilling opportunities and redeployment. Successful creation of new structures and opportunities for workers depends on increased labour-management cooperation, often difficult to achieve in an atmosphere of reduced financial resources and layoffs.

It is essential nevertheless that management fulfil their entire obligation to their employees by finding ways of cooperating. It is also essential that unions participate fully in joint activities with the potential to create new opportunities for members to gain skills and access to new jobs. For this process to succeed, management must be open and direct about change; hiding consequences will not work.

It will only erode trust. Bargaining agents and individual workers need to accept the inevitability of evolution and work to adapt.

Re-engineering health care services turns on the acceptability of reform. In turn, the acceptability depends upon each individual's perception of their own risk. This risk is accessed personally. Will I lose *my* job? Will *my* income be reduced? Successful management of reform requires good answers to these questions. Answers which must be found as a result of communication and sharing between management, employees and where applicable, bargaining agents.

These are troubled, tough, times for those leading change in health services delivery. Just surviving is difficult in an environment of turbulence and uncertainty. As a people–intensive business, health services are shaped, to a considerable degree, by perceptions of the individual health workers, as well as the realities of the situation. These are essential steps for those leading change:

- Clear vision and objectives
- Have a *plan* developed with lots of workforce participation and based on objective data that people can understand
- Take care of people in the process of change: address their loss and their needs for support in a period of adjustment
- Commit resources to training, education and communication
- Be consistent and visible in the implementation of change with a transparent timetable
- Meet at frequent intervals with the representatives of the bargaining agents or other worker representatives; a direct and informed discussion in advance of announcements will assist management of the change process; do not allow surprises
- Be honest and open about mistakes — they are inevitable — keep listening and learning

Leadership of people in health organizations must take into account several complexities. Health organizations assemble an array of professionals with varying degrees of professional autonomy. This complexity is deepened by a major professional group who derive most of their income from sources other than the organization's budget. Fee-for-service physicians participate in the financial and organizational structure of health care services on a different basis than most other health workers. This in turn, generates further layering in the management of change.

Our health institutions must become learning organizations if they are to survive and manage transition among their people in more effective ways during rapid transitions. Some of our hospitals pre-date the creation of Canada (and have life spans far longer than that of many corporations). They have already demonstrated one characteristic of a learning organization — an instinct for survival.

What is a learning organization?

Consultant and M.I.T. Professor Peter Senge sees five disciplines converging to innovate learning organizations. He views them as "component technologies" of the learning organization. They are:
- systems thinking
- personal mastery
- mental models
- building shared vision
- team learning

Of these disciplines, systems thinking acts as the fifth discipline, because it brings the others together.[1]

There is also a qualitative and power dimension to the human issues. Most vividly captured in recent actions to reduce sexual abuse of patients by health providers, the above mentioned cluster of issues is really about authority and responsibility.

Remember, There Is No New Money For Health Care

The best assumption for health care managers to make is that they must provide with existent dollars in the health care system. While reallocation of funds from low-priority to high-priority areas is inevitable, the overall picture in the resources available to health care will either shrink or maintain very slow growth. That makes all of our jobs tougher. The most reasonable national prognosis for the next three to five years is no real growth in health care spending and up to 3% per year real reduction. The form may vary greatly from province to province. Alberta is proceeding with real funding cuts of about 15%. Other provinces will freeze funding and let slow inflation grind away at the existing purchasing power already of the health care system. Whether radical surgery or a diet is the treatment, financial resources will diminsh or stay the same.

---

1   Peter Senge, *The Fifth Discipline — The Art & Practice of the Learning Organization* (New York: Doubleday, 1990), p.5-11. Peter Senge does a very fine job of explaining the learning organization. Read this book!

Pace of Change

Change is stressful. Pace of change is a real issue. A lot of health care leaders and providers are wearied by the pace of change and wish everything could just decelerate. Circumstances won't allow it. People are going to have to continue a juggling act of doing a superb job of managing their existing programmes while being involved in innovative redirection of programmes. That is stressful.

This overwhelming feeling is felt all the way up and down the line. We will need to be skilful in managing the 750,000 of us who work in the delivery of care and in the promotion of health in Canada, to arrive at a new and better place. We will need to support each other. This is a real opportunity to make change in a constructive way, while being aware of the mounting pressure to move rapidly. We are in the early stages of a major transformation of health work. Our working lives in health will be irreversibly altered and, if we are able to balance efficiency with compassion, improved.

Chapter 4
Restructuring Health Work

In his presentation to the 1993 *Financial Post* Conference on Re-structuring Health Care in Canada, Mr. Peter Ellis, CEO of Sunny-brook Hospital, vividly underscored the need to restructure health work. Utilizing the following table from a Booz Allen Hamilton Inc. U.S. study,[1] he noted that as little as 16% of hospital staff time is on actual patient care, less than one out of every six hours!

Traditional U.S. Hospital's Typical Allocation of Hospital Staff Time

Nearly twice as much time — 30% — is spent on documentation or

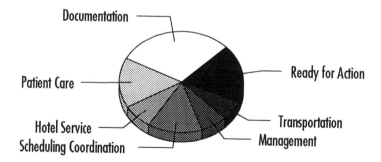

---

1   Booz Allen Hamilton study of American Hospitals from a presentation by Mr. Peter Ellis to the *Financial Post* Conference, 1993. Similar data is contained in other studies of time allocation in the hospital sector such as the work of Philip Lathrop, "Where Your Wage Dollar Goes," *Healthcare Forum Journal*, July/August, 1991, p.18. Philip Lathrop calculated that 24% of hospital employee time was direct patient care versus 29% on institutional and medical documentation.

paperwork. "Ready for Action," a positive way of indicating waiting, consumed 19% of total time. Peter Ellis reached the obvious conclusion: there is significant room for improvement.

In the context of restructuring health work, these are very powerful numbers. They provide a possible answer to the often-asked question "From where will the resources come to meet new health care needs?" Patient care time can be increased by finding more efficient means of handling documentation through new information technology. When nearly twice as many hours are spent on documentation as on patient care, there is an opportunity as well as a problem.

The objective of restructuring health work is two-fold: maximize the portion of health work allotted to providing patient care, and minimize all other work by health workers. This is a basis on which to re-engineer health work. It is important to start from a patient or consumer-centred view with a thorough process of examining how work is carried out.

New information and telecommunication technologies will be key enablers of the restructuring and re-engineering of health work. Because of our computer capacity to store and instantly retrieve information we have enormous potential to reduce the amount of time spent on documentation of patient records. Converting rooms full of files and paper records to data storage on computers can free up a significant portion of health care worker's time. This applies particularly to nurses, for whom paper-dominated record keeping has been a major misuse of their skills and time. As hand-held data entry computers replace the patient chart, nurses will have more time to nurse. Automation of records, and the ability to access them over telephone lines, will also allow physicians to utilize their time more effectively.

One of the activities undertaken by the Ontario Health Ministry in 1993 was movement to physician billings in a machine-readable form. By convincing Ontario physicians to submit their billings in this form, the Health Ministry redeployed nearly two hundred staff to other duties. There was also dramatic improvement in the percentage of claims free of processing errors.

The Ontario Health Ministry has conducted a pilot study with "smart cards," health cards with an embedded silicon chip containing full personal health records. While there were benefits to the use of the so-called smart card, the technology still proved too expensive for universal use. Automation, in addition to saving time and improving accuracy, also reduces inappropriate care and outright fraud within the health care system.

Any heath care organization should fully investigate the potential of information and telecommunication technology to assist them in re-engineering the processes of providing quality care. It is time to get going or risk being left behind. Many corporations have created the position of Chief Information Officer to underscore the importance of this expertise and to lead their investments in technology.

Multi-Skilling of Health Workers

Sunnybrook CEO Peter Ellis also noted that among the 1200 non-union staff at his hospital there had been 263 different job classifications. Compartmentalization is seen as a barrier to both care and performance in the hospital setting. Peter Ellis's remedy includes a matrix organization, multi-skilling of employees, a patient-centred care approach and larger service units.

Multi-skilling of health workers is a must as we move more services to the community and home. While many separate health providers visiting a patient's hospital bedside is inefficient, the inefficiencies grow dramatically when the many providers must travel to a patient's home. Without multi-skilling the move to greater in-home care will not achieve its full potential.

Teams and Super Teams

Self-managed teams is one useful approach to restructuring work and work organizations. Cross-functionality, an awkward word, is about connecting people in different jobs and functions, allowing them to problem-solve quickly and effectively. This contrasts sharply to a hierarchical organization, where decisions are delegated upward and instructions move downward. In a team-organized workplace, responsibility, accountability and decision-making rest with self-managed action teams.

Experience in the industrial sector shows the benefits of self-management. Over the last decade so-called super teams, between three and thirty workers who take responsibility for cross-functions and high performance, have been organized in about 7% of the U.S. workforce, according to a study of five hundred large American companies by the American Productivity and Quality Centre in

Houston.[2] Super teams make sense if a job entails a high level of dependency among three or more people. The more complex the job, the more it is suited to teams and super teams. The complexity and interdependence of health care work is indisputable. Teams and super teams could be the way forward in health care.

In companies that have introduced teamwork a dramatic improvement in quality and efficiency, an acceleration of decision-making and implementation have resulted. General Mills, a major food manufacturing company with all of its factories organized in super teams, reports productivity 40% higher than in traditional factories.

Plants with self-managed teams need fewer middle managers. De-layering is a part of the restructuring of work, but it needs to be accompanied by organizing, resourcing and empowering teams. Simply removing middle management layers will not realize the potential gains offered by a more comprehensive approach. In hospital settings or in community health care, significant movement towards interdisciplinary teams is afoot. Much more energy in that direction is needed if self-managed teams are to succeed. The relationships among different providers — physicians, nurses, physiotherapists, orderlies, in fact all those who have a role to play vis-à-vis service to the patient — will need to be carefully considered.

Allowing teams themselves to decide how to tackle the organization of work and other workforce challenges is essential. You cannot impose decisions from above and expect teams to own and be accountable for the results. Areas in which responsibility has been given to teams include work schedules, goal-setting and development of appropriate benchmarks to measure progress towards goals. Communication, flexibility and ownership of decisions made and their consequences, are key factors that make this approach more productive.

Among those involved in studying and implementing team concepts, there is a lively debate as to whether it is vital to tie compensation to the new team organization. Everyone agrees there must be recognition for teams and team members that do an excellent job. Whether the reward system must extend to compensation is unclear; there are strong views on both sides. Certainly, there ought to be motivation for the teams. Most involved in teamwork report enjoying

2 "Who Needs a Boss," *Fortune Magazine*, May 7, 1990, p.5.

it more than working in a hierarchy. One consequence of removing middle management is that there are fewer opportunities for advancement. This seems however, to be more than offset by career ladder shortening and opportunities for rewarding work.

Re-organizing from a hierarchical structure to a team approach is neither a panacea nor a short-term quick fix. It will require changes in everything from information available to employees, to the physical structure of the offices, including the furniture and how it creates relationships. And take a significant amount of time. In recognition of this innovative move in the work place, one large American furniture manufacturer now produces a line of "team" furniture which creates "neighbourhoods" or small areas for work teams, and a central work area with a meeting table, while desks nearby provide privacy.

These are some of the shapes of future work. Many of them are already evident in hospitals as leaders such as Peter Ellis at Sunnybrook Hospital and Jack Litvack at St. Boniface Hospital move their organizations towards a service unit approach.

Technology and Restructuring

Technology is restructuring work in the health sector by altering work activities. As in the industrial setting, the work of actually doing a task has been replaced by tending the machine that does it. In factories this evolution moved people from the shop floor into control booths. In the health care setting it has moved doctors from wielding the scalpel to overseeing machines.

An excellent example is the emergence of lithotripsy technology. A lithotripsy machine smashes kidney stones without surgical intervention. The patient sits in a bath of water. Sound waves bombard the kidney stones, breaking them into pieces small enough to be passed through the body. In the past, urologists would have performed surgery to remove stones to eliminate obstruction and the excruciating pain that would result. Now, some of these same surgeons spend part of their time watching the lithotripsy machine at work. Their role is machine-tending rather than active medical treatment. From performing to watching.

Generally, when machines take over functions there is a tendency to have the skilled worker of the past watch the working machine. Is this really necessary? Would a technician be just as competent? Naturally, in medicine, as in other fields, technology will de-skill particular tasks. This need not be negative, instead, coping with new technology will require retraining and a refocussing of effort.

Labour Relations

One problem in restructuring health work is a relatively dysfunctional labour relations system. There have been major upheavals in labour relations in the Canadian private sector, but the public sector need serious improvement. Historically, the roles of management and labour were clear, separate and apart. Labour relations was about dividing the "pie" between the two parties — labour and management. The labour relations system viewed its role only as distributing wealth, not creating it.

In the private sector, the Steelworkers Union — the United Steelworkers of America — has played a major leadership role in restructuring the American steel industry. They understand the trade-off between wages and jobs and the survival of the enterprise. They also comprehend the vital need to reskill their members. This is evident in Canadian Steel Trade Employment Congress (CSTEC), an innovative training initiative in which the United Steelworkers Union is an equal partner with the steel companies.

Job loss and rigidities in how work is organized are real consequences. Compartmentalization and fragmentation is not beneficial for workers or the health care system. To the extent that labour relations are unable to solve problems, they become part of the problem.

How do we change dysfunctional labour relations? Because the system is built around distributing wealth rather than creating it, bargaining agents must take some responsibility for the process that creates wealth. Management must be accountable for ensuring access to training and greater security for workers, as alternatives arise. Training security is essential to the survival of the enterprise and its success. This has happened well in some places and not so well in others. For example, when Canadair, the Montreal-based aircraft manufacturer, was purchased by Bombardier and they launched a new product, the president of the union at Canadair went to the Paris air show with the management team to help sell the plane. At Algoma Steel, the employees became owners to save the enterprise. The United Steelworkers Union played the decisive role in salvaging the company from bankruptcy. Historically, this has not been the role played by labour leaders. The old "no truck or trade with the bosses" approach to the world of labour relations is giving way to the new realities of technology, knowledge-based work and relentless financial pressure. There is enlightened leadership, in pockets, on both sides of the labour-management divide but also strong clinging at times to old confrontational approaches.

In labour relations, an adversarial system built around staying up all night, pounding tables, yelling and eventually, when everyone is sleep-deprived, coming to some sort of agreement is not constructive. Neither is an approach which looks to the past. Too often, bargaining starts with both parties soliciting criticisms with the existing agreement. This insures backward-looking. To begin with the premise that you want to deal with legacies from the last round rather than questioning where the enterprise must go is unhealthy.

Health care management needs to improve its attitudes towards unions and collective bargaining. Bargaining agents need to overhaul theirs toward the process and management as well.

New Roles For Managers

What about a new framework for the work of managers? This is absolutely essential to the overall healing of our system where the traditional barriers between workers and managers dissolve. As James Champy, co-author of *Re-Engineering The Corporation* observes in a recent article: "The role of managers becomes one of empowerment — providing workers with the information, training, authority and accountability to excel in a re-engineered business process."[3]

Champy cautions against three dangers for managers in this process.

1) Retain supervisory accountability:
   Work may be self-managed but it is not unmanaged. Instead, managers periodically must inspect the work, measure the performance of the process and its contributors, and coach the workers to even better performance.[4]

2) Leadership and vision:
   ...Managers must take on more leadership tasks — holding a vision for the business, articulating it to workers and customers, and creating an environment that truly empowers workers.[5]

3   James Champy, "Time to Re-Engineer the Manager," *Financial Times*, London, January 14, 1994, p. 16.
4   Ibid., p. 16.

3) New style:

...Shedding the traditional 'command and control' model for one of 'lead and enable' is proving a difficult transition for most managers.[6]

This is a transition of management style that not all managers can successfully achieve. Some individual managers, with self-awareness, will take themselves out of the line of fire. In other cases, board's will need to assess whether an executive or executive director is able to lead the change. Without vision and leadership, the restructuring of work in the health sector will be needlessly confrontational and painful.

Managers in health care have additional complexity in their working lives in that they deal with independently regulated professionals. Physicians are primarily not employees. Empowerment of workers must be balanced with physician accountability; a challenging task for managers.

Restructuring Health Work in Canada – Some Initial Progress

Formal Canadian experience with work restructuring in the health sector has been confined to a few hospitals. Many are in the early stages of planning. Much of the effort undertaken as quality improvement — either Continuous Quality Improvement(CQI), Total Quality Management(TQM), or as organizational redevelopment — has involved significant elements of work redesign. Often severe financial pressure has driven change. Frequently, incremental change has bogged down due to resistance.

In a recent presentation, Tom Closson, the Chief Operating Officer of Sunnybrook Health Sciences Centre, reached four conclusions on re-engineering hospitals.

Focus On The Customer
Think Big Changes
Use Data
Make Big Changes [7]

---

5   Ibid., p. 16.
6   Ibid., p. 16.
7   Tom Closson, "Gold Star Options: Lessons From Sunnybrook Health Science Centre," The Canadian Institute Conference, Re-engineering for Hospitals, Toronto, Ontario, April 11-12, 1994.

The sentiment expressed here of thinking big and making it big is reinforced by many in the work restructuring field. These are profound alterations to organizational culture and process. To avoid "vicious circles," where the organization cycles back to its previous inefficient or dysfunctional state, it is essential to make the shift permanent. Managing in a humane fashion will avoid unnecessary stress.

The best advice on work restructuring is to go and see for yourself. Visit the leaders in Canada: Sunnybrook in Toronto, St. Joseph's in London, St. Boniface and Health Sciences Centre in Winnipeg, University of Alberta Hospital in Edmonton, Foothills in Calgary. Talk to Jack Litvack, Don Schurman, Phil Hassen and others. Learn from their experiences. Work restructuring is going to be with us as a central challenge for the rest of the 1990s. It will carry different names, but it is a major trend. Learn the available approaches and select the right one for your organization. Better still, have your organization, itself, choose where it is going.

Good Stuff to Read

In Search of Excellence, Lessons from America's Best-Run Companies, by Thomas J. Peters and Robert H. Waterman Jr., Harper & Row, New York, 1982. The key book which began the new age of management change in the corporate sector. Because the health sector in Canada is about a decade behind the manufacturing industry in transforming itself, this is a very relevant book.

Meeting Materials, prepared by the Task Force on the Organization of Work, Ontario Premier's Council on Economic Renewal, May 21, 1993. Excellent background material from a joint labour-management perspective on the restructuring of work and workplace issues in their entirety. This material and further work on these themes may be obtained from the Premier's Council, 1 Dundas Street West, 25th Floor, Toronto, Ontario M7A 1Y7.

Chapter 5
Re-skilling Health Workers

It had struck us as peculiar that, on the one hand, everyone seems to agree that the pace of medical knowledge and medical technology is indeed pretty remarkable. Yet on the other hand, everyone seems relatively complacent about the fact that we train physicians over periods of five to ten years, then we set them loose on patients for up to forty years and sometimes longer without even requiring that they demonstrate that they are keeping on top of this constantly changing knowledge and skill-base. [1]

Morris Barer, 1993

Our basic challenge in skilling and re-skilling health workers is to ensure that all training is relevant to our population's current and emerging health needs and is consistent with technological progress. Re-skilling is fundamental to success. Once is not enough in health training. Evolution is far too rapid and profound to allow any health worker — nurse, technician or physician — to perform effectively for very long without acquiring significant new skills and knowledge. As health work is rearranged by efforts to enhance quality and reduce cost, new skills will be demanded.

What has been undertaken in Canada? Are we investing in new skills for health workers? Are they relevant skills health workers can adapt to new work in new settings? Let's consider a few examples of initiatives taken in Canada.

1   Morris Barer, National Media Briefing on Physician Resource Policies, February 18, 1993. Dr. Barer is director of the Centre for Health Services and Policy Research, University of British Columbia.

Physician Resource Policies — Barer-Stoddart and National Policy

The actors in the drama which created a new national physician resource included all thirteen of the ministers of health in Canada, their deputy ministers, two talented academic researchers, Greg Stoddart, Morris Barer and an assembled chorus of the provincial medical associations. The Royal Commission on Health Care headed by Justice Emmett Hall and the Banff Communiqué from January 1992 were two crucial papers in the overall discussion. The Barer-Stoddart Report and the articulate and forceful voice of health reform advocate Jane Fulton, were the other equally important components to the National Health policy devised. The central public question was "Does Canada have too many doctors?"

Barer-Stoddart Report

Two thoughtful and diligent academics, Morris L. Barer of the University of British Columbia Centre for Health Services and Policy Research and Professor Greg Stoddart of the Centre for Health Economics and Policy Analysis at McMaster University in Hamilton, were charged with completing an in-depth examination of physician resource policy. In their report, entitled, the Barer-Stoddart Report they devised a set of policy recommendations which caught the interest and commitment of Canada's previously mentioned assembled health elite. A number of factors led to it being openly embraced with the rapid implementation of its recommendations into policy.

The commissioning of the Barer-Stoddart report was rooted in a problem and a story. The first part of the problem is physicians are Canada's most expensive health workers. This is true not just in their remuneration for the practice of medicine, but also and more so for the cost of their training. As a nation, we invest very heavy subsidies to physician education. About 80% of the cost of educating a Canadian doctor — over $500,000 — is borne by the taxpayer. We fund physician practice through our single payer, taxpayer supported health insurance system. Unless on salary at a hospital or university, Canadian physicians are paid fee-for-service for their work, guaranteed by the government.

The second part of the problem was from the 1970s until very recently Canada was experiencing much more rapid growth in physician payments than in either population, even adjusted for aging, or in government ability to pay. A number of studies corroborated findings that when the number of physicians increased so, too, did the total billings to the government insurance system by those physicians. Contrary to the market logic of increased supply meeting or even saturating fixed demand, the addition of more physicians to any particular geographical area of Canada produced more supply and more demand. This phenomenon is not unknown in other areas of public policy. Building a new highway, for example, often generates more traffic rather than simply providing a means for existing traffic to move more swiftly. Say's law of economics, that supply creates its own demand, has particular application to physicians in an open-ended, fee-for-service environment. Governments in Canada, in particular deputy ministers of health, came to the view that managing the supply side of the system and its capacity would achieve more manageable costs. In commissioning Barer and Stoddart, they sought a comprehensive set of policies to implement supply-side management of physician resources.

The story which galvanized people to action, the over supply of physicians, was illuminated by Jane Fulton, a dynamic and controversial figure in Canadian health care policy. Jane Fulton is a public advocate for health care reform, an author and an extremely entertaining speaker. As Barer and Stoddart were preparing their report, Fulton brought to light that the original work of the Hall Commission had projected wrongly on Canada's population growth. Whereas the Hall Commission expected that by the early 1990s Canada's population would be 31.5 million people, it was only twenty-seven million. Physician requirements were calculated to supply services to 5.5 million extra Canadians, or a population 25% larger than it is. Fulton provided a solid explanation as to how the health care system's flawed planning created a situation of physician over-supply.

"... this issue of physician personnel is not something that arose simply during the 1980s. The issue really does go back thirty years. It goes back to the early 1960s and over that whole thirty year period there has been a steady increase in the number of physicians in Canada faster than the population and that is how we have come over that period to double physician supply in relative terms. Or put another way, there are only about 450 people per active civilian physician today compared with about 860 in the early 1960s. So we have gone through a long and extended period of massive increase in supply.

The second point is that this increase was an accident. It was not unplanned in one sense because the Hall Commission [the Royal Commission headed by Justice Emmett Hall which created the foundations for Canadian Medicare as a national programme] did present a plan. The Hall Commission put forward recommendations for a dramatic increase in the supply of medical school places and the remarkable thing is that twenty-five years later the number of places, first-year places, in Canada was still very close to what the Hall Commission recommended in the early 1960s. The problem was that the population was not. The Hall Commission reported just before the massive collapse in the birthrate in the mid-60s. So their 1991 estimate of Canadian population is 37 million and the actual is 27 million — 10 million did not show up. They also overestimated the amount of outflow, out-migration of physicians and underestimated the inflow and that is how we get the problem that the number of places they recommended as sufficiency to maintain the physician population ratio, in fact, led to a doubling of it."[2]

2   Professor Robert Evans, National Link of Experts in Several Canadian Cities, coordinated from Toronto, Media Briefing on Physician Resource Policies, University of British Columbia, February 18, 1993. He is director of Programmes for the Canadian Institute for Advanced Research and Professor at the University of B.C.

In their report, Barer and Stoddart avoided the obvious trap of developing a blueprint. Instead, they offered a set of linked policy proposals. Their preface states that: "Physician resource policy in Canada is plagued by historical and political inertia, professional and geographic territoriality, incomplete and inconsistent information, frustration and a great deal of nervous apprehension." It suggests, "we need to get over our collective Canadian-style fear of changing directions even when such redirection in clearly called for."[3] Barer and Stoddart identified priority areas in needed directions. They provided a clear and readable executive summary which, including fifty-three recommendations, totalled only twenty-nine pages. For busy ministers and deputy ministers, it was a welcome relief as documents go.

As a result of Barer-Stoddart being endorsed by deputy ministers of health, the provincial and territorial conference of ministers of health announced national strategic directions for Canadian physician resource management in a document entitled the "Banff Communiqué" of January 1992. Ministers accepted the fundamental findings of Barer and Stoddart that we should cease searching for the exact optimum number of physicians. Instead, we should recognize that annual increases in the numbers of physicians are in excess of population growth. The notion of matching needs and resources was fundamental to Barer-Stoddart and all of its recommendations. While disarmingly simple, this flies in the face of nearly two decades of governmental indecision on this aspect of health policy.

---

3   M. Barer, G. Stoddart, *Towards Integrated Medical Resource Policies for Canada*, Report prepared for the Federal/Provincial/Territorial Conference of Deputy Ministers of Health, 1991, preface p.v.

Excerpts from the Banff Communiqué:

NATIONAL PHYSICIAN'S STRATEGY ANNOUNCED

BANFF, Alberta — January 28, 1992

To strengthen the Canadian health care system and preserve the principles of the Canada Health Act, the Provincial/Territorial Conference of Ministers of Health today adopted a series of strategic directions for physician resource management.... The Ministers were in Banff to discuss the training, supply, distribution and payment of doctors within Canada's health care system. Across the country, governments are faced with spiralling health care costs and issues such as shortages of physicians in some areas and surpluses in others.... Physicians are one of the key players in Canada's health care system. Decisions they make have enormous impact on access to care and costs to the taxpayer. The Ministers recognize that working with the medical profession is essential and their plans include ongoing consultation between government, the health care professions and other partners.... Recognizing variations in health care priorities, each province and territory will develop its own plan in the context of this national agreement.

The Provincial/Territorial Conference of Ministers agreed:

National Policy Directions
1. To reduce by the fall of 1993 Canadian medical school entry class size by 10%. Future adjustments will reflect progress on other physician resource initiatives. The Ministers will ask the Canadian Council of Ministers of Education for endorsement.
2. To reduce national postgraduate medical training positions by 10%.

3. To reduce the recruitment of visa trainee graduates of foreign medical schools into Canada for postgraduate medical training.
4. To support the development and implementation of national clinical guidelines with an emphasis on health outcome research, that can serve as a basis for the funding and provision of both ambulatory and institutional medical services.

Coordinated Provincial/Territorial Policy Directions

1. To establish predictable medical care expenditures through a combination of regional and individual practitioner budgets.
2. To replace fee-for-service wherever that method of payment aligns poorly with the nature or objective of the services being provided.
3. To increase utilization of alternative service delivery models.
4. To restructure and rationalize the funding of academic medical centres to align with educational objectives based on identified community health status needs.
5. To introduce a series of initiatives to improve access to clinical services in rural communities.
6. To establish initiatives and processes to ensure the continuing competency of physicians.
7. To eliminate exclusive fields of practice and replace these by a more circumscribed set of exclusive acts and reserved titles through legislation.
8. To enhance the information base and share information for improved physician resource management, clinical practice and consumer education.[4]

---

4   Communiqué from the Provincial/Territorial Conference for Ministers of Health, Banff, Alberta, January 28, 1992.

The "Banff Communiqué" is a significant achievement of consensus among health ministers. Even more significant were the action's of provincial governments. Medical school enrolments have been reduced, in accordance with strategic directions. Consistent with Canadian Medicare, each province has taken a slightly different course. Provinces have worked together and two government officials, Dr. Stephen Gray from British Columbia and Bonnie Hoyt-Hallett from New Brunswick, have demonstrated incredible leadership in the transformation process. At various times, some of the provinces have backed off because of pressures in their own jurisdictions, however, the overall directives are being implemented and progress is happening.

In February 1993, a national media teleconference was organized where a number of deputy ministers of health as well as other health experts participated in a briefing. Throughout this process, one of the confidence builders for ministers was the sense that not only were they on the right track but there was enough detailed work being done involving all of the stakeholders, that progress could be achieved. One of the early steps endorsed by the ministers was the national conference on physician resources where all key health care partners were invited. Although there was some grumbling, particularly from provincial medical associations, there has been no fundamental challenge to the basic assertion of Barer and Stoddart. The Ministers accepted that we could do a much better job of getting the right number of physicians in the right place at the right time.

What will be the eventual result of this process approach? First, it's likely that a better overall match will be achieved between physician supply and physician requirements in Canada. Second, there will likely be better geographical and specialty matching. Third and most importantly, all of the crucial players — the teachers, the academic health sciences centres, governments and regulatory bodies — are working together with the expectation that sensible recommendations which emerge will be implemented.

An interesting dilemma was illustrated by Barer-Stoddart with the recommendation of 10% reduction in undergraduate medical enrolment in Ontario. Ontario has five medical schools. When Barer-Stoddart was released, the annual, first year enrolment for the five medical schools totalled 617; the target was to reduce it to 540. This could have been achieved in two ways. Either by closing one of the four smaller schools, McMaster, Ottawa, Queen's or Western, or the largest medical school, the University of Toronto, with an entering class of 250, could have been reduced in size. An across-the-board cut would have diminished the smaller medical schools to below the minimum feasible level. Arguments in favour of closing one of the smaller ones ran up against the unique qualities of each. Ottawa is the only place in Ontario for training French-speaking physicians to provide service to Franco-Ontarians. McMaster has a international reputation in population health and a significant portion of its graduates tend to enter teaching, research and public health careers. Similarly Queen's, in its rural and northern focus, and Western, in its service to southwestern Ontario, had appropriate claims to uniqueness. The policy dilemma became how to reduce the medical entering class at the University of Toronto by seventy-five students. A compromise was reached by University President Rob Prichard and Bernard Shapiro, then Deputy Minister of Colleges and Universities for Ontario, later principal of McGill University. It was decided that for a period of years, the government would protect the funding base of the University of Toronto Medical School. The University would reduce its Medical School enrolment, bringing Ontario in line with overall national goals and funds freed up from the teaching budget would be reallocated to a research fund. I am a strong advocate for increased investment in research. As we find ways of making the health care delivery system more efficient, and of growing healthier, lessening demands on physician services, the sensible redirection of funds is towards research. In downsizing the University of Toronto Medical School, reallocation of dollars to research proved an elegant means of meeting all objectives. Cost savings for the government, from the reduction in the number of physicians entering practice in Ontario, may total as much as $40 million a year. The funding transferred from physician education to research will average about $4 million per year.

Other provinces have shown likewise flexibility and creativity in policy implementation. The reshaping of the most entrenched and feudal of our educational institutions — the medical school — has begun. Surely we can add skills to other workers delivering health care.

Physician Supply, Priorities and Pogo

... What the data says is if you keep turning out physicians, each of them will remain, on average, at about the same level of employment and they will cost you proportionately more money. So you have in a sense mortgaged your budget to decisions that were made on mistakes 20 years old.

Now taking off from there you say, alright, if we don't know that the new supply is going to have a major impact on our health, we do know that it is having, has had, substantial budgetary impacts, so what follows from that? Well, one of the things that follows from it is that it distorts any efforts or prevents any efforts that you might be trying to make to reallocate resources within your existing health care budget. Every commission that has looked at the Canadian health care scene has said the priorities have changed. One of the reasons they have said that is because that is what people have told them loud and clear, that an aging population has different priorities for care than does the population of 30 years ago but you cannot re-deploy resources from one sector to another if you have already committed a continuous expansion of resources to the new physicians who are coming into the field. And yet, on the other hand, if you continue to increase the supply of physicians but then re-deploy the resources away from them the mathematics, the arithmetic of that very simply is that you are talking about trying to push physician income steadily down and that is going to be pretty contentious stuff too. So the political conflicts that you see arising now between physicians and provincial governments are a natural consequence of the inconsistencies of a policy of trying to re-deploy our resources from one sector of health care to another, combined with the continuing expansion of the numbers of people in that sector.

So that kind of growth distortion shows up in the great difficulty in trying to develop new kinds of personnel. Nursing associations all over the country have told us, and they are right, that there are many opportunities to use nurse practitioners, for example, to substitute for physicians. But if you are continuing to increase the supply of physicians then any nurse practitioner growth would be on top of that and, in fact, the nurse practitioner movement was killed off 20 years ago when we found that we were into a dramatic increase in the supply of physicians. If you look back, there were very strong pressures to introduce nurse practitioners at that time and they all died because of the physician growth.

And, finally, the bottom line distortion you get is that in a time of general economic contraction, very slow growth, if any, what we have found is that our health budgets continue to increase as a share of our national income, not because anybody has based a priority on them to this effect but because the overall economic base is not growing nearly as fast as it did prior to the eighties.

So, we are really now having to face up to questions that everybody knew were serious questions for the past 20 years, that the economic climate has become sufficiently severe that we are finally starting to think about what we should have been thinking a long time ago. And I think the relevant line may be from the Pogo cartoon strip which is that "man never reads the writing on the wall until his back's against it."[5]

Re-skilling Nurses for a Changing Environment

An important think tank on nursing and nursing research in the economic context was held in April 1992.[6] The organizers drew upon experts in the health economics and nursing economics field.

There has been a significant increase in the number of nurses in Canada. The ratio of nurses to population increased from one nurse for every 256 people in 1966 to about one nurse for every 120 people in 1989. Most nurses were still employed in hospitals, about 70%, but there has been a steady, accelerating shift toward greater nurse

5 Professor Robert Evans, national media briefing on Physician Resource Policies, Coordinated from Toronto, February 18, 1993.

6 Jan Dick, *Canadian Journal of Nursing Administration*, May/June, 1992, p. 7.

employment in community health and nursing homes. It is likely that, with reforms and restructuring, this trend will increase. As with other health professionals, nurses will need to acquire skills compatible with the new roles in the community and accommodate to greater community reliance on multi-disciplinary teams.

One issue is enormously important. Because nurses are largely employed by hospitals or other agencies funded by government on a transfer payment basis, their concerns occupy far less of the policy decision making time of ministers of health and their officials than those of physicians. This is a structural problem. Because ministries of health pay physicians directly, they spend a great deal more time battling with the physicians over the annual increase or decrease in fee schedules. Nurses are one step removed from the health ministry and receive correspondingly less policy attention. There are negotiations with the nurses' union, but these are typically centralized with the hospital association, at arm's length from the government. Nursing is central to quality care. Ministers and ministries of health need to incorporate nursing issues more centrally into the reform agenda. Nursing organizations are going to have to be aggressive, not simply about opposing change which they view as detrimental to their members, but in recommending constructive alternatives.

In this regard, the Canadian Nursing Association has been the leader for twenty years in advocating policies which look to a broader vision of health. We have much to learn by listening carefully to nurses when they give advice. We should take as much time or perhaps more to hear the economic issues raised by doctors as to the care issues raised by nurses.

An opinion poll done by Environics Research[7] occasionally tracks numbers as to the credibility of different professions. Nurses were at the top of the list with over 70% of the population surveyed saying they believe a nurse on an issue of public policy; some 55% had a similar view of physicians. Not surprisingly, given the times, political leaders ranked somewhere farther down the list somewhere near the single digits. The rest of us should listen more attentively to nurses. Nurses need to speak more forcefully than they have in the past.

Nursing leaders need to focus on the changes which health reform is bringing about and the fundamental economic reasons. The

---

7   Focus Ontario, Environics Research, Quarterly Report, 4th Quarter, 1992.

April 1992 conference previously mentioned, identified ten key areas of nursing economics.

Nursing Economic Issues

1. Current reporting structures hamper nursing input into decision making.
2. Cost benefit research is minimal in regard to nursing's value and cost effectiveness as a service profession.
3. Redefinition of staffing mix and human resource planning is needed.
4. Redefinition of the role of institutional and community nursing services is needed.
5. Multidisciplinary research amongst professionals is essential. This would include the economists, health care planners, and health professionals, including nursing.
6. There is no clearing house of nursing economics information available on a national scope for a repository of such information.
7. There is a need for lobbying strategies to influence policy.
8. There is a lack of nursing economics content in nursing education curriculum.
9. Revenue generation for all purposes related to nursing economic research is lacking.
10. Collaboration with the medical profession and other health disciplines in setting patient care standards is needed to a greater degree.[8]

Re-skilling Hospital Workers in Ontario

Like many innovations in health care management, The Ontario Hospital Training and Adjustment Panel (HTAP), was born of urgent necessity and politics, rather than scientific study and research. In

---

8   From editorial by Jan Dick, *Canadian Journal of Nursing Administration*, May/June, 1992, p. 7.

the fall of 1991, the fiscal situation of the Ontario Government led the Cabinet to determine a much lower rate of increase in transfer payments to the hospital sector for the fiscal year starting April 1, 1992, than in any previous time. After a decade of double digit annual funding growth — averaging above 10% per annum — hospital transfers would increase by only 2%.

Reactions were swift. In a flurry of emotional statements, reported as banner headlines in the daily newspapers, the Ontario Hospital Association forecast that this inadequate funding increase could cause 12,000 layoffs across the 223 hospitals in Ontario — almost 10% of the total workforce of 140,000. The Canadian Union of Public Employees (CUPE) forecast was slightly higher at 13,000. The Ministry of Health estimated job loss at a maximum of 2,500 or less than 2%. However, in a sector which had enjoyed two decades of nearly uninterrupted growth, this was uncharted territory. Whatever the actual number was, one reality was clear: there were no provisions for hospital worker retraining or redeployment and no infrastructure or mechanisms devoted to these. Some collective agreements contained extended notice periods, but collective bargaining in good times had focussed on dollars rather than on re-skilling or redeployment provisions.

In this atmosphere of concern and, at times, forceful disagreement, the Hospital Training and Adjustment Panel was created. Because there were no real models for a re-skilling and redeployment initiative in the Ontario public sector, HTAP was modelled on the successful joint labour-management initiative in the steel industry, the Canadian Steel Trade and Employment Congress (CSTEC). Then Health Minister Frances Lankin took three decisive steps to launch HTAP. First, Lankin approved $30 million to be transferred from unspent hospital funds in the Ministry of Health to HTAP as a three-year fund. Second, Lankin appointed Dr. Peter Warrian, the Executive Director of CSTEC, as the founding HTAP Board Chair to lead the start-up. Finally, Lankin invited the Ontario Hospital Association and the hospital workers unions (CUPE, OPSEU, SEIU, Allied Health)[9] to name representatives to the Panel. This was an offer they could not refuse. Anger at the government's funding decision did not preclude availing themselves of the opportunity to assist their member hospitals and hospital workers. HTAP was born.

9   CUPE-Canadian Union of Public Employees, OPSEU-Ontario Public Service
    Employees Union, Allied Health, SEIU-Service Employees International Union.

HTAP developed its policies and programmes at arm's-length from the Ministry of Health and with the active participation of these labour and management partners. Two years later, HTAP has created the following:

- joint management-employee committees in 210 of the 223 hospitals in Ontario
- over 650 displaced hospital workers in-training programmes
- a forum for labour-management discussion
- accurate information on layoffs in the system
- an agreement to expand the approach to the entire health sector.

HTAP Activity Summary as of December, 1993[10]

HTAP joint committees	**210**
Hospitals with reported layoffs	**160**
Committees accessing HTAP funding	**142**
Layoff notices* issues since October 1, 1991	**3800**
Workers accessing HTAP programme	**2100**
Approved training requests	**600**
Hirings through HTAP registry	**19**

* includes those whose hours were reduced by 75% or more[11]

One of the earliest and most important achievements of HTAP was actually a byproduct of its creation. HTAP's information system allowed a more accurate assessment of the hospital labour market. Instead of 12,000 or 13,000 or even 2,500 layoffs there were only a few hundred in the first year. Why? A number of reasons. Hospitals managed to make cuts that did not cause layoffs. Early retirements and normal retirements diminished the size of the labour force in a less painful fashion than layoffs. Significant reductions were made in hours of work for part-time hospital positions. The forecasted job loss "carnage" was replaced by a managed transition with support for re-skilling. A new mechanism, and a real commitment from government, management and labour found a better way.

10 HTAP unpublished material.
11 Ibid.

HTAP Works with You

The Ontario Hospital Training Adjustment Panel helps all public hospital employees, permanently laid off after October 1, 1991, to find employment. The panel oversees a programme, funded by the Ministry of Health, that fosters cooperation between unions and management through joint committees at individual hospitals.

The focus of the programme is local people working together. HTAP provides funds to hospitals through the joint committees, which are made up of equal numbers of management and employee/union representatives.

You Are Not Alone

HTAP has made a commitment to help you through your hospital's joint committee. The committee's first step is to develop a list of laid-off employees. To help you find other employment, HTAP provides assistance with:

- counselling
- determining your needs
- job placement assistance
- re-training and education
- family support
- retirement planning

HTAP's employment databank provides a valuable opportunity to access and share information. And, we're working with prospective employers in the public and private sector who are interested in hiring — and re-training — laid off hospital employees.

Funding Is Available

HTAP field staff will work with joint committees to develop a plan and budget for assisting laid off employees. Budgets are based on a formula of up to $500 per employee for first level assistance and up to $5,000 for training and relocation.

The funds are not paid directly to individuals. Once the plans are approved by the panel, joint committees will be granted lump sums. This funding structure is flexible — hospital joint committees may want to pool funds to maximize community resources.

Get Involved

To find out if there is a joint committee where you work, contact your hospital's administration office or your local union representative.

If you are a prospective employer call either HTAP or your local committee.[12]

Fortunately HTAP is not the only effort underway in Canada to re-skill and redeploy health workers. Many provincial jurisdictions have initiated activity in this field. The following chart provides an overview of these efforts

The Deborah Feltham Story

When Deborah Feltham received a letter last July telling her she was going to be laid off, she burst into tears. Her worst fear had come true.

"I'm a single mother with $1,000 to pay in rent each month," she said. "I was devastated. I felt betrayed and very alone."

Feltham worked full-time as an RN in gynaecology at Scarborough General Hospital. She spent years training to be a nurse and put in a lot of time. Two years later it was all over, and the prospects looked pretty grim.

Today, just seven months later, Feltham says being laid off is the best thing that could have happened to her. She is back at Scarborough General working part-time in critical care and taking home almost as much money as she made before.

---

12 HTAP brochure, published by HTAP in 1993.

"Thanks to HTAP, I was able to take a training course that changed the course of my career," she says. "A friend told me about HTAP during my last week of work. On my last day of work I went through the hospital's in service workshop for laid-off employees where I learned about what HTAP had to offer."

Two weeks later, an HTAP peer supporter contacted Feltham and discussed the programme with her. Within days she was enroled in the six-week, full-time East Metro Critical Care Education programme at Centennial College. Funding for tuition and books came through Scarborough General's HTAP joint committee.

"The peer supporter programme is wonderful," she says. "Before I spoke with the supporters, I felt if I was the only person in the world this had ever happened to. They gave me so much emotional support and good advice — it was just the boost I needed. I told a friend to go and she had the same experience."

While taking the course, Feltham managed to pick up a few shifts in emergency where she heard about a position available in coronary care. The day she graduated, she got the job. She started the following Monday.

Feltham says she wouldn't have gotten the job if she hadn't taken the course. And she never would have taken the course had she not fast-tracked through the HTAP programme and made use of the services available to laid-off employees.

"I never would have made the move to go back to school and improve my skills," she says. "Now, I'm planning to continue taking courses. I feel more positive about my future now than I did before."[13]

13 "*On the fast track to a bright future,*" *Communiqué*, Volume 1, Number 2, February/March, 1993.

Healing Medicare cannot be achieved by inflicting excessive hardship on a small minority of health workers. We need to continue to create schemes for re-skilling and redeployment. The HTAP story illustrates the need for problem definition and ownership of the problem by people with an ability to solve it. The Minister of Health could not successfully define the scale of the crisis and address it; she could only engage in a futile shouting match with the stakeholders. By creating HTAP, the key stakeholders were given both the structure to define what was happening and the tools to address it. There was also the capacity to achieve a win-win outcome for both labour and management. The Ontario Hospital Association and the hospital workers' bargaining agents delivered something positive to their respective members.

In its first two years, HTAP has achieved progress measured against its objectives. There has been significant, constructive investment of time and energy in problem-solving by the HTAP members, on behalf of their respective organizations. HTAP has broadened its mandate and focus from hospitals to the entire health sector in Ontario. As a result of the Ontario Social Contract Health Sector Agreement, the Panel, now known as HSTAP (Health Sector Training and Adjustment Panel), will also take on responsibility for the 140,000 or so health workers who do not work in hospitals. This includes workers in long-term care institutions such as nursing homes and homes for the aged.

Re-skilling and Redeploying Health Workers — Some Canadian Initiatives[14]

Program Name	British Columbia Healthcare Labour Adjustment Agency	Manitoba Provincial Health Labour Adjustment Committee	Quebec Health and Social Services Placement Service	Saskatchewan Health Reform Transition Program
Mandate	- placement of displaced employees - facilitation of employment security in hospitals	- address the needs of employees affected by health care reform (hospitals only, voluntary basis) - maximize redeployment, empower affected employees, provide information and guidance to employees and managers	- provide employment security to employees laid-off following bumping or closing of health care services - redeployment of laid-off workers - management of movement of employees, not restructuring of system	- provide funding for Career Assistance, Career Adjustment, and Severance Enhancement programs for employees laid off as a result of health care restructuring (ie setting up of 30 District Health Boards province wide as employers)

14 Adapted from HTAP Evaluation Report, 1994.

	British Columbia Healthcare Labour Adjustment Agency	Manitoba Provincial Health Labour Adjustment Committee	Quebec Health and Social Services Placement Service	Saskatchewan Health Reform Transition Program
Structure	- under Framework Agreement - Board of Directors — 6 organizational reps (3 union/3 employer), Chair by consent - Labour Adjustment Committee at facility level - Labour Adjustment Officers facilitate LACs, advise employees (each covers 2 regions and 40 hospitals) - HLAA is final arbiter of whether labour adjustment purpose is being served	- Letter of Understanding signed by participants - PHCLAC has 10 union reps, 10 employer reps, 2 co-chairs - government-appointed Chair - PHCLAC oversees program - facility Employment Adjustment Committees are being set up	- under S.C.F.P.— C.H.P. collective agreement - SPSSS administered by 1 MSSS person and 1 person designated by each association - general manager executes all decisions by SPSSS - Committee on Retraining has 4 employer reps and 4 FTQ reps - Parity Committee (SPSSS and 7 union reps) settle disputes under redeployment program	- Provincial Joint Committee — 11 members union/management, 1 gov. rep; 1/mo mtg.; sets policy guidelines - Sask. Assoc. of Health Organization (SAHO): administration of applications based on guidelines set by Prov. Cttee. Any non-standard applications go to Prov. Cttee for approval (in future District Health Boards — the new employers — may administrate program, but so far handling everything centrally is proving most expedient and manageable)
List of Services	- Priority placement - secondments - early retirement program - lay-off option - job sharing - voluntary transfer, relocation - funding of some retraining related to placement	- redeployment program/job line registry - employee/employer handbooks - supportive counselling, referrals	- placement service - lay-off indemnity (indefinite period) - continuity of benefits - retraining programs - moving expenses, relocation compensation	- Career Adjustment Program — funding for: training/retraining career counselling/job placement services relocation assistance alternate employment assistance - Enhanced Severance

Learning New Tricks

All the machinery for re-skilling and redeployment will not alter one reality. We're all going to need to cope personally with change. Whether we are writing health policy on a new and unfamiliar computer or learning a new surgical technique, it's made easier by a willingness to learn. Without it, change will be abrupt, jarring and damaging to health! With this willingness *and* the right machinery to connect people and opportunities, change may be bearable.

The U.S. Dept. of Labour, Bureau of Labour Statistics had estimated in 1975 that the average person would change careers once or twice in a lifetime, and jobs between four to five times. By 2010, the Bureau estimates that the average person will change careers four to five times and jobs ten times. To survive we must all learn a number of new tricks.

Whether we are professionals such as doctors, nurses and pharmacists, or the more numerous hospital orderlies and community health workers, two points are clear. Everyone is affected by the re-engineering of the Canadian heath care delivery system. *All* need new skills to cope successfully.

Employers, managers and funders of our health care system must ensure that investment in training and re-skilling are enhanced in this period of transition, not diminished.

The three key needs that prompted HTAP were the absence of accurate information on job impacts, the absence of a re-skilling "safety net" for hospital workers and the need for a new partnership, in which the government had a visible role. These concerns, and the development of new infrastructure to address them, have application to other groups of health workers.

There is no magic to training or re-skilling. It may take the form of a one-hour talk over lunch in your workplace, or a learning system embedded in the software on your computer work station, or a several year stint back in the classroom. The only universal truth is we need retraining to face the transformation we are undergoing.

Redeployment and Change

Significant redeployment measures are a necessary component of managing change. From HTAP to Sunnybrook Hospital to Vancouver, people in Canadian health care are leading and managing transitions for our most important resource — the people who work in health care. By building the new infrastructure of redeployment: committees, registries, linkages to re-skilling and accessible information on opportunities, we can achieve the needed affordability without sacrificing the humanity, morale and commitment of the health sector workplace.

Good Stuff to Read

The Fifth Discipline, The Art & Practice of the Learning Organization, by Peter Senge, Doubleday, New York, 1990. A brilliant book which has strong ideas on the management of organizational change. Senge is particularly good at explaining why change works in some organizations and not in others. A "must read" for those involved in managing change in health care.

Toward Integrated Medical Resource Policies for Canada, better known as the Barer-Stoddart Report in recognition of its co-authors Morris Barer and Greg Stoddart. This report was commissioned by the Federal/Provincial/Territorial Conference of Deputy Ministers of Health in 1990 and reported in June 1991. The Report is an excellent and comprehensive analysis of physician issues in Canadian Medicare. It is also one of the most significant health policy success stories in recent times. This report actually got implemented! Unlike a mountain of Royal Commissions, Task Forces etc., Ministers took the advice they sought. Available from Health Canada, Ottawa.

Unions and Economic Competitiveness, edited by Lawrence Mishel and Paula B. Voss, M.E. Sharpe Inc., New York, 1992. The section on Work Organization, Unions and Economic Performance by Ray Marshall is powerful and insightful in advocating a higher quality and productivity approach to the workplace. The message is one of a strong role for unions in competitiveness and productivity issues. The authors advocate greater union involvement in productivity improvement with a fair sharing of gains between workers and the employer.

Redeployment of Health Workers

Redeployment of health workers captures the increasing shift of health work from institutions to community, and the profound demand of rural and northern citizens for health services closer to their home. The enabling aspects of telecommunications technology have a role to play, but redeployment is based on the principle of workers following work. This voyage may be from institution to community or it may be a journey from a large city with doctor surplus to a rural or northern community without local physicians. The concept of redeployment also includes movement of health workers to non-health sectors where their skills are in demand. For example, the transfer of a displaced cook from a provincial psychiatric hospital to a vacant cook job in the provincial jail across the street.

The core belief embedded in redeployment is that workers are our most valuable resource not an expendable, throwaway commodity. Even in a period of rapid transition, people who have devoted their training and working lives to caring for others deserve more than a pink slip. People deserve, within the limits of reason, the opportunity to follow work as it is restructured by the financial, technological and public pressures. There is an obligation to uphold this opportunity principle. Everyone will need to be flexible and willing to learn new ways of working and proficiency in new areas. Job security will be a direct result of new work created from arrangements which support re-skilling and redeployment.

Sometimes, there are simple solutions to redeployment issues. At the Queen Street Mental Health Centre in Toronto, 25% of the psychiatric hospital workers have followed patient needs into the community. Over time, with the movement of programmes to an outpatient and community base, functions previously performed on the campus of hospital have relocated into the community. Workers have moved with the programmes and retain their benefits. Unfortunately, this model is not appropriate in every location.

Redeployment Possibilities

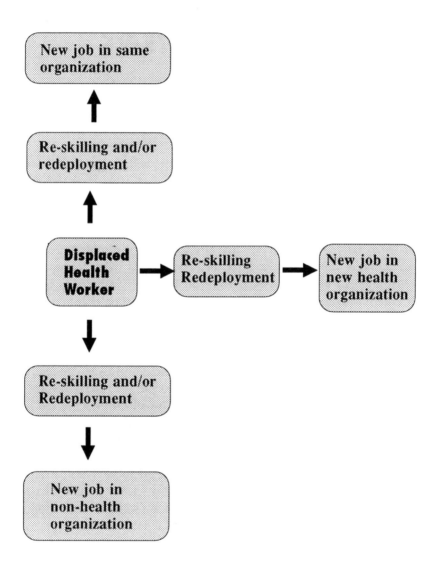

Getting Doctors in the Right Places

One preoccupation of national health policy has been to improve the distribution of doctors throughout the country. Historically and at present, Canada has a doctor surplus in the major cities such as Toronto and Vancouver, and shortages in the north and in southern rural communities. This is not unique to Canada. It's a situation which has consumed a great deal of time and energy on the part of policy makers and it has been a concern to the public, particularly to residents in southern rural and northern areas. Their assessment of the adequacy of the Medicare system is viewed largely through their experience of whether and what doctors are available. Doctors and hospital beds define health care services. It's not surprising that the inability of a community to secure a doctor or a sufficient number of doctors to meet a real or perceived need leads it to conclude that there is a fundamental problem with Medicare.

In all professions, whether law, accounting or medicine, professionals gravitate to larger centres. The fee-for-service system has produced the same situation for doctors. Often rural, northern or remote areas, because of relative scarcity of doctors, have larger numbers of patients, and therefore larger incomes than their colleagues. This is most true of general practice, and yet this has not been sufficient to assure a smooth geographical distribution of physicians. It's worth noting here that one would not want an absolute equal distribution of all physicians. There are specialty areas where the most appropriate situation is to have a few experts in the major centre and transport patients to them. This suggests that there should always be a greater endowment, particularly of specialists involved in tertiary care, in the major urban centres. On the other hand, specialization could be undertaken in regional centres were the medical and other personnel available to carry them out. For example, the Ontario Cancer and Treatment and Research Foundation (OCTRF) runs eight regional centres that deliver a high quality of care across Ontario in smaller cities such as Thunder Bay, Sudbury, as well as in Ottawa and Toronto. OCTRF operates on a different basis than the more open market, fee-for-service system.

Over the years a variety of methods have been attempted to secure physicians for less-serviced areas. In Manitoba, student loans to physicians have been forgiven at an accelerated rate if they move to an underserviced area. And the Manitoba fee schedule slightly favours service in more remote areas. That is, a doctor in rural

Manitoba would be paid a bit more for the same procedure than a Winnipeg colleague. Some other provinces such as Ontario have been unwilling to differentiate the fee schedule regionally. Quebec has undertaken the most prolonged and elaborate series of measures to bribe, cajole and force physicians to locate in underserviced areas. They include: limited access to facilities, fee differentials and compulsory service of various sorts. Ontario has stuck significantly to financial incentives rather than disincentives and has veered away from differentiating the fee schedule. In the most recent agreement between the medical profession and the provincial government, however, grants are provided for contract positions for physicians willing to locate in so-called under serviced communities.

As a result of the Barer-Stoddart Report on physician resources, described earlier, there have been a number of efforts made across the country to better match supply to needs. The following outlines Ontario's initial directions in this regard:

- better aligning the educational supply of physicians to the health care needs of the province
- modifying the medical education experience to better prepare physicians for the settings in which they will eventually practice
- exploring ways to better distribute physician human resources geographically and by health care setting
- creating a system of linked regional, multi-disciplinary referral networks to effect a mix and distribution of physicians that provides a more rational means of accessing health care providers[1]

Almost all measures have succeeded to some extent, although nothing has solved the problem. Our significant physician surplus has meant significant additional costs, with dubious additional medical value in larger centres, and continuing chronic problems in some of our smaller centres. Some rural, northern and isolated regions of the country have relied heavily on immigration of foreign-trained physicians to fill gaps. In light of the Banff agreement to manage physician resources, including restricting entry of foreign-trained doctors, this source will be curtailed somewhat.

Redeploying physicians depends significantly on changing the context in which they practice. In those parts of the country where

1   *Managing Health Care Resources*, Supplementary Paper, Ontario Budget, May 1992, p.20-21.

solo practice, particularly for a family practitioner, is the norm, the most frequent complaints from doctors working in underserviced areas are about compensation. There is a lack of backup support to take calls and a limited access to continuing medical education and other amenities. To solve the problems of under service, Canadian provincial health ministries will need new organizational structures, including more inclusive partnerships with physicians. Solo medical practice does not provide opportunities for work-sharing, nor does it provide for sufficient technological support. It is likely that physicians, like other groups, will need to form partnerships, even where individual practitioners are not in the same geographical location. Linking physicians together with information telecommunication technologies of various sorts will be a step in the right direction. So, too, will changing compensation arrangements so that physicians will be hired to work in the areas in which they are needed. They don't necessarily have to be employed by provincial governments, instead hospitals, community clinics or other health management organizations that emerge might take them on. The test of our ability to redeploy health workers must include a redeployment of the physician population to more appropriately meet the needs of all Canadians.

There are some encouraging signs. Recent graduates of faculties of medicine show very different attitudes from their predecessors. They are not assuming they will practice fee-for-service medicine as some divine right of physicians; rather, it is seen as an option to possibly pursue. Many others would prefer various compensation arrangements, particularly if they allowed the doctors more flexible hours. Real progress has been made in increasing the number of women in the medical profession. Women now constitute about 50% of graduates. Recognition of their approach to practice patterns can possibly lead to alterations in the overall approach of the profession to compensation issues. Younger physicians are generally more open to different models than just fee-for-service.

Another emerging direction in Canadian health care is a new look at academic health science centres. Previously, academic health science centres were seen significantly as locations for teaching and research. They were linked to teaching hospitals which were an integral part of the academic health science centre. Two interesting notions have recently emerged regarding academic health science centres. The first is that they could take on broader responsibilities for population health by harnessing broad expertise, including disciplines other than nursing, medicine or health (such as those in sociology, economics). The second notion is that academic science centres might take greater responsibility in the management of physicians in practice. There are already some isolated and successful examples of this. For a number of years the University of Manitoba Faculty of Medicine has operated a northern medical unit that educates young physicians and provides needed medical service to the north. In Ontario, a similar situation exists between the Mushkegot Tribal Council and Queen's University. The concept of academic health science centres taking greater responsibility for the delivery of care in under-serviced areas needs to be more fully explored. All partners, including physicians and future physicians, need to be involved in these discussions, if there is to be success.

Redeployment of Nurses

Canadian nurses have faced a rapid and uncomfortable shift from a nursing shortage to a surplus in a few short years. This happened so quickly that the Ontario government was still providing special bursaries to encourage nursing entrants when a moratorium on the programme was declared. In its second year, nurses graduating from the programme could not find placements. Four forces have simultaneously impacted on nurses: more appropriate payment for nursing services, the restructuring of everyone's work to free-up nurses to do only nursing work (this will be explored further in the next chapter), the shift from inpatient to outpatient services at the hospital level, and the shortened length of stay for inpatient services. The consequence of these forces is the reduction of nursing hours required in hospitals.

For nurses, redeployment will require creativity. There are opportunities for nurses in the community and home sector. There should also be openings in independent practice. Nursing clinics will require careful management, to ensure they are not a pure cost add-on to the system. The experience in the U.S. and elsewhere is that nurses can provide very good quality care in independent practice. Naturally, protocols for referral from nurses to other providers, such as physiotherapists or physicians, would be necessary. The second major opportunity for nurses may be in providing advice and helping to manage care over the telephone.

The Hospital for Sick Children in Toronto has operated two phone lines staffed by nurses since 1977. Their Poison Centre line handled 95,000 calls in 1993. The Medical Information line had 65,000 calls in 1993. It is estimated that these calls cost an average of $7.00 as compared to an average of $100 for an emergency room visit, though not every call substitutes for a hospital visit. Surveys have indicated that 75% of patients would have gone to the emergency room in the absence of the telephone line.[2] The benefits are not purely financial. Individuals worried about their health or the health of their children are greatly reassured by picking up a telephone and talking to a knowledgeable nurse. The benefits to the overall health system are significant in terms of improved patient confidence, improved quality of care and, particularly, more appropriate access to services.

Nurses will need to be organized and aggressive to seize the new opportunities and to ensure that as their work is restructured they can follow it through redeployment.

Good Stuff to Read

What Colour is Your Parachute, by Richard Bolles, Ten Speed Press, Berkeley, California, U.S.A. With over five million copies in print since its 1970 debut, and now in its 1994 edition, *What Colour is Your Parachute* is an excellent survival guide for the changing working world in which we live. It contains very useful tools to assess your real skills and interests. Investing in this book could help you on the road to a discovery of skills and interests hidden by the job or occupational label we all tend to stick on ourselves.

Updated annually, this is worthwhile companion for the voyage through a restructuring world of work.

---

2   *Journal of Nursing Administration*, March, 1993.

Chapter 7
Health Providers and Outcomes

Autonomy is not a right of professionals, nor a prerequisite to being a professional. It is a social reward, exchanged in recognition of the professionals' pursuit of knowledge for the purpose of better service to others. Professional autonomy is granted when society can trust practitioners to pursue goals which are consistent with the greater good of society.[1]

Ken Fyke, 1993

One of the consequences of Canadian Medicare's original great deal with physicians was the continuation of a provider-dominated health care delivery system. The political compromise necessary to bring in Medicare committed the government to act as insurer/payer and offer little "interference" with professional health providers. Consumers, no longer paying directly for their health care, became unaware of its actual cost. Government was only to pay the bills, not to manage the system. Taken together, these two conditions reinforced provider domination of delivery. The focus of health care debate for twenty-five years has been inputs: how many dollars are we spending on health care? How many hospitals can we build or rebuild? How many new health initiatives and programmes can governments launch? Evaluation of outcomes did not occur. The judgment of health care activities, on the basis of whether and how

---

1   Ken Fyke, "The Autonomy of the Medical Profession Must Be Earned," *Beyond Provider Dominance*, King's Fund, London, U.K. 1993, p. 48.

well they worked was always deferred because of the dominance of measuring inputs.

Physicians, although having had to endure some government restrictions in terms of practice in a hospital and incomes in the offices, have been in general, well protected from the effects of the recession. Compared to many other professionals such as lawyers, accountants, engineers, we have been able to maintain relatively stable income over the last four or five years. Many of us have friends, children and relatives who have suffered tremendously with the recession from job loss and reduction in pay to difficulty in obtaining meaningful work.

It is a difficult time for physicians but let's look around and we will see that it is a stressful time for a large number of Canadians. It is time for us to work together, to regroup, to replan and above all, to carry on our practice of medicine with great compassion and pursuit of scientific treatment. Difficult times bring forth the true art of medicine.

Profound changes will occur in the Canadian society and, in particular, in the delivery of health care in this country. We should be talking to each other, we should be adapting to these new situations and we should be, above all, keeping our cool in the face of adverse conditions of practice. Although it may appear that the grass is greener south of the border, I do not believe that Canadians need to embark on such a drastic course. Our country has a lot to offer, it has many challenges ahead and needs the participation of every man and woman to make it even greater. In terms of medicine, the trends will be to a diversified practice of medicine. We must be prepared to work with colleagues from other professions. We must discuss and plan new types of practice for the years to come. In general, governments agree that global budgets are the cornerstone of their financing for the next few years. With this in mind, we should be looking at new delivery methods of health care to our population. Group practice will become more and more important and through this, obstetricians and gynaecologists may be able to plan a better family life for themselves and better lifestyles in general.[2]

2   Andre Lalonde, ''From Time of Reflection,'' *SOGC News*, March, 1994, p 1.

Beyond Provider Dominance: Easy Theory, Hard Practice

There are Canadian examples of the tensions involved in the struggle to rebalance health care with a stronger consumer and citizen/payer role.

Lesson #1 — Witness — Quebec

In December, 1990, Quebec's then Health Minister Marc-Yvon Côté, launched provincial health and social services reform, focused on the consumer/citizen. These reforms identified the citizen as the focus, with three roles and nine 'orientations' with those roles:

For the citizen as consumer:
1. Citizens whose rights are recognized and respected;
2. Citizens who benefit from services adapted to their needs;
3. Citizens who receive services as close as possible to where they live;
4. Citizens who are welcomed, assisted and treated by staff dedicated to their task.

For the citizen as decision-maker:
5. Decision-making as close as possible to the action;
6. Citizens at the centre of the decision-making process;
7. Citizens accountable for their decisions.

For the citizen as payer:
8. Citizens who get their money's worth;
9. Citizens who must assume the cost of the services.[3]

By seeking to shift the authority within the system from providers — particularly physicians — to consumers, Minister Côté found himself in a noisy, difficult battle with physicians. Physicians advanced their critique of the reforms by portraying government as anti-health care quality, and themselves as in favour of it. The reforms were slowed down and amended because of the ability of

---

3   *A Reform Centred on the Citizen*, Report by Ministère de la Santé et des Services Sociaux, Gouvernement du Québec, December, 1990.

physicians to rally public support, or at least the appearance of public support, to their cause. This scenario has been all too common whenever health care reform, effecting physicians, is introduced.

As in all long campaigns, it's not the battles that are decisive but the general direction. Quebec is still leading a debate that will eventually be resolved in favour of greater citizen involvement.

Lesson #2 - Legislating a Tougher Regime for Patient Sexual Abuse — Ontario Bill 100

In 1991, the College of Physicians and Surgeons of Ontario (CPSO) became concerned about sexual abuse of patients by physicians. A task force, headed by a tough-minded Toronto lawyer, Marilou McPhedran, was appointed.

Based on survey work conducted by the Canada Health Monitor and Price Waterhouse Management Consultants, the McPhedran report estimated that 8% of Ontario women reported sexual harassment or abuse by doctors.[4] The Ontario task force advocated a philosophy of zero tolerance.

> We do not tolerate sexual abuse by physicians. We do not tolerate the ways sexual abuse by physicians is implicitly supported. We work towards the development of sufficient support for victims if they can come forward and they can heal. We work diligently towards educating doctors and the public about appropriate behaviour and attitudes so abuse cannot occur out of ignorance on the part of either doctor or patient. We continue to support touch as a crucial healing part of the practice of medicine when that touch is caring, nurturing and not sexually exploitive.[5]

Issues which go to the heart of power relationships in our society and to challenging past, implicit acceptance of abuse of power will always be controversial. A great deal of our energy as a society will involve assisting those damaged by the abuse of power by healers. Much of the healing is through various self-help networks and support groups, rather than the formal medical system. As Marilou McPhedran notes in the preface to the report:

4   *The Final Report*, Task Force on Sexual Abuse of Patients, Commissioned by the College of Physicians and Surgeons of Ontario, November 25, 1991, p. 4.
5   Ibid., p. 15.

Readers stay with us through the journey of this report, be open to the voices in it who speak urgently to us about doctors, lawyers, teachers, clergy, nurses, social workers, hospital administrators and others who have been vested with status, trust and power. If we allow ourselves to hear them, we will be able to move beyond the collective denial and resistance that have enabled abusers and allowed the suffering of patients for too long.[6]

I do not believe that the majority of professionals have abused their status, trust and power. It is clear on the evidence, however, that a minority have, and haven't been accountable for their actions. We have had a collective conspiracy of denial and silence in our society around sexual abuse. This is not, by any stretch of the imagination, exclusive to medical practitioners. Those without power, significantly women and children, have, for the most part been victimized, whether at Mount Cashel or in their family practitioner's examining room. A necessary part of both the personal healing and the social change is to bring this abuse out of secret denial. Acknowledge its existence. Our fundamental challenge is to ensure that none of it occurs in the future.

As a result of the CPSO initiatives, there is now a minimum penalty for any sexual offence by a doctor against a patient of a five-year suspension and a provision for a fine of up to $35,000. Recently, a parallel report to the McPhedran Report was done by a committee led by Dr. Anne-Maran Ponton for the Quebec Corporation of Physicians.[7] The president of that corporation, Dr. Augustin Roy, who has been criticized for both his comments and views previously, rejected the findings of the report. The Quebec proposals, which parallelled those in Ontario in measures such as penalties, more investigators and a toll-free hotline where patients can check doctors' records, were opposed and rejected.

At about the same time as the Quebec rejection a new national study found that 40% of gynaecologists and obstetricians answered "no" to the question "Do you think sexual involvement with a patient is always an abuse of power?"[8] Clearly we have a great distance yet to travel as a society to achieve understanding of this issue.

---

6   Ibid., p. 6.
7   André Picard, "Doctors in Quebec Reject Sterner Rules," *Globe and Mail*, January 14, 1994.
8   Ibid.

Provider dominance is a product of history and the structure of our health care system. It is not a permanent fixture. Although moving beyond provider dominance is a difficult struggle, we must. Determination and persistence will turn the tide to a healthier system.

Broadened Responsibilities — Prevention and Information

Health providers must take more responsibility for providing patients with high quality information. Providers have an important role to play in improving health status and in treating illness.

A 1993 study by the Kaiser Permanente Research Centre in Portland, Oregon developed some interesting insights on the smoking issue. Although smoking is the major preventable health danger for those who smoke, most physicians did not ask patients whether they smoked. Further, physicians did not record this vital health information on the patient's medical record. Kaiser's researchers developed an intervention where doctors asked patients whether they smoked. If the answer was yes, they asked if the person intended to quit. If the answer was yes to quitting, a date was set. Nurses followed up this very brief intervention by providing an informational video and a phone call at the planned "quit" date. This very modest and cost-effective intervention significantly increased the rate at which smokers successfully quit.

In Canada, we have been slow to provide sufficient information to patients. While patients have an obligation to take responsibility they can't do it unaided. We also have a great deal of room to expand multi-disciplinary approaches. This is not to suggest that health care providers will have the greatest role in decreasing tobacco consumption for example. Quite the contrary. Tough legislation, social marketing advertising and taxation all have an impact but health professionals can contribute both through advocacy and thoughtful interventions with patients. Even with the recent, and deplorable, reduction of tobacco taxation brought about by the Government of Canada, we have higher levels of tobacco taxation than other nations. As President Clinton increases U.S. levels of tobacco taxation to finance his health reform plan, Canada may have an opportunity to revisit its disastrous decision.

Canadian dentists have done an excellent job on patient education and prevention. The last time I took my son for his dental checkup the waiting room featured a very effective wall rack entitled, "The Dental Information System — Helpful Information for Patients." The display contained a series of excellent brochures on: *The Checkup* and *The Dental Office: Healthy and Safe*. *The Dental Information System* is provided by the Canadian Dental Association. It is a very thoughtful guide for people committed to better dental health. The physician's waiting room immediately adjacent to our dentist's had the usual collection of old magazines but no health information.

Good Stuff to Read

Beyond Provider Dominance: Managing Change and Transition by Fiona Hastings, stimulated by papers from a King's Fund International Seminar. Published by the King's Fund, London, 1993. Copies are obtainable from Bournemouth English Book Centre, P.O. Box 1496, Parkstone, Poole, Dorset, U.K., BH12 3YD. A provocative and intelligent series of papers addressing the questions of moving beyond provider dominance in the delivery of health services. The book is idea-rich and Fiona Hastings is able to wrap a thought provoking framework of Harvard guru Rosabeth Kantor's management insights (relevant books by Kantor noted in Chapter 4) around the health policy issues. It is both a good read and a road map to many of the tough questions among providers, consumers and payers. Questions that will occupy centre stage for the balance of the 1990s in all nations debating and implementing health care reforms.

The Final Report, Task Force on Sexual Abuse of Patients, an Independent Task Force commissioned by the College of Physicians and Surgeons of Ontario, November 25, 1991. Marilou McPhedran chaired this task force which brought to light the very serious extent of sexual abuse of patients by doctors. This report caused both a furore and new legislation on a very important issue which needs to be understood and resolved.

The Canadian College of Health Services Executives (CHESE) produces some excellent material for health care managers and others. Information is available to both CHESE members and non-members from CHESE, 350 Sparks Street, Suite 402, Ottawa, Ontario K1R 7S8. Material includes:
- *A Guide to Career Management for Health Services Executives*
- *Contracts and Compensation for Health Service Executives*

- *Management Control and Funding Systems* – Lawrence J. Nestman
- *Certification Preparation Materials – Self-Assessment and Certification Bibliography*
- *Ethical Dimensions of Health Administration* – Ed Chown
- *Case Studies in Health Services Management – Leadership and Caring Visions in an Environment of Constraints*
- *Seeds of Health – An Anthology on Health Promotion*

Promote Your Patient Care Focus Through Programme Management, a new video from the Canadian College of Health Services Executives with the support of Peel Memorial Hospital.

Viewing the patient as a customer has become crucial for health services since the mid 1980s when some hospitals began adopting a programme management approach. The key to ensuring efficient and effective quality services is to end the traditional hierarchical structure where departments work within their defined boundaries. We need to adopt a programme management approach where services are offered by cross-functional teams to best meet patient needs.

This video features presentations on programme management. Specific issues such as development, implementation and evaluation of programme management are addressed by a panel during a discussion sponsored by the College with the support of Peel Memorial Hospital, and held in conjunction with the Ontario Hospital Association Convention in November, 1993.

The panel included:
- Dr. Peggy Leatt, Professor and Chair, Faculty of Medicine, University of Toronto
- Marilyn J. Bruner, President, Markham Stouffville Hospital, Markham
- Bruce Harber, FCCHSE, President, Peel Memorial Hospital, Brampton
- William MacLeod, CHE, President and CEO, Women's College Hospital, Toronto
- David Martin, CHE, President and CEO, The Hospital for Sick Children, Toronto

Part 3

Taking Control of Health and Health Care

Is it beyond our ability as individuals to help save Medicare? Should it be left to the experts, the doctors, nurses, managers and health ministers? The experts need help in two very important ways:

- Stay healthy and be an informed consumer — use health services appropriately
- Be an active and informed citizen — help build a healthy community

One of the challenges in Canada is to become more involved as individuals, as consumers and as citizens, in our health and health care. When governments stepped in as the insurer for most medical and hospital services, we gained great security and benefit. The financial barrier to accessing care fell away. But Canadians, as consumers, lost a key role in the health care system. We were no longer individual purchasers. The marketplace process of consumer demand shifted responsibility to governments. Health ministers and ministries became the complaints department for the health care delivery system. Health care delivery issues became very political. Daily question period in every provincial legislature became the forum for consumer feedback.

Our reform efforts to date have concentrated on the supply side of the health care delivery system. Getting the right number of doctors, making our hospitals more efficient and shifting attention to outcomes are all essential to better care services. Healing Medicare requires us to go further and manage the demand side. Demand for health care services is not straightforward. We encounter the health care system for a variety of reasons. Sometimes we are ill. Other times we are fearful that we may be ill. Often we go seeking information. There are also times when the system provides care that we don't really need or want. To succeed in reforming Medicare we must take action to manage the citizens demands. We can accomplish this by enabling individuals to have much greater access to information about choice and control over their care.

How significant are the challenges in health terms? Consider the following data. Ontario will spend about $17 billion on health services, through the Ministry of Health in 1994. Many of these costs however, are generated by behaviour which could be changed. The

Addiction Research Foundation estimates that approximately 30% of this budget is due to excess expenses generated by legal or illegal alcohol and drug abuse.

Our health care system is situated in a social context which society shapes and affects. It can be assisted by our choices about our behaviour.

Chapter 8
Be An Informed Consumer

One of the most striking revolutions in our history as a species on this planet is the information revolution now upon us. If knowledge is power we are the most empowered group of humans in the history of our species. But do we act on the information? Do we take the time to consider how it affects our lives?

Staying Healthy

The most obvious way in which we can be informed consumers of health care is to reduce the need to use such services. By staying healthy we can defer or reduce our encounters with the care system. We can also enjoy life more.

What are the best steps you can take to stay healthy and enjoy a long life? When you scrape away the endless studies, a list of the top 10 ways to stay healthy is refreshingly straight-forward and sensible:

1. DON'T SMOKE
2. DON'T SMOKE
3. GET ENOUGH SLEEP
4. EXERCISE REGULARLY
5. EAT PROPERLY
6. LIVE SAFELY
7. PRACTICE SAFE SEX
8. DRINK MODERATELY
9. BUY A SAFE CAR AND WEAR YOUR SEAT BELT
10. DON'T SMOKE

If the list seems a little repetitive, don't worry. You only need to remember to stop smoking and seven others. Why the annoying repetition about smoking? Simply because smoking is many times more of a hazard to your life expectancy and health status than anything else within your personal control.

I am not the only list maker in the health world. The former U.S. Surgeon General is a fellow list addict.

Dr. Koop's Prescription for a Healthy Life

You can start to take care of yourself now. The prescription is simple:

- **Don't smoke.**
- **If you drink alcohol, do so only in moderation.**
- **Exercise and diet as appropriate to your age.**
- **Buckle up. It does not make sense to drive to the health food store without fastening your seat belt.**
- **Check your blood pressure and cholesterol. See your doctor if they are abnormal; then follow his or her advice.[1]**

By now we are all knowledgeable about the role of tobacco in causing cancer but how many of us understand the impact of smoking on increased numbers of heart attacks and strokes? Tobacco kills more Canadians each year than traffic accidents, suicides and AIDS combined. Almost five times more, according to Dr. Richard Schabas, Chief Medical Officer of Health for Ontario.

There is a silver lining in the lethal cloud of tobacco. If you quit you regain considerable health ground, some of it rapidly. Within one year of quitting your additional risk of heart disease drops by one-half. The risk of lung cancer takes ten years to drop in half, but by the end of fifteen years, your risk of death from lung cancer drops to an almost identical level with someone who never smoked.

It's also important to note that smoking rates are declining in

---

1 Dr. Everett Koop, *The Memories of American's Family Doctor* (New York: Random House, 1991). I don't support Dr. Koop's focus on cholesterol level measurement. If you take the rest of the advice you will also lower your cholesterol level.

Canada. About 27% of Canadian adult men and 28% of adult women are still smoking. This is a significant drop from 50%, or one in two men twenty-five years ago but a much smaller drop from 32%, or about one in three women, over the same period of time.

In planning a take-control approach to your own health you need to assess your starting point. A few key questions need to be answered:

What are your most likely health risks?
Do you smoke?
Drink to excess?
Exercise?
Eat a balanced diet?

Once you survive being born, as 993 of 1,000 do in Canada, your main and manageable risks are dealt with by the advice above.

Taking control of your own health is linked to becoming involved in the health of your community. No matter how well you eat or how thoroughly you exercise, a drunk driver can shorten your life. So can polluted air or water. Environment *is* a health issue. Our health as individuals is shaped by environmental factors, some of which are amenable to community action.

Staying healthy is not just a good idea for us as individuals. Studies document the overall cost to the system of a lack of individual responsibility. The lifetime health care costs in the U.S. average about $225,000 per person. The lifetime costs for smokers, despite their shorter lives, are as much as a third higher than for non-smokers. Increased physical activity is associated with fewer visits to doctors. A study by J.J. Sokalov indicated in a large corporate environment that claims costs for those who had three or more of the risk factors — including smoking, obesity, diabetes and hypertension — were double those who had no risk factors. This strongly suggests that staying healthy is not only good medicine for you but a vital part of healing Medicare.

It is also worth considering the costs imposed by these behaviours.

What It Costs Ontario Each Year Because of Alcohol and Other Drug Use

BILLIONS OF DOLLARS

	Alcohol	Illicit Drugs	High Level Use of Legal Drugs	Total
Excess Health Care	2.6	1.2	1.8	5.6
Excess Law Enforcement	.5	.3	.4	1.0
Value of Reduced Labour Productivity	1.2	.5	.7	2.4
TOTAL	4.3	2.0	2.9	9.2[2]

Be An Informed Consumer

Throughout the heyday of doctor-dominance in America, physicians kept a tight choke-hold on medical knowledge. Prescriptions were written in Latin, providing the profession with a semi-secret code, as it were, which kept most patients in ignorance. Medical journals and texts were restricted to professional readers. Medical conferences were closed to the laity. Doctors controlled medical school curricula and enrolments.

Contrast this with the situation today, when patients have astonishing access to medical knowledge. With a personal computer and a modem, anyone from home can access data bases like Index Medicus, and obtain scientific papers on everything from Addison's disease to zygomycosis, and, in fact, collect more information about a specific ailment or treatment than the ordinary doctor has time to read.[3]

Managing Your Own Care

Successful management of your own care is not a rejection of physicians, nurses, pharmacists or other very useful health care

---

2 Estimates based on research done by the Addiction Research Foundation, Toronto, 1989.
3 Alvin Toffler, *Powershift*, Knowledge, Wealth and Violence at the Edge of the 21st Century (New York: Bantam, 1990), p. 7-8.

providers. Self-management is the notion that you, the consumer, should not simply be a passive recipient of care. Multiple studies have shown savings from self-management. An article in the *New England Journal of Medicine*, in July 1993 estimated these savings from information and guidelines about self-management to be in the range of 7% to 17%.[4] This works two ways. Better information and increased confidence that much illness is self-limited. The *New England Journal* study also comments, in terms of self-management, that if confidence can be increased through education, there is a reduction in the cost of long-term health care even in people with chronic disease.[5]

Self-management is several parts Sherlock Holmes and a few parts your grandmother. Among the active steps needed are getting sound information from the beginning. Additionally, you need to build a home health kit with the following grandmother-inspired elements:

- Common cold kit
- First aid

Next, you need to understand informed patient choice as more than an idea. Finally, you need to make provision for health care in a situation where you cannot readily make decisions by writing a "living will."

If there were one right answer for each distinct health problem it would be easier to leave it to the experts. Your task would simply be to locate the best person. Unfortunately, there isn't one right answer or treatment for each condition. More often, there are a range of options with different consequences; potential risks and benefits are associated with each.

Getting Good Information

1. **Secure an information base.** This can be as simple as buying a book or visiting the library or as complex as linking to databases with your personal computer.
2. **Network of advisors.** Meet knowledgeable people you trust who can provide advice and link you to

4   Fried, Koop, Beadle et al., ''Reducing Health Care Costs by Reducing the Need and Demand for Medical Services,'' *New England Journal of Medicine*, Vol. 329, No. 5. June 29, 1993, p. 322.
5   Ibid.

appropriate care. Often there are support networks of those who are coping with the same disease or condition. Breast cancer support groups are an excellent example — they've been there. They know.

3. **Subscribe to ongoing information sources.**

These are the Sherlock Holmes steps.

It is probably advisable, in addition to books like *The Complete Canadian Health Guide* to subscribe to a health or wellness magazine. *The Berkeley Letter* is among the most popular, but there is a Canadian version available from the University of Toronto. A number of hospitals have health letters of various sorts as well. Their usefulness is that you are more likely to read something when it arrives than you are to browse through a health guide book. These letters are focused on new information, seasonal health tips and common issues. By devoting a small amount of your time and energy to making yourself informed, you will be able, in general, to manage your care. You will also be able to use services more appropriately when necessary, with a better understanding of what a particular health care service can provide.

In the case of treatment decisions involving significant medical surgical intervention, new information bases, supplemented by specific research on the condition or procedure, will vastly increase your confidence in asking relevant questions. Asking questions is an essential ingredient of getting more appropriate care. By asking questions you can state your preferences and also obtain more information.

Home Health Kit

Two or three components are suggested for your home health kit. One of the key ones is a simple first aid kit including bandages, gauze and ointment to prevent infections. Most homes would have a kit or a drawer with these items in it. Add to that, information on head injuries and cuts. You may wish to copy this information out of *The Complete Canadian Health Guide* or obtain it from other sources.

A second element is the very clever use of a "grandmother" approach of simplicity rather than high technology initiated by Kaiser Permanente, the largest U.S. health maintenance organization. In looking after their 6.6 million subscribers, Kaiser Permanente decided to take an active approach to enabling people to self-manage the common cold. The items in their common cold kit include:

- some chicken soup
- some generic aspirin
- a very good booklet on the common cold
- other cold treatments sold by your pharmacy over-the-counter

The point of the common cold kit, produced in both adult and children's versions, was to push back to the patient responsibility for a self-limiting illness. Colds come and go. The booklet contains the necessary precautions about going to the doctor if a fever or other symptoms persist. Generally your doctor can do little or nothing for the common cold. What she or he can do you can do just as well yourself.

Another useful ingredient for your home health kit is a diary in which to record illnesses, treatments for those illnesses and what seemed to heal you. With the proliferation of over-the-counter drugs and ointments, many common conditions can be appropriately treated by the individual. You can learn over a period of time about how your body reacts by keeping track of your minor illnesses and the successful treatments of them.

Informed Patient Choice

On several previous occasions in this book there has been discussion of informed patient choices as a means of making the health care system more effective. It's important to realize that informed patient choice is not only a good idea for the health care system, it's beneficial for you too. Take control of your own health care, understand the choices and participate in making them. We all have an understandable, human tendency, when faced with illness or a medical condition, to throw ourselves into the hands of the professional and say, "Whatever's necessary, doc, just do it." Part of our desire is denial. We don't like reminders that we are mortal. In many instances the advice offered by a health professional will be precisely the right advice, but how can you be sure?

Another major aspect to being an informed consumer is to seek within the health care system itself access to information. The Dartmouth technology of interactive video disks is one way. There are others like the CHEPA decision board. The main point here is to seek out more detail on the possible outcomes of various approaches to your conditions. In simple cases, such as a broken bone or an infection, there may be very few options. But in many other cases, the range may run from drug treatment to surgical intervention to a change in your lifestyle. The point is that you are a participant in that choice. Do you want back surgery or are you prepared to lose some weight and lead a more active life? Do you want to take drugs to lower your cholesterol level or are you willing to change your diet? Have you examined and felt fully informed about the consequences of particular interventions?

All of this is bound up in informed patient choice. The system can organize itself to better support patients but determination is needed on your part. If you are too passive you are unlikely to get access to full information.

Helping Patients Share Decisions with Their Doctors

The King's Fund Centre is piloting and evaluating an interactive video system designed to tell patients about the risks and benefits of treatment choices open to them. It makes information accessible to patients at the time they need to make decisions about treatment with their doctor. The system has two components—the hardware and the software.

The hardware consists of a personal computer (PC), a laser disk player, a video monitor, a video card for the PC and a printer. This compact collection of equipment fits on a desk in an outpatient clinic office.

The software 'asks' the patient to enter details about his/her age and symptoms. The system can then provide information about the risks and benefits associated with the treatment options available. The information is presented using a variety of formats—text, graphics, sound and full-motion video. The content of the programmes was assembled to answer specific questions about patient care raised as areas of concern by 'focus groups' of patients. Material is derived from work done by a patient outcomes research team (PORT) in the United States. This continuing initiative reviews research data from selected areas of health care to determine expected outcomes of treatments for common conditions.

The use of television and video can avoid the sense of confrontation and judgment sometimes associated with giving information through person-to-person contact. Interactive video programmes provide information which is standardised and consistent in presentation and content. An advantage of this technology over leaflets or conventional video is that patients don't need to apply their particular information to a more general population because the data is tailored to their own circumstances. This also means that the information can be personalized, using 'you' and 'your situation' instead of a general statement directed to the patient as part of a group.

The system is not applicable in all circumstances, for instance, patients in urgent need of treatment and where the choices are limited. Deciding whether a patient would benefit from the video is at the discretion of her or his doctor. Guidelines have been developed to help ensure that the information contained is relevant to the treatment choices.

The video does not make a decision about treatment for patients; it is designed to supplement the usual explanation given by the consultant or general practitioner in a way that means that the decision can be shared between doctor and patient. Programmes are available for the following conditions:

- benign prostatic hyperplasia (BPH)
- choices of surgery for early breast cancer
- chemotherapy after surgery for early breast cancer
- mild raised blood pressure
- the treatment of low back pain

The King's Fund Centre will evaluate all the programmes and assess the part this technology can play in the National Health Service. The evaluations involve studies of how patients and those involved in their care respond to this method of providing information.

Clinical trials have started on the BPH and hypertension videos in a hospital and in a general practice setting. How patients feel about the content of the video and how satisfied they are with the choices they make are of particular interest. The evaluations are being conducted in conjunction with the London School of Hygiene and

Tropical Medicine and the Health Services Research Unit at Oxford University.

The opinions of professional groups and patient organizations are being sought, as well as those of individual patients and doctors, to help decide whether the content of existing interactive videos needs adaptation before being introduced more widely into the NHS. A logical development is the production of British versions. Plans are being considered for this next stage.[6]

Managing Medications

Most of us already manage a range of medications. When we give our children an aspirin or rub ointment on a cut we are managing medication. Our role is certain to expand. Professor Michael Cooper, an insightful health thinker from New Zealand, offers his thoughts on self-medication:

Self-Medication

Virtually everyday of our lives we are subject to an array of discomforts the majority of which we either ignore or treat ourselves without attending a doctor. Surveys conducted in numerous countries suggest strongly that nine out of every ten people suffer from at least one condition of sickness during the course of any four week period. To be ill appears to be quite normal. Despite large variations in both scope and methodology a measure of consensus seems to emerge from the studies conducted to date which suggests that between 45–55% of all health conditions are largely ignored, 27–29% are self-medicated and 18–23% treated either by a doctor visit or by a prescription medicine already to hand from with the house. The percentage of conditions which prompt an immediate doctor visit, however, shows little uniformity ranging from 4% to 11% with one study suggesting that only 1 in 37 symptoms result in a doctor visit. Overall, it seems that at least 75% of all illness is

6   Adam Darkins, *KF News,* Vol. 26, No. 2, King's Fund, London, 1994.

coped with by the individual alone without recourse to a doctor....

...Self-medication is undoubtedly here to stay. It is as Rottenberg has put it, "a self-reliant attempt to solve a medical problem in the simplest, most economical way." In the UK, with medicine which is largely free at the time of consumption and low access costs to the general practitioner, market forces appear not to favour self-medication as strongly as overseas but the great majority of people are anxious to collaborate with their doctors and to use his services sparingly and to the best advantage. It is a tough job being a consumer, however, and we need assistance in determining when a consultation is appropriate, what conditions to self-treat, and how. As the Royal Commission studying medical education stated, "when adequate arrangements for health education and prophylaxis have been established, the typical patients of the future — who will be better educated and better informed about health dangers — can be expected to take more responsibility for the management of trivial and self-limiting complaints, provided that he is given the necessary encouragement and guidance by the medical profession.... The pharmacist, too, has an important role and one which must be more fully recognized. There can be no doubt that at present we fail to fully utilize his skill, knowledge and three years' training.

Much of future progress in health will come from what people are able to do for themselves in terms of collective and individual decision making about their life style and the socioeconomic environment. The rules of healthy living are fairly well known (if rather uninviting), and there is a rising tide of public opinion in support of the notion that people have become too dependent upon experts who make decisions on their behalf. Indeed, central to the future of primary care is the need for greater self-reliance and self-determination in matters relating to health. Responsible self-medication has an important role to play in this future.[7]

---

7   Professor Michael Cooper, "The Economics of Self-Medication," *Social Policy and Administration*, Vol., 19, No. 3, Autumn 1987, p. 238.

Make a Living Will

The fourth recommended step in utilizing care more appropriately is to provide direction about your care in case you are unable to give it directly.

Dr. Peter Singer describes a living will as:

> a written document containing your wishes about life-sustaining treatment. You make a living will when you can understand treatment choices and appreciate their consequences (i.e. when you are "capable"). A living will only takes effect when you can no longer understand and appreciate treatment choices (i.e. when you are "incapable"). There are two parts to a living will: an *instruction directive* and a *proxy directive*.
>
> An *instruction directive* specifies *what* life-sustaining treatments you would or would not want in various situations. A proxy directive specifies *who* you want to make treatment decisions on your behalf if you no longer can do so.[8]

Living wills are now legally recognized in Quebec, Nova Scotia and Manitoba. Recognition in Ontario is expected in 1994 and other provinces are likely to follow. Living wills go by a variety of names, including *health care directive* and power of attorney for *personal care*.

Dr. Singer notes that "a living will speaks for you when you are no longer able to speak for yourself."[9] An excellent description.

Why take this step? There are two types of burdens in treatment imposed by uncertainty. The first is a very human one. Your loved ones: spouse, children or others, must make decisions without knowing what you might really want. Many of us err on the side of more treatment for/to others than we might wish for ourselves. I lived through these decisions with a terminally ill father and probably insisted on too much treatment, the type that extended death rather than restored life. It's common for families to insist on heroic and often intrusive efforts because of a desire, a hope to prevent the inevitability of death.

The second burden is one of excessive costs. With 18-30% of health system costs incurred in the last year of life,[10] I would have

---

8   Dr. Peter Singer, *Living Will*, Centre for Bioethics University of Toronto, Toronto, 1993, p. 1.
9   Ibid., p. 2.

no desire to add to these costs by leaving choices to others. Recent studies indicate that 70% of people request no life-sustaining treatment for themselves when they are dying. 89% desire living wills, yet fewer than 10% have actually made an advance directive.[11] Clearly, the potential for vastly expanded use of these directives could allow both more appropriate care and a reduction in overly intensive terminal care.

The *instruction directive* requires you to think about possibilities and admit your own mortality. Making these decisions was not the most fun I've ever had. Nevertheless, upon serious reflection, the following are the choices I arrived at. These are not choices I want to burden my children with.

Bioethics Living Will Instruction Directive

Directions: Refer back to "Health Situations" and "Life-Sustaining Treatments" for the definitions of terms used in this directive. Write your treatment decision (YES, NO, or UNDECIDED) in the boxes below for each combination of health situation and treatment. For example, if you want tube feeding in severe dementia you would write "yes" in the bottom right hand box; if you do not want tube feeding in severe dementia, you would write "no" and if you are undecided, you would write "undecided." On the other side of this page, under "further instructions," you may express in your own words the situations in which you would or would not want various life-sustaining treatments.

10 Fuchs, V.R., "Though much is taken: reflections on aging, health and medical care," *Milbank Memorial Fund Quarterly,* Q Health Soc; 1984; 62:143-66.

11 Greco, P.J., "The Patient Self-Determination Act and the Future of Advance Directives," *Ana Intern Med* 1991;115:639-43. Emanuel LL, Barry MJ, Stoeckle JD, Ettelson LM, Emanuel EJ. "Advance directives for medical care -a case for greater use." *New England Journal Medicine* 1993; 24:889-95 Podrid PJ. "Resuscitation in the elderly: a blessing or a curse?" *Ana Intern Med* 1989;111;193-95

	CPR	Respirator	Dialysis	Life-saving Surgery	Blood Transfusion	Life-saving Antibiotics	Tube Feeding
Current Health	yes	yes	yes	yes	yes	yes	yes
Permanent Coma	no	no	no	no	no	no	no
Terminal Illness	yes	no	yes	yes	yes	yes	no
Mild Stroke	yes	yes	yes	yes	yes	yes	yes
Moderate Stroke	yes	yes	yes	yes	yes	yes	yes
Severe Stroke	yes	no	no	yes	no	no	no
Mild Dementia	yes	yes	yes	yes	yes	yes	yes
Moderate Dementia	no	no	no	no	no	no	no
Severe Dementia	no	no	no	no	no	no	no

Good Stuff to Read

The Complete Canadian Health Guide, Editor June Engel, University of Toronto & Key Porter Books, Toronto, 1993, $29.95. A marvellous new addition for your health "take control" library has just arrived. The University of Toronto Faculty, in cooperation with Key Porter Books, has just published a really, really fine guide, comprehensive in nature in a very open, readable style. Place this at the top of the highly recommended list. The Canadian content is also very helpful. The seventeen chapters cover the gamut from What Good Health Is All About? to Nutrition to Specific Diseases and Disorders.

Living Will, Centre for Bioethics, University of Toronto. Dr. Peter Singer, Associate Director of the Centre for Bioethics, has produced an actual Living Will. You complete it and it becomes a personal, legal document. The Living Will is available from the Centre for Bioethics for $5.00 per copy. It is a major step forward in allowing *you* to take control and make decisions now rather than someone else making them later. The document comes complete with directions and a form that can be completed and copied on legal-sized paper. You can get it by writing: Centre for Bioethics, University of Toronto, 88 College Street, Toronto, Ontario M5G 1L4, telephone: (416)978-2709, Fax: (416)978-1911.

Health News, University of Toronto Faculty of Medicine. Available for $18.95 per year. Six issues per year from Hilborni, The Newsletter Group, 205 – 109 Vanderhoof Ave., Toronto, Ont. M5S 1A8. A recent issue contained the following:
- review of birthing in the '90s
- first aid in the age of AIDS
- dry eyes and eyecare tips

Healthy Life Guide to Self-Care — An Apple A Day Isn't Enough. American Institute for Preventive Medicine, 30445 Northwestern Hwy., Suite 350, Farmington Hills, MI, USA 48334, Fax: (313) 539-1818. This is an excellent guide to key issues of self-care health.

Deadly Choices Coping With Health Risks in Everyday Life, by Dr. Jeffrey E. Harris, Basic Books, New York, 1993. A solid review of the most recent evidence on health risks at the personal level and what you can do about them. The use of individual cases makes it more readable.

Tobacco and Your Health, Report of the Chief Medical Officer of Health, Ministry of Health, Ontario, 1991. A short, extremely readable review of the available and horrifying data on the impact of tobacco on the health of Ontarians. A good report to share with adolescent children during a necessary parental talk on the effects of tobacco on every aspect of your children's health. If you can convince your children not to start smoking it may be the single most important contribution you can make to their good health and long life. Better than all those vitamins and beets! The report can be obtained free of charge by writing to: Communications Branch Ministry of Health, 8th Floor, Hepburn Block, 80 Grosvenor Street, Queen's Park, Toronto, Ontario.

The 1992 and 1993 Reports by Ontario's Chief Medical Officer of Health can also be obtained from this address.

Mayo Clinic Family Health Book. First class medical reference available on CD-ROM from Interactive Publications.

The *Get Well Quick Kit*, by Linda Allison and Tom Fergusen M.D., Addison-Wesley. For children ages seven and up. A good health primer and modest "kit" of useful stuff.

Chapter 9
Be An Active Informed Citizen

Why is this important? Does it really matter how involved we are in health care? Why not leave it to the experts and the leaders we elect? The best answer is that both the experts and our elected leaders sincerely need your help. The changes necessary to make us live longer in good health and to re-engineer our health services cannot simply be imposed by legislation. Active involvement is essential. Without your help progress will be too slow, services will be discontinued and resources wasted on ineffective and inappropriate endeavours. From a personal standpoint, you may lose years of potential good health.

Helping Make Healthy Public Policy

To succeed in reforming Canadian Medicare we need health goals. We also need healthy public policy.

There are two key ingredients to healthy public policy:
- leadership and vision;
- new ways of making public policy.

Fortunately, both seem to be in evidence in Canada in the 1990s. Health goals however are meaningless without the means to achieve them.

There is, it is often said, only one group of taxpayers — us — and therefore the magic solution to access significantly more revenue is non-existent. Another dimension of public policy-making in health is the emergence of not one but two major advocacy coalitions. These are the Coalition to Keep Medicare Healthy, largely spearheaded by the Canadian Union of Public Employees with some

400,000 members, (100,000 of whom work in health care), and the Health Action Lobby (HEAL) coalition, with some 500,000 members (largely providers, although the Consumer Association of Canada is part of HEAL).

The Coalition to Keep Medicare Healthy has a seven-point plan. This coalition, with its roots in hospital workers' unions feels that we need to:

1. Stop the fee-for-service treadmill
2. Give non-physician staff a larger role in patient care
3. Eliminate health care for profit
4. Elect hospital boards and democratize health-care institutions
5. Reduce dependency on prescription drugs and make them more affordable
6. Guarantee that health care is of the highest quality, whether it is provided in the home, the community or an institution
7. Encourage preventive care

The HEAL group has ten principles or goals with three specific requests to health ministers. One is to ensure that consultations with consumers and providers, in developing health goals, are meaningful and occur at early opportunities; they want to be involved. The second request is to establish a stable financial planning horizon to consider transition funding and invite HEAL to participate in the forthcoming review of major federal transfers to the provinces. Thirdly, they want to establish a national task force to clarify the five Medicare criteria and develop more effective methods to ensure its attainment. HEAL and the Coalition have met with five of the provincial ministers, to agree on which of the two groups (or none or both) to hear. The federal ministers have met with HEAL, and provincial ministers have met with each of the two groups. Not everyone is quite at the same table yet, but movement is afoot. The National Health Forum proposed by the Government of Canada may improve the dialogue. Already many of the provinces have engaged their citizens, at the community level, in constructive conversation about health and health care.

There is an odd verbal puzzle to health care reform debates. First, everybody agrees that the status quo is not working, that we are in a period of change. Two, everybody puts the rhetorical umbrellas of health care reform and quality over the changes that are taking place. The crunch comes because there is fundamental disagreement inside that umbrella about what is meant by health care reform. Meanings are not necessarily diametrically opposed, but certainly the prescriptions of the Coalition to Keep Medicare Healthy and those of HEAL, diverge significantly. It is understandable that provider organizations, which are largely what the two coalitions represent, are concerned with protecting the interests of their constituent members. The national organizations have embraced change at the level of their statements, speeches and policies more generously than their provincial constituent organizations. That is understandable. It's not the federal minister that explains why a certain procedure isn't being performed or why a certain patient is leaving the country, the ten provincial and two territorial ministers have that privilege. As Nye Bevan once said of the National Health Service in England: "If a ward nurse dropped a bed pan in a public hospital anywhere in England, the sound resonated through the Parliament of Westminster." The complaints department for the health-care system is unfortunately the provincial legislature and the daily newspaper. So, too, the leader of the national organizations are less involved in the day-to-day struggle for dollars than their provincial counterparts. Canadian health reform is a struggle of ideas at the national level and a battle of financial interests as well as ideas at the provincial and local level.

New Ways to Make Public Policy

Traditional public policy-making in Canada is failing to keep pace with needed change. The old ways of Royal Commissions, hierarchical government departments and academic institutions are unable to contend with the onslaught of television, lobbyists and public expectations of speed. How can a Royal Commission be credible after five years when all the same experts gave their identical views on television the night it was launched and again when it concluded? Particularly when five years and twenty-five million dollars have failed to deliver any new insights! How can government officials successfully advise elected leaders on the complexity of issues in a thirty second television clip?

Speed has come to dominate our channel changing, fast food, ATM, fax and cellular phone society. It cannot leave public policy unscathed. New ways of merging competing interest and obtaining intelligent advice are arising. So too, are innovative decision-making forums. How are we making public health policy in the 1990s?

Several new ways policies are being made, are delineated briefly below. They range from new approaches to provider (physician/hospital) negotiations, to devolution from provinces to regions, to greater consumer involvement. None has gained hegemony in the discussion of how to achieve transformation of our system. All are being experimented with or being implemented in various Canadian jurisdictions at this very moment.

More Interventionist Public Policy Leadership by Governments

Governments are shifting from an insurance role to a more directive managerial role. In a number of instances, governments in Canada are acting unilaterally, through legislation or policy to accomplish change. This new role is much more intrusive than governments have played in the past. As noted above, Saskatchewan, Alberta and New Brunswick have taken particular action in the case of hospital restructuring and governance. The British Columbia government legislated a cap on total payments to physicians after failing to reach a negotiated settlement, which led to further talks and eventual agreement.

Governments managing under severe fiscal constraints are taking more explicit decisions and finding, if not full public support, at least not the same degree of opposition that existed in the past. The view that hard choices will need to be made to preserve Medicare has gained considerable weight throughout the country, although there are still suspicions, largely among provider groups, that some of these actions constitute a dismantling of Medicare. In Alberta where the government is reducing funding by 17% over three years the debate is very heated.

In some instances governments have announced targets or decisions and then negotiated with providers within the limits. For example, in its 1991 Budget, the Government of Ontario proposed to reduce fees paid to private laboratories by 5% across-the-board. Instead, it reached agreement with the laboratory association to reduce fees for eighteen particular tests by a larger percentage achieving the same result.

Governments have also undertaken to publish supplementary budget documents and health action plans, which set out specific directions and allocation of resources. These documents represent the translation of health policy into the concrete reality of dollars allocated among health programmes.

Negotiations between Governments and Providers

Negotiations are taking improved forms, and diversified/alternative bargaining structures are being established. Historically, government-provider negotiations dealt almost exclusively with price of services. After several years of failure to agree on anything significant, the Government of Ontario and the physicians' organization, the Ontario Medical Association (OMA), reached a landmark Framework Agreement in the Spring of 1991. Under this agreement, a Joint Management Committee was established with representation from both the OMA and the Ministry of Health. Other features included the so-called Rand formula (a compulsory dues payment to the association) and the awarding of representation rights for all physicians in the province to the association. The scope of the agreement was also unusual in that it involved the physicians' organization in physician human resource planning, utilization and affordability. In short, it represents simultaneously the coming of age of the physicians' association as a union on one hand, and the acceptance by that organization of significant responsibility for management on the other.

It's too early to tell how well this agreement will work. It is however evident that a number of features of the agreement, including the Joint Management Committee, have been adopted by other Canadian provincial jurisdictions. As well, arbitration has been granted to Ontario physicians as a way of settling fee disputes. A third innovation in negotiations is a much greater focus not just on physician and laboratory utilization, but overall services. Rather than conducting narrow discussions focused only on price, all governments are seeking some control and management over the volume of procedures and billings.

Collective or Stakeholder Processes

There is greater interest by government and the public in consultative processes involving all stakeholders. The evolution of the discussions on better management of physician human resources provides an important example. Following the Barer-Stoddart Report, described earlier, ministers of health endorsed a national action strategy and plan. A national conference was subsequently held involving all stakeholders, and a wide array of consultations with individual provinces was conducted. This process produced a more constructive policy process, although not yet total agreement, by all of the players on what decisions are to be made.

Collective or stakeholder process does not absolve governments of their responsibilities for resource allocation. It does, however, blunt criticism and enhance understanding of the complexities of issues.

Greater Consumer Involvement in Choices

There are three important dimensions to greater consumer involvement. The first is emphasis on Total Quality Management (TQM) or Continuous Quality Improvement (CQI) techniques which involve a more consumer-centred approach to reform. The second thrust is informed consumer choice. The work of Dr. Jack Wennberg, of Dartmouth Medical School, has gained considerable interest and following in Canada. Finally, rebalancing governance and advisory structures to include more consumers and fewer providers is necessary.

As more hospitals and other health service deliverers adopt TQM or CQI techniques there will be a greater focus on the individual consumer. Early results are promising with significant reductions in waiting times, amelioration in service efficiency and, most importantly, improvements in quality of service perceived by the consumer. In 1992, Canadian health ministers adopted "a vision of quality statement" to guide intergovernmental efforts in the health care delivery system; pursue quality, through greater consumer involvement.

There is a range of methods underway to involve individual patients more directly in their care choices. An informed patient is a must. The techniques of informed patient choice are discussed at greater length below.

A third area where greater consumer involvement is needed is on the boards, commissions and other governance structures. Major re-examination of the historical appointments to citizen boards is underway. Traditionally board members have been chosen to deal with such tasks as private fund-raising for institutions, generally for capital requirements. The consumer movement is gaining considerable authority.

In many Canadian jurisdictions, a specific percentage of consumer representatives (in the 30-50% range) is now gaining prominence as a norm. With more citizens on boards historical provider dominance is offset and more balanced decisions are made.

From the consumer point of view greater involvement means greater emphasis on service. One-stop shopping, convenience and absence of waiting — features normally associated with customer service — are becoming more central in health care delivery. The era of a patient passively awaiting physician's time and accepting physician's conclusions seems to be ending rapidly. Consumers are much more informed in health and medical matters, through the media and publications, than they were in the past. Much of the "black box" technology of medicine is giving way in the face of an enlightened and informed consumer.

Restructuring of governances in several provinces is also underway. A major Senior Citizens' Consumer Alliance played a pivotal role in altering the Government of Ontario's thinking on long-term care. The Consumer Alliance insisted on greater involvement in decision-making and a non-bureaucratic structuring of the long-term care delivery system, with much more of a community emphasis.

Each of these three dimensions of consumer involvement: board appointments, being informed, and restructuring governance, will significantly alter decisions and choices and improve the quality of the health care system.

The Canadian Consumers' Association has been active in promoting these changes and in participating in the national Health Action Lobby (HEAL).

Where You Can Get Involved

As a Governor
- **Board of health**
- **Boards of hospital**
- **District health councils**
- **Community health organizations**
- **Volunteer health association**
- **Research organizations**

As a Voter
- **Ask candidates about their health views**
- **Help organize community discussions on health and health reform**

- Participate in all candidate meetings and other public forums and ask questions about health and health care
- Insist on common sense about health and health care, not tired old clichés

As a Volunteer
- Volunteer nearly anywhere (there are hundreds of groups extending from local Meals on Wheels, to the Cancer Society)

As a public servant
- Provide clear, factual information to the public

Your Role — All of This Only Works If *You* Get Involved.

Where can citizens get involved? There are the traditional board structures, community health centres, hospital boards or C.L.S.C.s. There are also new local authorities, some elected and some appointed. None of these have any chance of success without your active participation. If the only people rolling up their sleeves are providers, we will not shift to a more consumer-based system. Some 30,000 Canadians already volunteer as governors of our health system as hospital trustees and members of boards of health.

More Evidence-Based Policy Making

Several Canadian provinces have opened institutes to bring together notable expertise in clinical epidemiology and related fields. This is the institutionalization of the ad hoc Royal Commission and Task Forces of the 1970s and 1980s which flourished in most Canadian jurisdictions.

The Institute for Clinical Evaluative Sciences (ICES), established under the Joint Management Committee (JMC) by the Government of Ontario and the Ontario Medical Association, will have consequential effect. The mandate of the Institute is to conduct research to assist the JMC in improving the quality and effectiveness of medical services. ICES replaces an earlier Joint Task Force on utilization, with the major differences being scale and permanence. ICES has a $4.5 million per annum budget and a permanent core staff. The Task Force was smaller and not as well financed.

The Government of Manitoba established the Manitoba Centre for Health Policy & Evaluation with university-based researchers, who function at arm's length from the government, through the Department of Community Health Sciences, at the University of Manitoba. The Centre, although small, with two career scientists and associates of the Canadian Institute of Advanced Research, is examining health expenditures, outcomes and service effectiveness. The Advisory Board of the Centre has substantial national and international expertise.

The Government of Saskatchewan founded the Saskatchewan Health Services Utilization and Research Commission with a mandate to produce information on effectiveness, efficiency and relative usefulness of various programmes, procedures and intervention. This new commission subsumes the earlier Saskatchewan Health Research Board.

The challenge for each of these centres of analysis, research and expertise will be to alter behaviour and to help us understand and react to a dynamic system. The translation of research work into clinical guidelines, decision algorithms and protocols requires new insights into physician-patient interactions. Altered behaviour requires much more than insight. It also needs incentives or disincentives.

Producing evidence of inappropriate or unnecessary procedures does not, in and of itself, determine any reduction of such activity or change its pattern. The infrastructure to reconfigure incentives is in a fledgling state. Its evolution will largely determine whether the range of newly-established institutes simply contribute to advancing knowledge or more directly influencing service delivery.

The emerging network of institutes will compile data, information and analysis. How rapidly and how successfully this is brought to bear on clinical practice remains an open question. But, compelled by fiscal pressures, governments will seek to bring about some practical applications.

One challenge for evidence from solid research is to serve as a counter balance to the "complaints department" — the daily Question Period in each Provincial and territorial assembly — nature of health care management with more diverse health goals. The aforementioned Nye Bevan's experience is common to parliamentary democracies based on the British model. Question Period is a powerful influence on health decision making. Perhaps, magnified by television and the other media, too powerful. The influence of the case is greatest when it pits the individual's human interest against the indifference of THE SYSTEM. Sometimes these individual heart-wrenching cases are symptoms of underlying and profound problems. More often they are the statistical reality of errors in a large system. The buffeting that Ministers take, shortens their effective time as Ministers; they are moved to other portfolios more rapidly than is sensible or they lose momentum. The most insidious impact of the complaints department mentality is to divert attention and resources from real problems to firefighting of media or political emergencies.

How then can we build the importance and profile of broad health goals? One reality is clear. We have no ability to diminish the complaints department. It fulfils a valuable, if distorting, role in enhancing the responsibility and accountability of the health care delivery system. Instead, we need to continue elevating debate about the real determinants of health.

One very successful device utilized in the United States has been public, high profile reports by the surgeons general. The elevation of this position to that of a senior spokesperson on health issues and health hazards has been valuable. In Canada, some medical officers have taken leadership in issuing broad policy reports as well as in tackling public education at the local level. The Chief Medical Officer in Ontario, Dr. Richard Schabas has issued three powerful reports in recent years and intends to continue.

Devolution

Another approach taken by many provinces is to create advisory bodies or consultative forums of a broad sort to provide advice, not only on *health* policy, but on *healthy* public policy. The Premier's Council on Health Strategy in Ontario expanded its focus to become The Premier's Council on Health, Well Being and Social Justice. The Alberta Roundtable on Health held in Red Deer in August, 1993, brought together 160 people to "chart a fundamentally new direction for health and health care in Alberta."[1]

As noted previously, the Province of Quebec has devolved a significant range of decisions in health and social services to local boards. This trend continues there, with further devolution, as well

---

1 *Alberta Roundtable Report*, Alberta Health, Government of Alberta, August, 1993, p. 6.

as democratization of local boards. In fact, Quebec is creating a new level of government for health and social services.

The most recent Quebec initiative is contained in Bill 120 — *An Act Respecting Health Services and Social Services* which set out the following key changes:

- the creation of a regional level of government responsible for the development and organization of health and social services
- the abolition of the present councils on health and social services
- to replace them, the creation of a health and social services authority in each administrative region of Quebec

The new sharing of responsibilities envisioned in Bill 120 permits a clear delegation of powers to regional authorities. The regions have 2 main responsibilities:

- to carry out the services within their jurisdiction
- to allocate to that end the available financial resources[2]

Two other provinces, Saskatchewan and New Brunswick, have combined regional or district restructuring in a devolved model. Saskatchewan describes its efforts to create new health districts and mandate them.

It is expected that the new health districts will:

- conduct health needs assessments and develop district health plans
- integrate and co-ordinate health services within the district; this will include establishing arrangements to safeguard the rights and missions of privately-owned health facilities
- manage all health services within the district
- develop 'community health centres'; these centres may take a variety of forms to be determined by the district, such as "health and social centres," co-operative health centres, "community clinics" or "wellness centres"
- ensure that all health services within the district meet specific provincial guidelines and standards
- be governed by a single health board[3]

2   *The Policy on Health and Well-Being*, Government of Quebec, Ministry of Health and Social Services, 1992.
3   Hon. Louise Simard, "A Saskatchewan Vision for Health, A Framework for Change," Minister of Health, Regina, August, 1992, p. 17.

New Brunswick has also moved recently to a legislated integration of previously independent hospitals under regional governance structures.

Advocates of devolution argue for the greater convergence of local or regional needs and resources. There has also been a view that devolution would allow provincial governments to transfer fixed "envelopes" of money for allocation by local or regional bodies. Whether this strategy will enable provincial governments to avoid demands for more funding remains to be seen. It's likely that devolution of significant management authority will lead to better integration of health and community services at the service delivery level.

The report of the Comprehensive Health System Planning Commission in Ontario proposed a fully integrated regional health planning and management authority for the southwest region with 1.4 million population.[4] It presented Ontario with a full devolution opportunity already taken up in several other Canadian provinces. To date it has not been accepted. Devolution without citizen involvement is not a solution. With your help it may be part of the answer.

Good Stuff To Read

Reports of the U.S. Surgeon General.

Reports of the Chief Medical Officer of Health, Ontario.

Tobacco and Your Health, Queen's Printer, Toronto, 1991.

The Policy on Health and Well Being, Government of Quebec, Ministry of Health and Social Services, 1992.

---

4   Earl Orser, "Report of the Comprehensive Health System Commission," a report to the Minister of Health for Ontario, 1992.

Chapter 10
Managing Demand for Services

Most of the activity in Canadian health care reform has been on the supply side. Although this is essential, it's not enough. Unless we also influence the demand for services, we will fail because the problems are too big to be solved purely on the supply side. Individuals seek health care for a wide variety of reasons, not just because of need. We often visit health providers — doctors and emergency rooms — because we need information. Why does this hurt? Should I apply heat or cold? With the collapse of extended families and the loss of grandmother-held-health-knowledge we have been driven into the formal health system.

Much of what we do to take control of health and health care rests with each of us as individuals. But, we need leadership and innovation from the formal health system to help us take that control. The list of ways this can be accomplished is not yet as long as the list of how we can re-engineer hospitals but is just as important. As we develop our tool kit on the demand side and learn new techniques the list will grow.

Making Costs Transparent to Providers

One of the unintended consequences of single payer, government insurance of hospital services and global budgets was the elimination of detailed accounting in hospitals in the 1950s and 1960s. With investments in information systems, hospitals are regaining their ability to track costs at the provider level. This allows managers to make known the cost of various activities to providers.

Sunnybrook Health Sciences Centre in Toronto is a leader in this trend. By making comparative resource data available to physicians, Sunnybrook is influencing behaviour. Physicians who know how their resource use compares to their peers are more willing to consider alternatives. For professionals who are trained to react to evidence, the necessary change in behaviour is best accomplished with data and evidence.

One of my younger brothers, an energetic family practitioner in a rural community, told me about a visiting expert who explained the huge cost difference between intravenous and oral antibiotics. Will this influence how my brother practices? Yes, I believe it will. Cost must not become the sole determinant in health care decisions, nor should cost information be so totally absent that there is an inability to consider it as an aspect of managing care.

Making Costs Transparent to Consumers

The flip side of the cost transparency issue is making patients and the public aware, as consumers, of the costs involved in health services. The Canadian health care system is the second most expensive in the world, exceeded only by the United States. This fact has been obscured by twenty-five years of invisible cost information and political attachment to a confusing vocabulary. Payment for services as a collective responsibility creates the erroneous conclusion that health care is free. By restoring cost information to patients, they can gain greater insight into more appropriate use of hospital services. Lest the reader draw the wrong conclusion — that this type of transparency is step one on the inexorable road to billing patients — it should be noted that billing patients is a direction I fully and vigorously oppose. I am advocating that people know exactly what they are getting and at what cost. Transparency of costs will cause a lot of very good questions and probably a few bad ones to be raised along the way. We must be careful to place this initiative of cost transparencies in the context of patient education. The goal and outcome must be to avoid scapegoating or frightening ill and elderly patients.

Sunnybrook Hospital in Toronto has developed its information system to permit it to issue full cost reports to each patient. Whether other hospitals and governments will follow remains to be seen. It would be an excellent and sobering idea for each of us to know what our activities as health consumers cost us as taxpayers.

Managing Demand for Hospital Services[1]

One area where we can learn from the United States is in managing more appropriate use of hospital services. Educating the patient in a variety of ways has been a central task of well-managed U.S. health maintenance organizations such as Kaiser Permanente. Canadian health care managers are gradually understanding the potential of actions which affect the demand side. Most of our health reform effort remains on the supply side, but more balance is needed. If we do not utilize available techniques and technologies to affect demand for health services through public and patient education, we are giving up half the leverage for necessary change. We are also perpetuating a system judged by many observers to be inappropriately dominated by providers. A few ideas on the demand side:
- nurse call lines
- video cassettes for patient education
- advertising campaigns to convince common cold sufferers to visit a pharmacy not a doctor or a hospital

Shared Decision-Making: Informed Patient Choice

Perhaps the best known advocate of this change is Dr. Jack Wennberg, from Dartmouth Medical School, who in conjunction with Sony Corporation, is making available a continuing series of video discs dealing with informed patient choice. These video discs focus on a particular procedure and are based on the view that there is no one correct course of treatment. For example, Dr. Wennberg's rather well-known work on prostate treatments indicate that there are three general courses of action. These are watchful waiting, surgery or treatment with drugs. Depending on one's tolerance for risk and one's particular circumstances, one could reasonably choose any of these three options.

---

1 An excellent article on demand management "Reducing Health Care Costs by Reducing the Need and Demand for Medical Services," *New England Journal of Medicine*, Vol 329, No. 5, July 29, 1993, p. 321-325. Authored by former US Surgeon General Everett Koop, Mary Jane England, The Health Project Consortium et al. It identified a number of measures to manage demand for health services and to reduce need for care.

Kaiser Permanente's work in the United States has indicated a significant reduction in the percentage of patients choosing surgery when confronted with all of the available information and evidence on their other choices. The Government of Ontario is supporting production of a video disc for cardiovascular surgery being developed by the University of Toronto. It is likely that more and more specific information will be made available to patients capable of making a choice. Of particular emphasis would be procedures which involve significant resource usage.

What is Expected from Interactive Video Disks?

The rationale for using interactive video disks is most often tied to concerns about utilization and an interest in patient utilities, quality of life, health education and the dynamics of medical decision-making. The reasons varied from place to place, but the most common were:

- CONSUMER EDUCATION — giving individuals a consistent, thorough review of treatment options is a meaningful step toward consumer empowerment. Anyone facing a surgical decision needs information about the disease and available treatments and an opportunity to balance personal preferences against probable health outcomes. Detailed information is presented in an understandable way that helps consumers ask questions and participate in the treatment decision.

- PATIENT UTILITIES — personal values and preferences of a consumer facing serious treatment decisions are not always discussed with the physician. Whether through embarrassment, timidity or lack of opportunity, consumers often keep their fears and opinions under wraps. The interactive video disk openly presents a range of considerations and preferences that can be explored.

- REDUCED UTILIZATION — inappropriate utilization is driven by physicians and consumers. Surgeons see people who were referred to them for a reason and feel an obligation to fix the problem. Consumers sometimes demand treatments that are excessive. Interactive video disks push both sides to rethink their assumptions. The Foundation claims that prostate surgeries decrease by up to 50% when the disks are used as part of the decision-making process.

- INFORMED CONSENT — in the litigious environment of U.S. health care, informed consent is a significant issue. After viewing a disk, the consumer receives a print-out of the interaction: the personal information that was recorded before the disk started and the material that was reviewed in the program. A signature line on the print-out turns the form into legal protection for the physician.
- OUTCOMES RESEARCH — as a research tool, the disks capture consumer demographics, disease condition, preferences and decisions. Follow-up questionnaires capture patient satisfaction with the information provided and the decisions made. The potential exists for research that establishes utilization changes, patient preferences at various points of disease progression and outcomes from various decisions.[2]

Another technology with the same objective is the decision board developed by the Centre for Health Economic Policy Analysis (CHEPA) at McMaster University in Hamilton. The CHEPA decision board tool is a portable foamcore board, easily transported to an office, home or bedside. The fundamental assumption of the board is that patients are capable of making a decision that is right for them if they have the necessary information.

How informed are the patient choices made in your hospital? How available is information for the patient and their family? Could you improve the situation?

Patient Education

If you are a parent, chances are high that at one time you have made the journey to the hospital emergency ward because your child bumped his or her head on the sidewalk, fell off a bicycle or engaged in some other regular childhood mishap. Chances are also high that

2   Colleen Savage, "A Interactive Video Disks as Shared Decision-Making Programs in Health Care," Report for the Health Strategies Office Ontario Ministry of Health, June 1993, p. 6-7.

you returned home after a long or short wait in the emergency department clutching a piece of paper labelled "head injury sheet." This valuable paper informed you of the danger signs indicative of a possible concussion. Many parents' anxieties have been diminished by simple informational tools such as cold kits or head injury sheets.

Public Education

Public education is essential to healthy public policy and management of demand for health services. Government leaders have a role in changing public attitudes and perceptions. For two decades in Canada, governments have tended to say: "Isn't our health care system wonderful: it's free, it's accessible, it's universal." The reality has been that it is not free. It's the second most expensive health care system in the world and the public has been encouraged in a belief that everything is solvable, that death can not only be postponed but may be eliminated altogether if only enough treatments are applied. Moreover, the public has not been given much help as consumers in how to appropriately use the system.

A good analogy is energy conservation. People were not told, "Stop using energy. Turn off the heat and freeze to death in your houses." They were told that they could adjust how they used energy and how to have a more affordable situation which was equally good in quality terms. We are starting nationally, in Ontario, and in other jurisdictions, to look at how health ministries talk to the public. Is the public informed about self-limiting illnesses? About appropriate use of emergency rooms? Are people given guidance to better manage the system? There is a lot of distance to be made up here. We need the health equivalent of a dimmer switch to replace the on-off mechanism.

The physicians have been put in the middle of an unpleasant sandwich by being told on the one hand, "People can come to your office and if they are not really sick, by the time you determine that, you have already invested your professional time in that determination." On the other hand, governments get upset and say "Why is the single biggest expense in physician services in Ontario the common cold? Why is that the major reason for office visits?"

One of the major reasons is that the public has not been told, through public education, that visiting the physician for a common cold is not going to get them much benefit in the process. Nor has much investment been made, until recently, in getting an informed and knowledgeable patient.

Health care providers have not been extraordinarily forthcoming about everything involved in treatment either. Contrast that with choosing a place to go to for a ski holiday. Making this choice, thanks to the marketing efforts of a number of very aggressive American resorts, you can sit for an evening watching videos from half a dozen American ski resorts and choose the one you like. Having in a sense pre-skied the major runs, one can make a more intelligent choice. Through various technologies, care providers can create, as allies, consumers who are informed participants. This education is going to require active involvement at the workplace and community levels. The public will need to be educated where they live and work. Health care professionals are going to have to manage better and more openly.

The success of the health care system will be determined by the ability to marry very difficult contending objectives. We will succeed because none of us wants to look our grandchildren in the eye a few years hence, admit we had a health care system envied all over the planet, one that we let get away from us. We are already on track, but there will be roads we venture down that are in the wrong direction. We will have to be honest enough, on all sides, to admit that seemed like a good idea at the time but it wasn't. We may have to step back and find another way of achieving the objective. The objective is clear: we want a quality system and one we can afford. Those are two non-contending and achievable goals.

Chapter 11

Community and Public Health Services

People died while public health authorities and the political leaders who guided them refused to take the tough measures necessary to curb the epidemic's spread, opting for political expediency over the public health.... In those early years, the federal government [US] viewed AIDS as a budget problem, local public health leaders saw it as a political problem, gay leaders considered AIDS a public relations problem, and the news media regarded it as a homosexual problem that wouldn't interest anybody else. Consequently, few confronted AIDS for what it was, a profoundly threatening medical crisis.... It is a tale that bears telling, so that it will never happen again, to any people, anywhere.[1]

Randy Shilts, 1987

No single event in matters of health during our lifetime has captured the public interest and attention as thoroughly as the AIDS epidemic. It is a pervasive reality of life in the 1990s and is likely to remain so, well into the next century. In a series of blows to an evolving human mastery over disease or at least over plagues, the AIDS pandemic has revealed our inability to prevent premature death. It has shaken our faith in many health institutions. In many industrialized countries public fear about AIDS related blood safety has

---

1   Randy Shilts, *And The Band Played On* (New York: St. Martin's Press, 1987), p. xxiii.

become a central issue. In France senior health officials are in jail for their negligence and inaction in the face of the AIDS prevalence. In the United States, the Federal Drug Administration had the American Red Cross blood activities placed under court administration due to safety concerns. The Krever Commission provides a daily forum for the debate of safety issues pertaining to Canada's blood system, past, present and future. As we sort our path through the HIV/AIDS issue, we rediscover the roots of public health.

Public Health

Three key public health issues: tobacco, AIDS, and vaccines and immunization are critical to our success in achieving and maintaining a healthy nation. We have lessons to learn from our experiences in each case, from both successes and failures.

Tobacco

Tobacco is a key public health issue. The World Bank estimates that tobacco related deaths will increase from two million per annum at present to twelve million per annum by 2050 if present consumption trends continue.

Prominent public health officials do not primarily advocate for more treatment services in health. For example, the 1991 report in Ontario by the Chief Medical Officer of Health stated:

> ...we must prevent our children from becoming tobacco users. We must help current smokers quit. And we must protect non-smokers from exposure to tobacco smoke.[2]

Legislation introduced by the Ontario Health Minister in November, 1993, was created to reduce children's access to cigarettes. The Federal Government is considering a generic packaging requirement which would further hinder marketing efforts by the tobacco industry. Yet, despite all we know about tobacco as the number one preventable killer of Canadians, the Federal government, for a host of dreadful reasons, collapsed on tobacco taxation in 1994. It seems that knowing the facts is insufficient.

---

2   Dr. Richard Schabas, *Tobacco and Your Health*, Report of the Chief Medical Officer of Health, Ontario, 1993, p. 7.

World Bank Policy
on Tobacco

In 1992, in recognition of the adverse effects of tobacco consumption on health, the World Bank articulated a formal policy on tobacco. The policy contains five main points.

- The World Bank's activities in the health sector — including sector work, policy dialogue, and lending — discourage the use of tobacco products.
- The World Bank does not lend directly for, invest in, or guarantee investments or loans for tobacco production, processing, or marketing. However, in the few countries that are heavily dependent on tobacco as a source of income and of foreign exchange earnings (for example, those where tobacco accounts for more than 10% of exports) and especially as a source of income for poor farmers and farmworkers, the World Bank treats the subject within the context of responding most effectively to these countries' development requirements. The World Bank seeks to help these countries diversify away from tobacco.
- To the extent practicable, the World Bank does not lend indirectly for tobacco production activities, although some indirect support of the tobacco economy may occur as an inseparable part of a project that has a broader set of objectives and outcomes (for example, rural roads).
- Unmanufactured and manufactured tobacco, tobacco-processing machinery and equipment, and related services are included on the negative list of imports in loan agreements and so cannot be included among imports financed under loans.
- Tobacco and tobacco-related producer or consumer imports may be exempt from borrowers' agreements with the Bank to liberalize trade and reduce tariff levels.[3]

---

3   World Bank Development Report, "Investing in Health," World Bank, New York, July 1993, p. 89.

Canadian governments and banks should consider following the World Bank's approach to tobacco as well. Instead the Government of Canada lead a shameful retreat on the tobacco taxation issue, causing a significant increase in tobacco consumption with the attendant future deaths.

AIDS

Much has been written about AIDS and much more will be written. No recent tragedy captures more fully the apparent helplessness in the face of the unknown. What is particularly depressing about the pandemic is how little action in public health measures we took in the early stages against the spread of the disease. In a failure there are always a myriad of villains upon whom some blame falls. Randy Shilts captures the breadth of the failure in his books and others have recount it in articles and television documentaries. Our challenge is to learn from our experiences with HIV/AIDS both so that we can improve present actions and to prevent a replication of this tragedy in the future.

The fundamental lesson to be learned is that the basic public health principles that we have painfully learned over the past one hundred years should not be abandoned for any reason. Although the advocacy for protection of AIDS patients and the gay community from discrimination was powerful in the early stages of the AIDS situation, it should not have eclipsed, as it did, proper public health. We need to take steps to limit infectious diseases not on the basis of which community, or individual is infected but on the basis of protecting others and limiting the spread of the disease. This notion has been central to public health since its inception.

The classic public health story is the tale of the removal of the pump handle and saving countless thousands from water borne disease. There is a clear parallel to the AIDS story. Action was eventually taken in regards to HIV/AIDS to treat the blood supply, to close bath houses and to properly warn the whole population as well as those in high risk groups. But these actions lagged far behind the certain knowledge of the deadliness of the disease.

Even now, the pendulum seems to have swung too far. Instead of directing our efforts to those at risk we may be spreading our energy too widely. Public education, programmes of testing and the tightening of all preventive measures took a very long time to come to pass in Canada. There are further steps to be taken: needle exchange programmes and distribution of condoms in prison. No one likes to admit the realities behind these necessities. Even if inaction is jeopardizing human lives, there are still some who don't want to believe that drugs are present in prisons or that risky sexual practices go on behind bars. Our only option is to ensure all preventive efforts are taken.

If we are prepared to learn about the AIDS tragedy there are some positive lessons. We have seen the community as a group of consumers bringing great advocacy and thoughtfulness to bear on the pandemic. This dialogue between health consumers and providers has been at times an extreme and aggravating one, but it has taught providers some general lessons about the need to involve consumers more directly. As well, options for palliative care, hospices and other less acute care settings than the hospital have sprung up to provide options for those dying of AIDS. Among these options is important leadership in terms of the evolution of palliative care for many others with incurable or untreatable conditions. There are also lessons about the appropriateness of different types of care.

Not all of the lessons are positive. It may come to pass that we learn that rushing untested or not fully tested drugs through into general use has produced harmful consequences and side effects. It may also emerge that, with all the advocacy in the world, scientific discovery may not be rapid enough or successful enough to solve the problem. We may have to come to terms with a pace at which dollars can be invested in worthwhile AIDS research. I take no position on our current level of investment but, it does seem possible that we invested too little in the early stages and may be in danger of overloading the research capacity in response. We need better tracking of emerging threats to public health. We need to act on them early and in a comprehensive fashion.

Evolution of the HIV-AIDS Epidemic

Region	HIV incidence (millions)		HIV prevalence (millions)		AIDS-related (millions)	
	1990	2000[a]	1990	2000[b]	1990	2000[c]
Demographically developing group	**1.6**	**2.5**	**7.4**	**25**	**0.3**	**1.7**
Sub-Saharan Africa	**1.1**	**1.0**	**5.8**	**12**	**0.3**	**0.9**
Asia	**0.3**	**1.3**	**0.4**	**9**	*****	**0.6**
EME and FSE[d]	**0.1**	*****	**1.4**	**1**	**0.1**	**0.1**

* Less than 0.05 million
Note: Incidence refers to new infections in a given year, prevalence refers to the total number of persons infected.
a. Conservative estimates
b. The countries of the demographic regions Sub-Saharan Africa, India, China, Other Asia and islands, Latin America and the Caribbean, and Middle Eastern crescent.
c. India, China, and the demographic region Other Asia and islands.
d. EME, established market economies; FSE, formerly socialist economies of Europe.
Source: World Health Organization data.[4]

As the AIDS epidemic decimates the poorer nations we must be careful to learn the important lessons that public health has to teach us.

Vaccines and Immunization

Investments in vaccines and immunization are easily our best health care and health status bargain, in terms of preventive medicine. Immunization programmes based on vaccines have been the most cost-effective intervention. Our progress against particular diseases has been based very much on the availability of vaccines and immunization.

4   Ibid., p. 95.

Shortly after I joined the Ministry of Health in 1991 I was approached by Dr. Richard Schabas, Chief Medical Officer of Health in Ontario. He set out to convince me that we should add the vaccine for haemophilias B to our programme. We could not obtain new funds to pay for this vaccine. However, Dr. Schabas and I agreed that he could squeeze the money out of his existing operation and proceed with the vaccine.

In 1994, a few months after leaving the ministry I spoke to the meeting of the Ontario Campaign for Action on Tobacco. At the end of the lecture Dr. Schabas approached me to disclose the very impressive results that adding this new vaccine had achieved. The table below details those results.

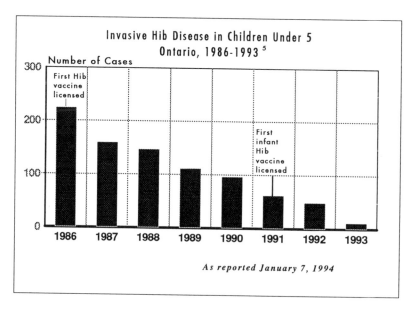

Invasive Hib Disease in Children Under 5
Ontario, 1986-1993 [5]

As reported January 7, 1994

In Ontario, the Ministry of Health budget totals over $17 billion per annum. Of this amount, total spending on the public health system was about $230 million, or about 1.5%. Within public health, vaccines accounted for only about $25 million of spending, although the cost of implementing vaccine programmes adds to that. Still, it is worth considering that our single best public investment in the future health of Ontario children and adults was drawing only .15% of the

5   Provided by Dr. Richard Schabas, Chief Medical Officer of Health in Ontario, 1994.

Ministry budget. Or, simplified, only one dollar out of every $680 was being spent by the Ministry on vaccinations. By contrast, the Ontario Medical Association estimated that we were spending $200 million on the common cold paying physicians for office visits by cold sufferers.[6]

Imunization with vaccines are key determinants of the state of public health on a global basis. The World Bank notes, "Vaccines to prevent tuberculosis, measles, diphtheria, pertussis, tetanus and polio have revolutionized preventive medicine over the past two decades. Costs are less than $10 per DALY[7] immunization and less than $25 for polio plus diphtheria and tetanus."[8] The Expanded Programme on Immunization (EPI) pursued by the World Health Organization now reaches about 80% of children in developing companies. It is estimated that this programme alone averts an estimated 3.2 million deaths per year. An increase in immunization in developing countries from 5% in 1977 to 30% by 1985 and 90% for all children by 1990 has been achieved. Estimates are that if this massive improvement in vaccination levels had occurred, preventable disease would total 23% of the global burden of disease among children. The table below illustrates the scope geographically.

The World Health Organization projects that polio will be eradicated by the year 2000. The World Bank argues for the extension of the Expanded Programme in Immunization (EPI) in two directions. First, coverage should be moved up from 85 to 95% of all children born. The total cost would be between $500 and $750 million a year but the gains would dramatically outweigh the cost. The second direction is adding additional items to the package, hepatitis B and yellow fever vaccines for selected countries, micro nutrients in regions where deficiencies are highly prevalent. These additions would improve health substantially.

The following table from the World Bank Report indicates that fifty-five million disability-adjusted life years (DALYS) could be saved by the recommended EPI expansion. The total annual costs of less than 2% are a fraction of the amount that is spent on public health in the developing countries. While we have made great progress we have a way to go to achieve the 95% level. Within the

6   Ontario Medical Association unpublished work by Darrel Weinkauf, 1991.
7   What the heck is a DALY? A DALY is a Disability Adjusted Life Year—or a year of healthy life added. DALYs are the best measure of bang-for-the-buck in health investment.
8   "Investing in Health," World Bank, New York 1993, p. 72.

developed countries, maintaining, or, in the case of the United States, achieving the 95% immunization level will continue to be a challenge.

Burden of Childhood Diseases Preventable by the Expanded Programme on Immunization (EPI) by Demographic Region, 1990

Region	BURDEN (millions of DALYs per year)	share of the total burden in children under age 5 (percent)	burden per 1,000 children under age 5 (DALYs)
Sub-Saharan Africa	23	15	242
India	16	12	137
China	1	3	8
Other Asia and Islands	7	10	81
Latin America and the Caribbean	1	3	18
Middle Eastern Crescent	7	10	86
Formerly Socialist Economies of Europe	*	*	1
Established Market Economies	*	*	1
World	55	10	87

* Less than 1.

Note: The EPI includes immunizations for pertussis, polio, diphtheria, measles, tetanus, and tuberculosis. These estimates exclude the burden from tuberculosis because most of it falls on adults.[9]

Source: Calculated from Murray and Lopez, background paper.

Connaught, one of the world's major producers of vaccines, is introducing multiple vaccines. At the time of writing, Connaught is working on a pentavalant vaccine which would combine polio with four other major vaccines in a single injection. The advantages of this, both in cost-effectiveness and health terms, are significant. Research that combines vaccines into single applications will improve the cost-effectiveness and the health outcome of the World Health Organization's Extended Immunization Programme and similar projects.

9 Ibid., p. 73.

Canada should not be smug or complacent. Although we have reached near universality in vaccination programmes, we face risks in two areas. Immigration to Canada from countries without similar vaccination programmes means new arrivals to Canada could be in a risk situation. We need to provide vaccination to these people as part of their settlement process. Second, we have difficulties reaching all those in the First Nations communities. This will require developing a full partnership with First Nations governments to ensure that all Aboriginal children in Canada are also protected against the diseases we hope to eradicate from the world.

Research investments, which will be discussed further in a subsequent section, have enormous application to vaccines and immunization. We need progress not only on vaccines themselves, but also on more cost effective and safe means of delivering them. As the Provincial Auditor of Ontario recently pointed out, there has been significant wastage in the vaccine distribution system in Ontario. Total quality management in each Canadian jurisdiction would help direct money to the most cost-effective distribution mechanism. In some parts of the country, we may be relying too much on physician-based delivery systems when broader public health approaches, such as school vaccinations delivered by nurses, are more appropriate. This should turn on the age at which the vaccine is necessarily given. As well, it should take into account the cost-effectiveness of the various delivery methods.

In terms of disease, we are truly becoming a global village. We need to direct our attention to the immunization and vaccination of all those who dwell in the village. The United States has the worst track record of any developed nation in immunization and vaccination. This is a policy area which will receive significant attention from the Clinton health reforms. The rapid movement of the world's population among countries, whether for a short or long stay for immigration, whether as refugees or for holidays in warmer climates, gives us all a stake in the health of the world's population, a stake that our own humanity dramatically underscores. Drug resistant strains of tuberculosis are appearing with increasing frequency not only in New York City but also in Toronto. It is also evident in the history of the transmission of HIV/AIDS that travel had a large role in the spread of the disease.

Mandatory Public Health Programmes – The Ontario Experience

An interesting revitalization of public health services has been prompted by the introduction of the Mandatory Health Programs and Service Guidelines in 1989 by the Ontario Health Ministry. The document[10] which set out the new approach, identified four health goals and twenty specific programs. The goals included: development, community level health promotion, communicable disease reduction and environmental health. The programs covered a broad range from Tobacco Use Prevention to Sexual Health, from Healthy Children to Healthy Elderly. The legislative authority for the Mandatory Programs was under the *Health Protection and Promotion Act*, funded 100% by provincial government sources. This provided an incentive to the municipal public health system which is generally in a cost-sharing relationship with the province.

The roots of this approach are in broad population health. Dr. Schabas, Chief Medical Officer of Health in Ontario notes the following key issues around development of the mandatory programs.

1. The entire process was health goals based. The first thing we did was to establish health goals and objectives. Program discussions were then based on whether or not the programs actually addressed a health goal and whether they did it in an effective way. This approach forced us to address issues that had previously received insufficient attention. It also called into question many traditional public health programs.

2. The health goals, and therefore the entire process, was population health focused. Looking at health outcomes and health behaviours on a population-wide basis invited us to consider both high risk interventions and population-wide interventions. Perhaps the most important shift represented in the mandatory programs was the recognition that the latter approach, population-wide strategies, are critically important in addressing our health goals.

3. The entire process of developing the Mandatory

---

10 *Mandatory Health Programs and Services Guidelines*, Ministry of Health Ontario, Queen's Printer, April, 1989.

Programs was highly consultative. This meant that the membership on all of the committees that put together the health goals as well as the program guidelines was overwhelmingly non-ministry. The role of the ministry was to provide coordination for the process.[11]

The introduction of this new, strengthened and health goal linked approach represents progress in revitalizing public health. Evaluation of the Ontario effort will provide important lessons for that province and the rest of the country.

Community Health

In all provinces except Quebec, community health in Canada is a collection of disparate and remarkable organizations epitomised by community health clinics. In Quebec the organized CLSC system[12] operates. In a recent paper former Quebec Health Minister Claude Forget and Monique Jerome-Forget, the head of the Institute for Research on Public Policy (IRPP), capture the difficulties Quebec has experienced in endeavouring to implement the CLSCs as the mainstream health care mechanism.

In 1971, Quebec introduced the concept of the CLSC (or local community service centre), drawing inspiration from Swedish and Czechoslovakian models and incorporating a full range of medical and social services, with salaried medical staff, thereby creating a primary care gateway to the whole system. The Quebec government found itself unable to implement the changes in the form desired. In retrospect, the reason for that failure are apparent — the neglect of preexisting institutional arrangements. Quebec physicians had, at the time, little experience of, and even less appetite for, group practice. The general public, as well as the medical profession, had little understanding of the complementarity between primary medical care and a host of social services. Finally, while CLSCs were promoted in parallel with the introduction of medicare (instead of being able to bank on its existence and a medical profession familiarity with it), the notion of a salary for physicians was

11 Dr. Richard Schabas letter to the author, May 9, 1994.
12 The CLSCs are community health and social services organizations.

widely seen (not just by physicians) as a tactic to reduce medical income levels under a new publicly financed system.[13]

CLSCs remain a key element of Quebec's health reform strategy. We should consider for a moment some of the examples of community health activities in other parts of Canada before contemplating what sort of framework into which they could be amalgamated or organized. In particular it is essential to understand that community health centres have grown from community activism and the crusading leadership of individuals. They have not been sparked by external forces, nor could a successful community based organization evolve without strong community support.

Among the examples are the approximately fifty community health centres in Ontario, including the South Riverdale Community Health Centre, the long-standing Group Health Centre in Sault Ste. Marie, which is heading towards a role as a comprehensive health organization, and Mount Carmel Klinic in Winnipeg, Manitoba. Like hospitals before them, many of these community health initiatives have sprung up with governance from the community and, more recently, funding from government. In many cases, government funding has gradually displaced voluntary charitable funding for these organizations. Most frequently a dynamic individual or a community-based organization provided the spark, determination and drive. Anne Ross lead the Mount Carmel Clinic against all odds for decades in Winnipeg's north end. The United Steelworkers Union supported the creation of the Group Health Centre in Sault Ste. Marie and remain its defenders and protectors. While governments can encourage the development of community health centres, the experience of Quebec CLSCs and community health centres elsewhere suggest that grassroots community support is essential for success.

Health in the Workplace

Shortly before I left my position as Deputy Minister of Health for the Province of Ontario in November of 1993, I had a visit from Mr. Frank Stronach, the dynamic founder and Chair of the Board of Magna. Mr. Stronach has built and rebuilt a huge and successful autoparts manufacturing concern which employs roughly 11,000

---

13 Monique Jerome-Forget and Claude Forget, ''Too Smug for Comfort?,'' IRPP/Brookings International Conference, Montreal, May 15-16, 1994, p. 6.

Canadian workers and will produce upwards of $3 billion worth of products this year. Why would he seek to meet the government's Senior Health Official? His concern was the health and well being of his employees. Accompanied by Dr. Arif Bhimji, his progressive chief medical advisor, Mr. Stronach was very keen on exploring a Comprehensive Health Organization (CHO) model for Magna employees and the communities in which they live. His unique Magna Employee's Charter contains a commitment to a safe and healthful workplace. The objectives for a Magna CHO are:

- set an example for others in industry to follow
- shift the emphasis in health care to health promotion and disease prevention
- establish a partnership between providers and consumers
- change the focus to preventive health practice from institutional care
- allow for effective and appropriate use of allied health personnel
- permit the best use of resources and institutions
- improve health outcomes and the health status of all consumers involved.[14]

Mr. Stronach told a personal story about his early days as a young factory labourer, in either Austria or Canada, I can't recall. The essence of it was that he had drilled a sizable hole in his finger with the drill due to carelessness. Rather than seek medical help and forfeit a starting position on the soccer team, the young Stronach stuck his finger in a bottle of iodine, wrapped it in a bandage and went off to play. Today a workplace accident of this sort would trigger an orgy of forms, investigations and medical treatment.

Neither Mr. Stronach nor I would advocate the return to the "good-old" days before improvements to workplace health and safety laws and regulations. We did find common ground, however, on the subject of greater workplace education and more individual responsibility. Neither of us were expressing simple altruism in the exchange.

Mr. Stronach's competitive company depends on healthy, productive workers. The economic survival of any health ministry and Medicare depends on convincing employers and individuals to focus on wellness rather than generating, either passively or actively, more business for the care delivery system. Mr. Stronach and I had a strong

---

14 Proposal by Magna for a Comprehensive Health Organization, October, 1993.

shared interest. Employers in Canada have a key role to play in employee health and wellness.

Two very important avenues for engaging Canadians in achieving greater wellness and health status are healthier communities and healthier workplaces. They are by no means mutually exclusive for there would be little point in creating healthier communities if the people who lived in them went off each day to work in unsafe or unhealthy working environments. Similarly, the safest and healthiest working environment will not compensate for a violent, dangerous and unhealthy community. We must work on both if we are truly to achieve progress.

Healthy Communities Movement

One of the most innovative aspects of revitalized public health is the rediscovery of the powers of local governments to improve the environment and health of cities. While our senior levels of government debate health care, as a federal or provincial problem, our cities are moving forward on health issues at the local level. Toronto has been a leader in the Healthy Cities Movement as the following material demonstrates. Other Canadian cities have much to learn from Toronto in this regard.

Excerpts from Healthy Toronto 2000

Many would be surprised to learn that the greatest contribution to the health of the nation over the past 150 years was made, not by doctors and hospitals, but by local government.
Dr. Jessie Parfit
The Health of a City:
Oxford 1770 to 1974

To make Toronto the healthiest city possible, we must ensure that health is a principal concern on everyone's agenda and that the health impacts of our decisions are recognized and taken into account. This is the central message of Health Toronto 2000.

Some Fundamental Concepts and Values

We see health as a resource for everyday life. People wish to be healthy in order to lead rich and fulfilling lives, and to attain their maximum potential. In this context, health is more than just physical health—we have to pay much more attention to mental and social well-being.

We recognize that the level of health of our community is a reflection of the quality of our community and that a high level of health for all in our community must be our aspiration. Therefore the basic prerequisites for health must be available to everyone.

Health is a complex phenomenon involving physical, mental and social well-being and is determined by many factors. We therefore need a sophisticated understanding of health, one which illuminates the complex interactions and the holistic nature of the determinants of health and can guide us in our actions.

We have come to recognize certain fundamental public health values. These include:

- Promotion of health and prevention of disease are better than cure.
- Social interventions to enhance the common health of the community are appropriate and may take precedence over individual concerns.
- Inequalities in health must be reduced and their roots in social inequities must be addressed.
- We must treat our natural ecosystem with respect, both for our own benefit and for the benefit of future, generations and we must provide for them a clean, green, quiet, healthy and sustainable environment.
- Our community must be human-centred and human scale, a caring, sharing, cooperative and supportive community that places people above material things.
- Each individual in society needs a meaningful role and the ability and the opportunity to participate actively in the community and in decisions affecting their health.

A Health Promotion Strategy

The five strategies of the Ottawa Charter should be used as the basis for developing the Healthy City Initiative.

Thus, as a City and as a Department we must:
- establish public policies that support health;

- create or help in the creation of environments supportive of health;
- strengthen and facilitate community action for health;
- develop or aid in the development of personal skills for health;
- reorient health services towards health promotion and a community-based health services system.

Health Goals for the City

The following broad health goals, which correspond to proposed health goals for Ontario, are not primarily the responsibility of the Department of Public Health; they require the commitment of City Government as a whole.
1. Reduce inequities in health opportunities in Toronto.
2. Create physical environments supportive of health.
3. Create social environments supportive of health.
4. Advocate for a community-based health services system.[15]

Does your city or community have healthy community policies? What could you do to spark change? How could the Ottawa Charter improve the health of your community?

Workplace Wellness: a Proposal

Healthier communities and workplaces can move us towards better health as a nation. If employers take a keen interest in the health of their employees much benefit can be shared by all.

Workplaces are sources of injury and ill health as well as a major positive part of giving our lives and relationships meaning. Our images of which workplaces as hazardous to health are often dated. The images of filthy factories and unsafe construction sites need to make room for a few realities for those who work in the health care sector. Accidents and injuries in hospitals and nursing homes are frequent.

Most provinces are now collecting an employer payroll tax or levy on the basis that employers should contribute to health care

---

15 Excerpts from ''Healthy Toronto 2000,'' City of Toronto.

costs of Medicare. Perhaps it is time to base the levy on employers willingness to take steps to improve employee wellness. A charter of workplace wellness drafted collaboratively by health experts, employers, bargaining agents and governments might serve as a foundation to a new initiative. A discount in the levy or employer health tax for employers willing to abide by such a charter is a worthwhile idea.

Good Stuff To Read

And the Band Played On — Politics, People and the AIDS Epidemic by Randy Shilts, St. Martin's Press 1987, or Penguin paperback 1988. As a journalist, Randy Shilts covered the plague from its initial days. If there can be such a creation as a wonderful book describing one of the great and preventable tragedies of our era — this is it. The Shilts' chronicle of the failure of both will and systems is a gripping unfolding of tragedy. A must-read for all of those who want to ensure that it is never allowed to happen again. Public health must be vigilant and unmoved by the politics of the moment if it is to protect us all.

The Memoirs of America's Family Doctor, by Dr. Everett Koop, the former U.S. Surgeon General, Random House, New York, N.Y., 1991. An interesting, quite personal memoir which provides a glimpse behind the scenes at health policy making and lack thereof in the Reagan era in Washington. Dr. Koop played a major role in the smoking and AIDS issues. A useful read for those intrigued by the politics of health policy. Dr. Koop's case histories of his surgery on babies and young children are also fascinating.

Tobacco and Your Health, Report of the Chief Medical Officer, Ministry of Health, 1991. A short, easy to read, presentation of the grisly facts on tobacco as the major preventable cause of illness and death. Good graphics add to the impact of the numbers.

Part 4

World Health
Economic Development
in the Global Village

The short-hand story, then, is that despite their diversity, health care systems in every society have all evolved without mechanisms to assure accountability for effectiveness, efficiency, and appropriateness of care provided. The response of providers to every issue, every problem, every question, has been, 'We must meet needs — Give us more.'[1]

Robert Evans, 1993

Health is an essential human desire. The activity of seeking health and providing health care represent a major economic endeavour for our species.

In health and health care, the global village presents Canada with opportunities for learning and prospering. Two developments in 1993 on the global scene are worthy of special attention. The unprecedented commitment of an American President, Bill Clinton, to health and health care for all Americans is noteworthy; the United States is the last major industrial nation to make this commitment. The publication of the World Bank Development Report, "Investing In Health," entirely devoted to health issues, is also unprecedented. With these two events, health and health care have moved to the global centre stage. Confronted simultaneously with twin realizations that much progress has been accomplished and we know how to achieve much more, it is time for an important reformation of health and health care on a global basis. Ideas about reform may vary from country to country but they are taking hold in many, many systems.

Health economic development is the link between health care endeavour as nations, the care of ourselves and our neighbours, and business opportunities and research which all add enormous value to our health and economy.

For Canada, health economic development can be a strong support to Medicare and to our economic well-being, if directed properly, or it can be the leading edge of a misguided privatization and eventual destruction of our Canadian success. The public administra-

---

1 Robert Evans, ''Our Bill of Health,'' *Alberta Health*, 1993, p. 17.

tion and not-for-profit nature of Canadian Medicare is one of its essential and necessary qualities. It must be maintained. However, we need the continuing creative energy of the Canadian private sector in several important ways. These do not include insurance of basic, necessary health care services or ownership and management of health care delivery. These should remain not-for-profit and publicly administered.

As Canadians, we need to focus on three aspects of health economic development that support our ability-to-benefit approach. Increasing our exports of health goods and services, increasing research in Canada and expanding the Canadian production of more affordable goods and services which supply our health care delivery system. These endeavours are inter-related. Strengthening our exports provides larger markets and revenues to support domestic research. Efficiencies achieved through greater volumes will assist affordability of products in Canada. Most importantly, because our wealth as a nation is a direct result of our health as a nation, our health economic development side will have direct health benefits in reduced unemployment and increased income for Canadians.

Learning from other nations is essential for our progress. We contribute to world progress in health by teaching others what we know. If we are to benefit fully, our role in the global village must be as both student and teacher.

Chapter 12

We Have Much to Learn from Each Other

Among the six countries surveyed Canada's health care services get the best overall marks from its citizens. Canadians are especially satisfied with the quality, personal control, not having to wait too long to see a doctor and minimizing personal costs of care.[1]

Canada has much to teach and much to learn. We need only to look at the experiences of our neighbours on the planet, both those with whom we share a border and those with whom we share values and historical roots. A cautionary note on ideas from elsewhere: two approaches should to be avoided. The first is a winner-take-all or "Stanley Cup" notion of comparative health care systems where we argue about who has the best system and then everyone else copies the winner.[2] This approach is fatally flawed. Health care systems are rooted in national histories and are not simply transportable. The other extreme view is just as wrong, that we can learn nothing from other places because everything is unique and different here. Lessons can cross national borders, but we must think critically about which

---

1 "An International Comparison of Health Care Systems," Harvard Community Health Plan, Annual Report, 1990, p. 6.
2 I am grateful to Ted Marmor of Yale University for this idea which he effectively presented. In Professor Marmor's formulation the World Series was referenced, but since Toronto seems to win the World Series frequently I needed a more appropriate example!

are general and which are only country-specific. Bad ideas travel just as easily as good ones.

Canada and the United States

After twenty-five years of relative stability, Canadian Medicare is facing twin challenges posed by the demand from our nation's bankers and taxpayers of affordability and a parallel consumer demand for quality. President Clinton has embarked upon the most ambitious re-engineering of health care delivery in many decades, perhaps even in the history of the United States.

There is much mythology about these two countries approaches to health care. Many of the advocates in one nation believe the grass is greener on the other side of the longest undefended border in the world. Often the debate stirs more negative aspects.

Dispelling Some Myths About Canadian Medicine

Myth No. 1:

Canadian doctors are employees of a socialist state which tells them how to practise medicine and ration care.

Reality:

Canadian doctors are overwhelmingly (90%+) self-employed, fee for service practitioners. The ten provincial health plans pay for medically necessary services on a fee schedule negotiated annually between the government and the professional association. In comparison to the United States we have little to no utilization management or prior approvals. Doctors are able to bill separately on a fee schedule they get for non-essential, largely cosmetic, procedures, for treating non-Canadians and for third party services (insurance medicals and the like).

Canadian doctors have far less intrusion into their medical practice than U.S. doctors. (Some believe too little intrusion, but that is a separate issue.) No Canadian doctor needs to discuss ability to pay with a patient. Nor do they face bad debts from patients or expensive malpractice insurance. Many doctors find this appealing.

Myth No. 2:

Canadian doctors are migrating to the United States to escape socialized medicine.

Reality:

Out of a total physician population of about 22,000, Ontario loses about one hundred doctors a year to the United States (or .5%). Of those one hundred doctors, about half return to Canada within five years.

Canada is a middle country in medical migration. We recruit in Commonwealth countries such as the U.K., Australia, New Zealand, Hong Kong. We do lose some of our best and brightest to the United States, but Canada remains a very good place to be a doctor.

Myth No.3:

Waiting lists characterize the Canadian health care system and provide proof of rationing.

Reality:

Judged on the basis of number of major procedures to population, Ontario compares to either California or New York. We do as many or more by-passes, gall bladders, etc. We have waiting lists for some procedures as a means of better organizing our system. For example, in cardiac surgery, Ontario has a provincial registry and network. A patient can decide to either wait for their surgeon or to be on the registry and take the first available one.

A recent study concluded that mortality rates on the Ontario waiting list were at the same level as mortality rates during surgery in New York State. Often patients wish to have surgery scheduled sometime in the future. We have the same global shortage of radiation oncologists as other countries.

Myth No. 4:

Canada has the same affordability problems and financial pressures as the United States.

Reality:

Affordability — Comparing Costs

How has a single-payer publicly-insured system affected affordability? If we use health spending as a percentage of GNP as our measure, the following data is revealing.

Pre-Medicare Period:

1960   U.S.   **5.5%**
             Canada   **5.5%**

1970   U.S.   **7.3%**
             Canada   **7.0%**

For the pre-Medicare period, health spending grew from the same level and at the same rate in both countries as a share of GNP. In both, the share increased from 5.5% to a little over 7%. In the nearly twenty-five years of Canadian Medicare (1968-93) the rate of growth has sharply diverged. U.S. spending has risen from a little over 7% of GNP to almost 14%. This doubling of the GNP share in the U.S. compares to a much more modest growth in Canada from 7% to about 10% in the same period.

Medicare Period:

1993   U.S.   **From 7% to about 14%**

             Canada   **From 7% to about 10%**

Canada's system has achieved a greater containment of costs. While we face a continuing affordability challenge, it is on a slower growth path.

Myth No. 5:

The United States achieves a better health status by spending 40% more on health care services.
      What does spending 40% more of its GNP on health care yield the United States?

Reality:

Better Outcomes

According to the Harvard Community Health Plan International Comparison carried out by the Louis Harris Co.:

	Canada	U.S.
Life Expectancy	79.2 years	75.6 years
Infant Mortality	7.3 deaths per 1000 live births under 1 year	10.4 deaths per 1000 live births under 1 year
Satisfaction	No. 1 – Canadians satisfied with quality, personal control, not waiting too long and minimizing personal costs of care	No. 2 – Americans satisfied with access to advanced tests, drugs and not waiting too long
Dissatisfaction	Canadians dissatisfied with access to high technology, Medicare and elective surgery. Although less dissatisfied than other nations.	Americans dissatisfied with quality, cost and equal care.

In summary Canadians have somewhat better health status than Americans. It is important to note that social and policy determinants such as poverty and frequent violent acts such as shootings cause the U.S. result. The important point is that spending more on health care services does not offset these social determinants. Harvard's study concludes that Americans rank the opportunity to receive top quality care, regardless of income, as first in importance, last in satisfaction.[3]

3   Michael Decter, "We Have Much to Learn from Each Other," 18th Annual Garland Lecture, Boston Medical Library, November, 1993.

Shared Lessons

Health systems are rooted in culture, values shaped by history, and not wholly or simply shipped across national borders. The United States needs a "made-in-the-U.S.A." health care system. President Clinton and Congress are embarked on creating, or remaking such a system. In Canada as a nation we have a constitution based on the concept "peace, order and good government." Our starting point in health is ability-to-benefit. The United States Declaration of Independence has as its principles life, liberty and the pursuit of happiness. The American starting point in health has been ability-to-pay.

Nevertheless, much can be learned from comparative health studies. In all countries, citizens would rather see resources going to support services than overheads. The human body is not a fundamentally different entity in Toronto than in Buffalo. And so the great challenge — what can the United States learn from Canada about the operation of a health care system at a macro level? Conversely what knowledge can Canada acquire from the United States about the operation of a health care system at the micro level?

Some Lessons from Canada

Canada is a very good teacher. It *IS* possible to provide health care for *ALL*. It is not easy nor will it be achieved without conflict, but it is possible.

Watch Those Overhead Costs: lean is better in health administration. If competing insurers means creating significant overhead, a single payer approach has cost advantages. Canadian provinces manage care for anywhere from 100,000 to 10.8 million "lives" to use the American insurance lingo. The efficiencies of both scale and simplicity are significant. Some of these scale efficiencies are captured by large U.S. health maintenance organizations such as Kaiser Permanente and California Blue Cross. The U.S. General Accounting Office (GAO) has studied overhead costs. Its conclusion is that the U.S. could find the funds to pay for health care for the thirty-five million uninsured by achieving the Canadian level of administrative efficiencies. Some aspects of the proposed Clinton health reform would improve efficiencies in the American health care system, but as long as there are over one thousand different health plans in place, that complexity imposes a very high administrative cost.

There are deals to be had through bargaining and bulk purchasing: one of the strengths of the Canadian approach is the "bulk" purchase by government of most services offered by the physicians. Negotiations with doctors can be noisy and contentious. They also produce savings.

Litigation Can Be Avoided: Canada has a very modest amount of litigation in health care. Perhaps the United States should consider a compensation-based approach rather than a litigation-based means of settling malpractice claims. Canada considered this approach, however, the anticipated increase in Canadian medical litigation has not occurred. Defensive medicine, with over-testing, does impose a cost burden in both countries, albeit a higher burden in the United States.

Generic Drugs Offer Significant Room in Affordability of Drug Plans: by legislating the principle of interchangeability Canadian provincial governments saved themselves and their taxpayers billions of dollars. At both the state and private insurer level, Americans could learn some aspects of cost-containment in the drug area from Canadians.

Some Lessons from the U.S.

Micro efficiencies are possible at the delivery level: put dramatically, if Canada could achieve the same efficiency in the use of hospital beds as the United States, we could close up to 30% to 40% of our existing hospital beds and shift resources to day surgery, outpatient and community care.

Larger Physician Practices: the Kaiser Permanente Health maintenance organization has some five thousand physicians employed in its organization. In Canada, most doctors are still in solo practice. Group practice offers many advantages in terms of quality of care, peer learning, as well as efficiencies. Canadian clinical resource management techniques and technologies are areas to be improved as well.

Broader definition of insured services: Canada set artificial distinctions when it locked "medical services" into various legislation. We need to broaden our definition of health services and embrace a larger range of health providers on a more level playing field. Outcomes should be the guiding light. A good example is the psychiatry/psychology distinction, vast in Canada, but much less so south of the border.

Alternate Site Delivery: the American system has made great

advances in technology, shifting services to the community and the home. Canada needs to invest in technology to enable more care to be unbundled from the hospital setting.

Strategies for Learning

How can Canada and the United States learn from each other? First, we need to acknowledge that both countries have problems and solutions. The winner-take-all mentality needs to give way to a willingness to share lessons and learning. Second, Canadians need to become more aggressive about marketing our expertise in health to the American market. The American corporate health sector is already very active in selling expertise and products to Canada.

Lessons from other Nations

The Finance Ministry, the most powerful arm of Government, operates a near monopoly in the production and sale of cigarettes in one of the world's largest and most lucrative tobacco markets. The Government-owned company, Japan Tobacco Inc., generates a cascade of taxes — $15 billion last year — making it the largest corporate taxpayer in Japan.[4]

There are lessons for Canada to be aware of from the experiences of other nations. In Japan, the profitability of a government tobacco monopoly has distorted public policy to such a degree that, in the words of Dr. Hirayama, director of the Institute of Preventive Oncology, "Eventually, this is going to create a catastrophe in the health care system."[5] This is an excellent example of what not to do.

We have set out our stall in terms of promises to the public in the Patient's Charter. We intend to cut down waiting times, develop a more responsive service, treat people as customers, provide a more personal service, measure the public reaction to see how we are doing and measure the hard bits, the waiting times and so on. Then to publish those, show who is doing well and give an account to the public on services.[6]

4   *New York Times*, October 17, 1993.
5   Ibid.
6   Interview with Sir Duncan Nicholl, CEO, National Health Service, U.K. *Management Today* , October, 1993, p. 40.

On the more positive side of the international learning curve, the example of the British National Health Service, long regarded as unresponsive and bureaucratic, becoming more consumer-centred, points to important issues for Canada. The measurement of quality must become a more public affair. We must move from the complaints department approach to true measurement of consumer reaction and satisfaction or dissatisfaction.

Early in December, 1993, I attended an international symposium on "Managing Health System Change at the District Level." Dr. Vic Neufeld of McMaster University, a leader in health care education who served as theme chairman, put forward the following thoughts on this topic.

This theme is driven by the realization that innovative restructuring of the design, delivery and financing of human services is needed at the community level, in order to maintain and improve our quality of life. The focus is on the health system and its interaction with and impact on other human services. Several assumptions underlie our exploration of this theme:

- the Canadian health system is highly valued by its citizens
- the current system is threatened by factors such as the prolonged economic recession; entrenched thinking; and unawareness of rapid global change
- new ideas are needed for managing health system change, to contain costs, while maintaining satisfactory services, and ultimately enhancing the quality of life of Canadian citizens. Creative solutions are needed at a community (district/regional) level, as well as other levels
- innovative models, and other knowledge and experience is available in Canada, and elsewhere around the world; this includes countries in "the South" where much can be learned about "how to do more with less[7]

One of the participants in the symposium came from the Benin Republic in Western Africa, one of the poorest nations on earth. Sourou Gbangbade described an award winning community health

---

7   Dr. Vic Neufeld, presentation to Health System Change Symposium, McMaster University, Hamilton, December, 1993.

and development project, CREDESA,[8] in his country. The CRE-DESA approach uses health as a starting point for engaging communities on wider development issues.

The CREDESA approach is a holistic development model with an integrated view of community development at its core. This method has significant potential ramifications for smaller Canadian rural and northern communities as well as for First Nation communities.

The Credesa Approach

Key aspects of the approach include:

VILLAGE HEALTH WORKERS	**- Development committee**
	- Village meeting
ADULT EDUCATION	
COMMUNITY PARTICIPATION	
HEALTH ACTIVITIES	**- Health workers**
COMMUNITY ACTIVITIES	**- Curative care**
INTERSECTORAL	**- Preventive care**
FINANCING AND DEVELOPMENT	
DIRECT ACTIVITIES	
FOOD SECURITY AND INCOME GENERATING ACTIVITIES	**- Supervision**
	- Training
	- Planning
DEVELOPMENT WORKERS	**- Monitoring**
COMMUNITY BANK	
EDUCATION	
SUPPORT ACTIVITIES	

CREDESA represents an integrated grass-roots development process with health as the jumping off point. There is an arrogance to our first world notion that international development is a one way

---

8 Eusebe Alihonou, Sourou Gbangbade, ''Improving Health of the Community at District Level — An Experience from Credesa in Benin, Republic (Western Africa),'' Centre Regional Pour le Developpement et La Sante, (CREDEA).

street with Canada and the other industrialized nations sharing expertise with the less developed nations. In fact, Canada has much to learn from the less developed nations; CREDESA is but one small example of where we might start our learning.

Chapter 13
Exporting Our Health Expertise

In recent years, vast amounts of money have been spent on health services worldwide, and this situation is likely to continue. Many developing countries are in need of basic health systems and other aspects of care. Like other developed countries Canada — and the province of Ontario — have the expertise to satisfy the demands of these countries.[1]

Canada is a nation of twenty-seven million people struggling to preserve a very high standard of living in an increasingly difficult and competitive world economy. There are five billion other people with whom we share the planet, or for each Canadian there are two hundred other people. To sustain our wealthy and healthy nation, we need to offer something of value to the rest of the world's people.

For the first 125 years of Canada's existence, and before that as a colony, we sold natural resources. We began with fish and furs and advanced through wheat, minerals, timber, and oil and gas. The world economy has changed dramatically. Raw resources no longer command high prices. We must sell our knowledge as product and as services. Health care services and commodities products can provide a powerful, new economic driver.

Looking at health as a global market, our position is favourable:

---

1   *Strategies for Managing Export Opportunities in Ontario Health Industries,*
    "Outward Bound," Report of the Advisory Committee to the Ontario Minister of
    Health, 1993.

1. Canada's health care system and expertise is much admired by other nations.
2. All peoples and nations, as they gain income and wealth, invest in their own health and their nation's health.
3. Canada spends about 10% of its total gross national product (GNP) on health care, over 750,000 Canadians work in health care or health care related activities.
4. The world economy expends about 8% of its GNP on health care. A 1% share of the world market in health care products and services translates to $17 billion of income and 300,000 jobs for Canadians. Even 0.1% could support 30,000 jobs in Canada.

We have a number of obstacles to overcome in pursuing international markets for our expertise and products. The opportunity is enormous, but so are the challenges. A history of selling commodities has left us with a price-takers attitude and lacking in aggressive sales tactics. We have historically emphasized expertise in mining or drilling in the production end rather than in the selling. Other obstacles include:

- Lack of health care goods production. We do not make many of the products our health care system uses. About 80% of the health care products (everything from bedpans to syringes to drugs) we use are directly imported from the U.S. We do, however, make some very high quality products in fields as diverse as diagnostic imaging and generic drugs and have the capacity to produce many more.
- Absence of marketing expertise for services. Because our health care delivery system operates on a not-for-profit, publicly-administered basis, marketing expertise has not been developed. We do hire consultants, among others as intermediaries.
- Companies are not geared to export. Many of our companies, in health care products or related fields, are small and not yet focused on exporting goods.

Whether these obstacles are too profound or fundamental to be overcome is an important question. The evidence suggests otherwise. Two key realities underscore our ability to jump the barriers. The first, and most important, is the outstanding progress of several

Canadian firms active both in Canada and internationally in the health products and services field. Three Canadian success stories range from a small Canadian-owned private company, RMC, to a large, diverse Canadian-owned public company, MDS, to a large subsidiary of a major health multinational corporation, Connaught. Each can teach Canadians about export.

RMC

RMC: Resource Management Consultants is a dynamic Canadian consulting firm founded in 1967 and led by Walter Kudryk. RMC has consulting projects across Canada in health care and other sectors. Despite this, corporate headquarters is a modest brick building in a residential part of Toronto.

RMC's expanding role and possible opportunities are most evident in Poland where they have an important role in a major World Bank Project. That country is struggling to evolve an affordable health care system. RMC is providing advisory services to the Ministry of Health in policy formulation and strategic planning. Through RMC $200 U.S. million is being invested by the World Bank with the Polish Ministry of Health benefitting from Canadian expertise. The next phase of the work in Poland is likely to be an examination of National Health Insurance.

RMC has undertaken work in a range of other countries including The Bahamas and Uganda, work that has followed some twenty-five years of Canadian consulting experience in health care and other fields. It is important to note that scale is not an absolutely essential ingredient. Through expertise and quality work, RMC has succeeded internationally, in competition with much larger firms. Canada's reputation for quality in health care has also assisted. Our financial participation in world development organizations such as the United Nations, the World Health Organization and the World Bank is another advantage.

The important lesson for Canadian consulting and health service firms is that size is only one factor in international success. Persistence and active marketing are equally as critical. RMC and a growing number of other Canadian consulting firms are successfully transporting our health expertise to other markets around the world.

MDS Health Group

The MDS Health Group is the largest for-profit health care business in Canada, which employs more than six thousand people in its diversified endeavours.

Canadian-owned, its employees own a significant share of the company. Other Canadians, such as police officers, fire fighters, teachers and office workers are investors in MDS through their pension funds. The Ontario Municipal Employees Retirement System (OMERS) is also a major shareholder group. While known primarily for laboratory operations, MDS exports to over one hundred countries. Its Nordion subsidiary is a major international supplier of isotope products.

In 1993, MDS decided to actively pursue the export of its lab management expertise through a new company. Success in the form of a major American contract was not long in coming.

Mayo Clinic Orders Robotic System

TORONTO, ONTARIO — MDS Health Group Limited and MDS Health Ventures announced today that it has signed an order to provide the world renowned Mayo Clinic with an Automated Specimen Handling System ("ASHS"). The Mayo Clinic conducted an extensive evaluation of more than nineteen companies in North America and Asia. It selected a system developed in Toronto at MDS Health Group facilities in partnership with AutoMed Inc., wholly owned by MDS Health Group Limited and MDS Health Ventures.

The Mayo Clinic anticipates that the implementation of this system will lower overall costs to its patients. MDS sees its system as a contribution from the private sector while responding to the need to decrease health care costs in hospitals and commercial laboratories.

The ASHS, a fully automated system, allows laboratories to triple productivity in specimen handling while virtually eliminating sorting errors. It addresses health and safety issues for technologists by eliminating risks of breakage, spillage of blood tubes and resulting contamination.[2]

2 MDS Health Group, press release, Friday, April 30, 1993, p. 1-2.

MDS anticipates growth of its new AUTOLAB venture within a $500 million dollar market segment and expects up to five hundred Canadian jobs will be created through this enterprise.

Connaught

As ownership consolidates on a global basis, to achieve scale and efficiencies in distribution, the interests of individual nations will be affected. Connaught's recent history provides an excellent example of the current trend toward ownership consolidation in the global economy. In 1989, Institut Merieux, a French vaccine maker, purchased Connaught with assistance from Rhone-Poulenc, a larger French pharmaceutical company. In 1993, Rhone-Poulenc consolidated its ownership in Institut Merieux by increasing its shareholding from 51% to 100%. Will Connaught, now French-owned, remain a good corporate citizen of Canada? With links between Connaught and the Canadian research community, as well as a continued securing of world product mandates by Connaught from its parent company, the answer can be a strong yes. If Canada and Ontario pay insufficient attention to forging partnerships with Connaught in research and development and in marketing vaccines, then there are long-term risks to Connaught's contribution to Canada. As with other multinationals, the issues will be strategic alliances and world product mandates. The world vaccine manufacturing industry has consolidated into four major areas. Yet, there are still opportunities for Canada. We should continue to regard Connaught as a Canadian-based, if not Canadian-owned, manufacturer.

In December, 1993, Connaught announced a contract with Merck under which Connaught will manufacture Hepatitis A vaccine for purchase worldwide. Sales of $16 million per year are forecast, once the vaccine is introduced in 1995/96. This approach links Merck's research, development and marketing ability to Connaught's manufacturing expertise. Michael Trainow, president of Merck Frost, Merck's Canadian subsidiary, commented: "The men and women of Connaught do what they do better than anybody in the world. Canadians can and will compete given the chance."[3]

This comment underscores precisely the reality of Canadian expertise and the opportunities we must pursue to realize our health economic development.

---

3 *Toronto Star*, December 11, 1993.

Despite the large scale of numerous, global pharmaceutical companies, there is enormous scope for a consolidation of the world pharmaceutical industry. Merck, the largest firm, has, in total, only 4% of the world market. The three next biggest firms share less than 10% of the world market. There are thousands of active companies in the pharmaceutical industry. In a speech to the 1993 *Financial Post* Conference, Dr. Martin Barkin, Chief Executive Officer of Deprenyl Research presented the following data:

Country	*Number of Active Pharmaceutical Companies*
Japan	**1500**
Germany	**1000**
U.S.A.	**800**
France	**350**

As cost containment in the pharmaceutical sector takes hold in the United States, there is accelerated pressure for global consolidation of the pharmaceutical industry. American policy changes, proposed by the Clinton administration, will impact upon the United States. Because the United States is the largest single country market it will shape the evolution of the global industry. As noted previously, the shift of investment from new products to delivery systems, evident in the Merck acquisition of Medco, points to a new reality.

Canada has, through its experience with Connaught, an insight into emerging world-wide trends. As part of a strategy of increasing Canadian health exports, we will need to actively pursue international product mandates for subsidiaries of multi-national corporations housed in Canada. From MDS and its experience with Autolab we gain a glimpse of the export potential of expertise; from RMC we learn that persistence succeeds in distant markets. Global consolidation presents both threats and opportunities to Canada in the health care sector. We will need to be strategic in what we pursue, and nimble in that pursuit, to succeed.

Firms on the Health Care Export Horizon

RMC, MDS and Connaught, the three firms described above, are each leaders. There are many others with export activity or potential. Among the most interesting are:

- Diagnostic Chemicals Ltd., a PEI-based company supplies diagnostic testing kit chemicals. Sales to twenty countries generate 70% of the $7 million in sales.
- Alellix is developing biotechnology products.
- EFOS exports most of its production of light-activated dental equipment.
- ISG is a world leader in computer graphics to assist complicated surgery.
- LacMac is a manufacturer of hospital gowns and linens to world markets.
- Medtronic is developing low cost, reliable pacemakers.
- The Ottawa Heart Institute, lead by Dr. Wilbert Keon, is best known for its excellence in cardiac surgery and research. Now, the Ottawa Heart Institute is developing an artificial heart with CAE and CME.
- Sherritt, originally Sherritt Gordon, a Canadian mining company, has evolved into a technology leader through its Westaim operation in Alberta. The company is developing anti-microbial systems to prevent infections utilizing advanced industrial materials. Sherritt presents an interesting rebirth of a company rooted in the old economy of resources emerging into the new economy of knowledge-based production.
- Torcan is developing fine chemical processes for major international pharmaceutical companies.
- Vascath supplys cardiovascular devices to world markets.

As the brief profiles of these firms illustrate, there are great opportunities for Canadian expertise in the larger world market. And these openings are not confined to the for-profit sector. Another important reality is Canada's commitment to international development, both through the efforts of the Canadian International Development Agency and hundreds of volunteer organizations. Canada has been a constructive advocate of international development and cooperation among nations. We needn't choose between continuing our humanitarian efforts or becoming more active on a commercial basis. We must do both.

Our approach to marketing Canadian expertise must be in response to different nations' needs for our goods and services. The following chart illustrates the differing requirements.

Nations' Needs — Opportunities

Countries & Annual Income Levels	Health Care Market Opportunities
Lowest income countries with less than $500 GNP per capita - Asia - Africa	preventive programmes public health health promotion sector planning/management basic infrastructure
Lower income countries with from $500 to $1,500 GNP per capita	preventive programmes public health health promotion sector planning/management basic infrastructure training primary care
Middle income countries with more than $1,500 GNP per capita	hospital management services laboratory services health policy
Highest income countries with more than $15,000 GNP per capita - Western Europe - U.S. - Japan - Australia	cost containment technologies long-term care facilities large-scale health system management high technology

The emphasis of the World Bank and other international financial institutions is on financing preventive and health promotion programmes in developing nations. Canada has proficiency in health promotion, prevention programmes and public health. Most of this is lodged in public health units, departments of health and universities. To successfully export this expertise, we need new partnerships and joint ventures between the public and private sectors.

Canadian International Development Agency (CIDA)

CIDA's role is not only development aid and education, it also provides a very important potential entry point for Canadian enterprise. I spent five weeks during the summer of 1990 touring China, conducting an evaluation of the Open Cities Project which CIDA had sponsored with the Federation of Canadian Municipalities and the Special Economic Zones Office of the Government of China. As one of its initiatives, the project had brought very senior Chinese civic officials mayors and vice-mayors of the largest cities in China to Canada.[4] The Chinese leaders were not only extremely impressed by our cities and how we manage them, but they also expected Canadians to return to China and sell them some good old Canadian know-how. Instead Americans, whose cities have many difficult problems, have been selling the good old Yankee know-how at very handsome prices. Why? We had not been back to follow up CIDA's good work. Less developed countries want fair trade, quality health and health care for their citizens, as much as they want aid. We can contribute enormously, without exploitation, by establishing and expanding trade and selling our health products and services to the developing countries of the world.

Efforts are already underway in Canada to increase our international activities. Can we compete with the best? Yes, we can if we are determined.

The Manitoba Health Industry Initiatives

My earliest acquaintance with health economic development and the

---

4   A note on Chinese government and business structures. Chinese city governments appoint the managers of most of the enterprises within their boundaries. The Mayor of Shanghai is the Canadian equivalent of the Mayor of Toronto, Premier of Ontario and the top 100 business managers in Ontario all rolled into one. And, Shanghai has about 1 million more residents than the Toronto Metropolitan area.

ability of government to make a difference arose during the period from 1981 to 1986. I served as Cabinet Secretary in the Manitoba government as well as Deputy Minister for Intergovernmental Relations at that time. A good portion of this job was trying to pry federal dollars from Ottawa. During the period when Lloyd Axworthy was the Manitoba Minister, we enjoyed a great deal of success. Mr. Axworthy was a determined regional minister and the only prominent elected Liberal between the Manitoba-Ontario border and the Pacific Ocean. With his help, Manitoba was able to secure Canada's first Economic Regional Development Agreement (ERDA). It not only covered funds for traditional expenditures like physical infrastructure — roads in the north, water and sewer — but it created opportunities in Mr. Axworthy's transportation portfolio to benefit the province (and the country) economically. In 1984, when the Government of Canada changed, Jake Epp became Minister of Health and Welfare and also the regional minister for Manitoba. Our challenge was to figure out how Mr. Epp could be helpful to Manitoba, even though he had strongly and publicly opposed Mr. Axworthy's largesse to the province. On the health side of Mr. Epp's portfolio, there were significant allotments for issues such as research. The Manitoba government decided to attempt to construct a partnership between the two levels of government, to expand the health sector in Manitoba.

Our starting point was that Manitoba was blessed, as is much of Canada, with formidable resources in health. Winnipeg had the University of Manitoba with a faculty of medicine, two teaching hospitals — the Health Sciences Centre and St. Boniface — as well as some industry related to health care. What began then as a voyage of discovery has continued since as a strong initiative of the Manitoba government: public investment in the form of actual monies to research laboratories. Private sector investment has meant drug and device manufacturers have set up in Manitoba, largely because Manitoba has the right ingredients to support them: a hard working and skilled labour force with research skills, relatively low cost for land and business operations, and a first-class health infrastructure. The focus that the Manitoba health industries initiative brought was important to the overall success of investment in that province. Those active in health care in Manitoba became aware of business with implications for jobs and technology.

Manitoba's success was not because of unwarranted federal or provincial government spending. It succeeded because of a focus on the public sector investment and strong ties forged to the private sector. The Canadian landscape is littered with badly conceived regional development efforts that attempted to fly in the face of the real economy: heavy water plants, and car manufacturing plants, in the Atlantic region; white elephants in all areas of the country. What fundamentally distinguished Manitoba's health initiatives from misguided attempts was that they built on strengths already present in the Manitoba economy.

Companies subsidized by government rarely succeed. Michael Porter argues persuasively and with a massive weight of empirical evidence in his book, *The Competitive Advantage of Nations*. Nations succeed because industries succeed. Governments can play a role in the success of particular industries and sectors, as long as they avoid the ruinous activity of trying to select individual corporate winners. The public sector can make a difference by reinforcing the infrastructure of a particular industry or sector. Reinforcing health infrastructure, whether in support of research or in other ways, has strengthened the health sector in Manitoba. This in turn led to the creation of jobs and greater economic health and activity.

The Quebec Sector Strategy Approach

Quebec uses a cluster approach in their industrial economic strategy. The province draws very heavily on the work of Michael Porter and others, who in turn follow A.O. Hirschman and Vasily Leontief. Harvard Professor Hirschman developed theories of forward and backward linkages; Vasily Leontief won the Nobel Prize for his work on input/output tables. Their work, refined further by Michael Porter, goes to the heart of how economies function and grow, recognizing the existent connections among various industries.

The Quebec strategy has focused heavily on the pharmaceutical industry and on biotechnology. Through tax policies and the management of its drug formulary, Quebec has managed to attract significant pharmaceutical industry investment into the Montreal region. Some of this may have been at the expense of other regions of the country, and, these investments might have taken place in an absence of subsidy, at the expense of federal and Quebec taxpayers. A difficult one to fully assess. What is clear is that Quebec's concentration on particular clusters has allowed linkages to develop between the plants attracted and Quebec suppliers. Quebec's view of the relationship between biotechnology and pharmaceuticals is that it connects to the rest of the Quebec economy which is deepening and strengthening.

Ontario's Health Industry Initiatives

When I became Deputy Minister of Health for Ontario in 1991 I began working on how the Ontario Health Ministry might contribute to the renewal of the Ontario economy. The Ontario economy had undergone a dramatic job loss over the previous two years. Some 300,000 jobs vanished, many of them in the manufacturing sector.

The Free Trade Agreement and the accompanying recession accelerated the pace of an economic restructuring driven by Canada's need to be globally competitive in a more open world. Economic renewal was essential to Ontario.

What contribution could the health sector make? On the delivery of care side, it was clear, from 1991 on, that the care delivery system, as it restructured for effectiveness and survival, would shed some employment. And it could not be counted on for additional jobs. That left the supply side of the equation: companies supplying input to health care and the export market. Ontario had a rich array of health resources, including a number of major companies and a myriad of consulting firms selling health expertise. Some of these were architectural and engineering firms capable of designing and building health facilities. Others were consultants active in the evaluation of health policy. Mr. Graham Scott, a lawyer and public servant who served in the early 1980s as Deputy Minister of Health, was asked to chair a committee which, in an excellent report, *Outward Bound*, recommended the creation of Interhealth.

Interhealth is a consortium approach to marketing, both Ontario, and Canadian expertise, outside the country. During the writing of this book I remained involved with Interhealth, chairing an implementation committee. As of this writing, the basic direction has been established on the basis of the Interhealth recommendations and accepted by the Government of Ontario. The Government has pledged an investment of $3.5 million to be matched by the private sector. A committee of twenty is working on the corporate structure, financing and policies. The committee will turn the full responsibility over to a Board of Directors and Chief Executive for Interhealth.

Other aspects of Ontario's health initiatives include a Health Industry Advisory Committee (HIAC) chaired by Mr. Bill Blundell, the retired chief executive officer of General Electric Canada. The enthusiasm with which individual companies are active, for a short or a long period of time, in international markets greet a more organized approach to these markets is encouraging. It will be essential for Canada to present a united front internationally; other nations have already taken this approach. For many international projects there is a French or a German national bid. We need structure and organization in order to succeed. Many disparate proposals for the same work will not go forward. In the international market, some of which is heavily shaped by the decisions of the World Bank, Canada must have, in addition to its good reputation, a strong organized approach to obtaining business.

Interhealth Canada Limited Proposal

It is proposed that Ontario health companies and public sector organizations in the health field join to spearhead a renewed competitive thrust in the export market. The committee is unanimous in its belief in and its commitment to a joint endeavour, tentatively named Interhealth Canada Limited ("Interhealth"). It is conceived as an Ontario corporation with shareholders, drawn from firms across the health private sector and from health organizations in the Ontario public sector. Membership would provide individual firms, associations and universities with an added degree of strength, which they would not have on their own. It would also enhance their reputations and standing in those markets they seek to penetrate.

Mission

Interhealth is committed to a disciplined, flexible, multidimensional approach that seeks to maximize profitable opportunities for Canadian companies engaged in health goods and services consulting activities in key markets worldwide.

Value Statement

Interhealth will seek to promote, encourage and sustain the quality of life through the delivery of efficient, culturally-appropriate quality health services in all countries where international projects are undertaken.

Role and Function

As the primary focus for Ontario's health export initiative, the company would have a variety of roles and functions as follows:

- Market intelligence gathering/international networking. Responsibility for gathering, evaluating and acting on current market intelligence to develop a competitive position in overseas markets. Linkages would be formed and maintained with existing organizations, such as the Ontario International Corporation, Ontario Ministry of Health, Health Canada, Industry, Science and Technology Canada, External Affairs and other provincial governments to allow the company to exploit fully this existing intelligence network.

- Project management. When projects are awarded to the company, it would have both the legal authority and the lead role for managing them from beginning to end. There should be a management structure in place to ensure that each project is given full attention and the best combination of expertise the membership has to offer. Clearly, the role of the project manager is critical, as he or she will be responsible for all the major decisions of the undertaking.

The establishment of project teams, preparation of bids and submissions, securing and managing contracts, and arranging export financing must reflect the best the company has to offer. As a result, this may often call for secondment of individuals from shareholder companies.

In addition, one of Interhealth's strengths would be the combination of health products and services. As Interhealth bids on major international health consulting projects, it could offer a full range of products to support the front-end consulting work.

- **Marketing opportunities.** The company would be responsible for a variety of activities in support of securing international projects. These may involve the development of an infrastructure in the local markets to encourage effective client liaison, including language translation, background on business habits and cultural assessment and understanding.
- **Administrative support.** There are also numerous administrative functions to be carried out, including the provision of member and shareholder services, public and investor relations and public education, financial management, and general office administration [5]

Earning Our Way

Canadians have the talent to work anywhere in the world. We have a rich, internationally-linked multicultural talent bank from which to draw. In addition to our health skills, we have, within our borders, almost every language spoken on earth. We are becoming organized to tackle these markets in a thoughtful and successful manner. If we are to reach beyond our historic role of exporting our resources, to a twenty-first century role of marketing our expertise, the health sector has a huge role to play. Governments will need to provide leadership and use their international connections. The Government of Canada, in particular, will need to use its High Commissions and Embassies around the world in a cooperative way to support the efforts of individual provinces and the private sector to market Canadian endeavours.

We must also reinforce the infrastructure within Canada. Our health services must be of the highest quality and that we can demonstrate their effectiveness. This is necessary, first of all, to ensure that Canadians are getting excellent health care and good value for their tax dollar. We also need quality insurance to meet the test of the world marketplace in convincing our customers that what they buy is truly the best.

Many of the investments needed in Canada to create necessary infrastructure will support both making more products here and exporting them. The amalgamation of capital to support innovation

5 *Outward Bound Report, Strategies for Maximizing Export Opportunities in the Ontario Health Industries,* a report to the Ontario Minister of Health, 1993, p. 9-10.

will also support expansion of marketing activities beyond Canada's border. Investments by government, in research and particularly in ways of commercializing research, will enhance our production and exports. Finally, a focus by the health industry sector, on recognizing itself as a sector, sharing information and opportunities within that sector will allow much stronger linkages and more powerful marketing to global markets.

The sheer scale of the global market for health care and the success to date of some of our firms are sound reasons for optimism. Much effort will be required to realise our full potential in exporting Canadian health expertise to the rest of the world.

Good Stuff to Read

The Competitive Advantage of Nations by Michael Porter. The most powerful recent analysis of what drives competitive advantage among nations and industries. Harvard Professor Michael Porter's Studies reveal that industries with strong pressures in their local markets and competition become strong initiated competitors — the Japanese car industry and Italian tiles are excellent examples.

Outward Bound — Strategies For Maximizing Export Opportunities in the Ontario Health Industry. Available from the Health Economic Development Office, Ontario Ministry of Health, 56 Wellesley Street West, Toronto, Ontario M5S 2S3. Fax: (416) 314-5916.

Chapter 14
Canadian Health Economic Development

Increasing Canadian exports is only one challenge to be taken up in the health economic development field. Creating more health products and services in Canada and increasing our research are also vital. We need to combine the ingredients of research, production and marketing. Our health economic development has enormous potential to create jobs and economic activity of a long-term sustainable nature.

Making More Stuff Here

Healthy & Wealthy,[1] the Health Industries Advisory Committee (HIAC) report to the Ontario Government provided an interesting profile on health industries. The gap of $2 billion per annum, between Canada's $5 billion production of health care products and our consumption of $7 billion, provides one target for making more health products here. So, too, is the 40,000 jobs which the report estimates could be created in this field.

The relationship between public policy and health economic development opportunity is well illustrated by an examination of the origins of two of Canada's most successful health-related companies, Novopharm and Apotex. In 1974, the Ontario government established the Ontario Drug Benefit Programme (ODB). The legislation

---

1 "Healthy & Wealthy — a Growth Prescription for Ontario's Health Industries," *The Report of the Health Industries Advisory Committee to the Minister of Health*, March 1994, p. 12.

which created the ODB contained the legal principle of interchangeability. Simply stated, interchangeability meant that the pharmacist was required to dispense the lower cost generic drug in place of the more expensive "brand name" drug where the two drugs were of the same chemical compound. In addition to saving the government tens of millions of dollars on ODB, interchangeability, coupled with the Federal government policy of compulsory licensing, created a rapidly growing market for Apotex and Novopharm, both manufacturers of generic drugs. Both of these companies have grown to be significant employers and exporters. They are described below.

Apotex

In September, 1992, *Profit Magazine* named Dr. Barry Sherman as one of Canada's Top 10 Entrepreneurs of the Decade. They described him as "The Robin Hood of Pharmaceuticals" and noted the growth of Apotex Inc. from a 1974 start-up to a conglomerate with revenues of $500 million per year. Some 40% of revenues are still from generic drugs, despite strong diversification. The Apotex Healthcare Group of companies has diversified into development, manufacturing and distribution of non-prescription medicines, vitamins, diagnostic products, laboratory equipment and supplies, disposable plastic products for medical use, and hospital waste management systems.

From its two-employee, 5,000 square foot birth, the company has grown to employ 2,000 people in research, development and manufacturing. Canadian operations now occupy over 800,000 square feet in Toronto, Montreal, Winnipeg and Vancouver. Apotex produces more than one hundred generic pharmaceuticals which, in Canada, are used to fill almost fifteen million prescriptions a year.

Dr. Sherman has been an aggressive litigator defending and expanding markets for his products. He has also been a spectacularly successful Canadian businessman. Apotex exports to over 80 countries around the globe with export markets representing an ever-growing portion of the total sales. Apotex has also established a presence through subsidiaries, joint ventures or licensing agreements, in Morocco, France, the Czech and Slovak Republics, Mexico, Peru, Costa Rica, New Zealand, Australia and Russia.

Novopharm

It's difficult to find a contrast in personalities and business styles greater than those between Novopharm founder and Chief Executive Leslie Dan and Apotex founder Barry Sherman. Although their generic drug manufacturing firms have grown side by side, Barry Sherman's litigation-oriented, aggressive style is the antithesis of Leslie Dan's calm, quiet approach.

Leslie Dan is a Hungarian by birth. Driven from his native country by war and prejudice, he, like millions of others, settled in Canada. Through decades of toil and investment, Mr. Dan has built Novopharm into a huge generic drug manufacturer with sales of several hundred million dollars per year.

In January, 1994, Novopharm announced it had acquired a large minority position in the Hungarian state-owned pharmaceutical manufacturer Human Serum and Pharmaceutical Co. of Godallo. Human Serum employees 950 people and its business includes injectable pharmaceuticals, vaccines, insulin and blood-derivative products. Through this acquisition, Canadian expertise will allow Novopharm to expand Human Serum's business in Eastern Europe.

Why did the Hungarian government approach Leslie Dan as a partner/purchaser of their state company? For the previous two years Novopharm and Human Serum had successfully operated Human-pharma Ltd., a joint venture manufacturing pills and tablets. Trust and a well-earned reputation for putting quality first were the attributes which convinced the Hungarian government to build their partnership with Novopharm.

The success stories of Apotex and Novopharm, Canada's two largest generic drug manufacturers, illustrate the benefits of increasing Canadian production of inputs to our own health system. Canada has gained two world class and globally competitive companies with their homebase and ownership in Canada. We *can* "home-grow" new firms to produce new products. But, home-growing firms with public policy support is only one means of furthering health economic development. Canadian governments can also encourage existing health-related businesses to expand their product lines by entering new product markets. Canadian businesses, not currently involved in the health products sector, can expand by entering into it. Canadian governments can encourage multi-national firms to establish production facilities here, and to grant world product mandates to their Canadian subsidiaries, so they may export, as well as sell in

Canada. These approaches are not mutually exclusive. All four activities can be combined into a strategy. But, to succeed this strategy needs fuel in the form of private investment dollars to finance research, product development and marketing. Such financing is not always easy to obtain in Canada. The business and labour communities, and the health sector, will need to advocate and support this effort.

Financing Health Ideas

Fraser Mustard is one of Canada's leading thinkers and advocates on matters of health and wealth. As one of the founders, and the driving force behind the Canadian Institute for Advanced Research (CIAR), he has pushed Canadian political and business leaders, as well as policy-makers, to confront realities beyond the conventional wisdom upon which much flawed policy is based. One of his recent crusades is that Canadian financial institutions, particularly our chartered banks, should lend money for ideas, as well as for bricks and mortar. Dr. Mustard points out that the rise of Japan has been accomplished with significant lending and investment inside the Japanese business organizations — Keritsu — which combine finance and ideas.

Dr. Mustard's dominant concern has been that a decline in our country's wealth would also erode our standard of health. In every study health-wealth are fundamentally married. He is also certain that future Canadian prosperity does not rest on the resource-based economy which generated Canada's initial wealth as a nation. A financial sector heavily-oriented to lending against hard, tangible assets, rather than against the more ethereal intellectual property of ideas, is a legacy of Canada's pioneer economy. What if our chartered banks had shifted a few billion dollars of lending away from the red hot Toronto property market in the late 1980s and into small, idea-driven enterprises? Perhaps we would have had less carnage in the real estate market and more dynamism in the economy.

We are a nation well-supplied, perhaps over-supplied, with shopping centres and office towers. While this may be admirable, investment in the world of intellectual property will allow us to continue a high standard of living through a high valued-added economy. Our financial community, particularly the banks, must expand their understanding and support small business, in general, and small knowledge-based businesses above all others.

There are encouraging signs. Some modest pools of capital have formed, specifically to invest in health economic development. As well, a number of venture capital companies consider health-related investments among their priorities. Interesting examples are the MDS Health Ventures and the BioCapital Biotechnology Investment Fund. Other similar health investments include Vencap Equities in Alberta, which has an informal target of investing 20% of its total portfolio in the health sector. But what types of companies do these pools of capital seek? What are their investments for the future?

A few examples are helpful in understanding the range and diversity of the investments.

MDS Health Investments

Diagnostic Products and Other Services

ADI Diagnostics Inc. is a manufacturer of rapid human diagnostic kits for the major screening markets: reference laboratories, blood banks and public health institutions.

CME Telemetrix Inc. is involved in the development of a proprietary non-invasive instrument for the measurement of blood analyses including glucose, cholesterol, lactates and alcohol.

Tokos Medical of Canada Inc. is investigating the availability of government funding which will enable it to sell products and services to the women's health care market in Canada that Tokos Inc. markets in the United States. Tokos Inc.'s principal product is used in the assessment and treatment of pregnant women at home for symptoms associated with pre-term labour.

Pharmaceutical and Biotechnology Products and Services

Allelix Biopharmaceuticals Inc., a publicly-traded company is involved in the discovery and development of novel biopharmaceutical products for tissue repair and inflammation.

Ethical Pharmaceuticals Ltd. (U.K.) is the parent company of a specialized group of pharmaceutical development companies offering products, technologies and services with a special emphasis on delivery systems.

Ethical Pharmaceuticals North America Inc. is a 15/85

joint venture between Ethical Pharmaceuticals (UK) and MDS Ventures. They have rights to develop, manufacture and sell, in Canada, all products and technologies owned by Ethical Pharmaceuticals (UK). In addition, Ethical Pharmaceuticals North America retains certain royalty rights on sales of products and technologies of Ethical Pharmaceuticals (UK) in the United States.

Hemosol Inc. is actively engaged in the development of a human blood substitute based on hemoglobin.

Rehabilitation Products and Other Services

3c Rehabilitation Technologies is involved in developing pain relief treatment devices and services.

Columbia Health Group Inc. is developing a network of acute and chronic care clinics in Canada and the United States.

Medical Information and Robotics

Andronic Devices Ltd. is developing automated products for the laboratory and operating room both to facilitate surgical procedures and to assist in automating the manual aspects of the laboratory and the operating room.

AutoMed Associates is a partnership between AutoMed Inc. and Automated Specimen Handling, Inc. which is developing a series of modules for automation of the specimen handling aspect of a laboratory. Automated Specimen Handling, Inc. is 50% owned by MDS Health Group Inc., a U.S. subsidiary of MDS, and MDS Ventures.

I.S.G. Technologies Inc. is a publicly-traded company which designs, manufactures and markets full-solution medical-imaging workstations to construct three-dimensional images of patient anatomy from Computerized Tomography ("CT") Scan and Magnetic Resonance Imager (MRI) data.

Access Health Marketing Inc. is a health care marketing services company that designs, markets, implements and supports information based marketing and telemarketing programmes in the health care industry.

Homecare Products and Other Services

Disys Corporation, formerly Dicon Systems Limited, is a publicly-traded company and a leading manufacturer and marketer of equipment for the detection of smoke, gas and intrusion in the home.

Thompson & Nielsen Electronics Ltd. is a manufacturer of instruments for radiation protection in medical, environmental and industrial fields.[2]

The BioCapital Biotechnology Investment Fund

In May 1990, Balthazard, Coupal et Associés inc. (BC et Associés), in collaboration with the Fonds de solidarité des travailleurs du Québec (FTQ), created a focused investment fund called the Fonds d'investissement en biotechnologie BioCapital. The goal of this fund is to support the growth of this sector, mainly in Quebec, by establishing close cooperation between companies and the financial and scientific communities. BioCapital highlights the innovative potential of the many research teams working in the industrial, academic and hospital environments.

Since its creation, the Fund has received more than 200 projects, including about 100 from Quebec. Up to now, BioCapital has invested in 12 companies in the biotechnology sector, providing them with the support necessary for the scientific comprehension of their projects and the development of their operations. Investments by the Fund totalled $6.6 million as of April 30, 1992.

BioCapital is a venture capital fund specializing in biotechnology and managed by a company held by BC et Associés. This fund has $10.5 million (Cdn.) in capital, subscribed mainly by the Fonds de solidarité des travailleurs du Québec (FTQ), the Société d'investissement de la Province de Namur (S.I.B.S.), The Generics Group plc and by Gestion BioCapital Inc.

The fund invests in innovative companies offering

2   MDS Health Ventures, Corporate Material, 1993.

high growth potential and operating in strategic fields related to biotechnology.

1.   Aggressive Investment and Action

BioCapital is a fund committed to making profits from venture capital investments. BioCapital relies on methodology supplied by a well-established network of expertise which offers the best possibilities for success.

Selection of Innovative Firms

- Identification and devaluation of companies by committees of national and international experts in science, technology and business;
- Selection of 15 to 20 companies in the start-up or development stages; specializing in biotechnology;
- Technical and management support for companies;
- Ongoing supervision of companies;
- Geographical distribution (70% in Quebec).

2.   A Diversified Portfolio of Companies Specializing in Biotechnology

BioCapital offers fund sponsors a diversified portfolio of innovative companies featuring high growth potential.

Holding Companies

- Lipopharm
- Médi-Force
- Biomatrix Médical Canada
- Quantum Biotechnologies
- Polychol
- IBS
- Diagnostics Biovet
- Serrener
- UniSyn Technologies
- Bio-Systèmes Biosys
- Haemacure Biotech
- Ventana Growth Fund II

3.   **Tax Advantages that Favour Technological Development in Quebec**

BC et Associés has developed, with BioCapital, the expertise necessary to take advantage of government financial vehicles and programmes aimed at facilitating the financing of biotechnology R & D projects. These assistance programmes substantially reduce the sponsors' investment risks.

4.   **A National and International Network of Expertise**
BioCapital has access to a national and international network of expertise which includes the Fonds de solidarité des travailleurs de Québec (FTQ); The Generics Group plc of London, England; the Ventana Growth Fund II of San Diego, California; S.I.B.S. de Namur of Belgium; Biosurvey s.a. of Belgium, as well as members of the consultative committees.[3]

Capital linked to ideas also changes the role of our research institutes. The institute must strengthen the bridges to intermediate structures with a capacity for commercialization. More output here will require more investment in health economic development. Our dilemma is joining our research to commercial ventures. In Ontario, alone, there are eighty research institutes and associations in the health care field; most are affiliated with a hospital, a university or both. Others are connected to a particular disease or condition. Together they constitute a key resource and powerful engine for the production of valuable intellectual property. A major challenge, which investment pools are helping to address, is harnessing this engine to the creation of high value-added jobs and exports.

Building on Our Research Strength

"Research is essential to any strategy to improve health."[4]

"The major challenge for both developing and developed nations

---

3   BioCapital Corporation Material, 1993.
4   *Health of the Nation*, U.K. Government, 1992.

is how to strike the correct balance between basic medical research, with the longer term perspective that this entails, and research into our more immediate requirements in the provision of health care. While the latter is less newsworthy, recent advances in epidemiology and statistical methods have given it the potential to be of enormous benefit to our patients.[5]

Canada has developed a varied and rapidly growing array of research institutions. We also have elaborate structures in place through which funding flows to research institutions, and a formidable collection of fundraising organizations. Our overall research enterprise as a nation is a complex and valuable endeavour. In a world where knowledge and information command premiums which once accrued by natural resources, Canada badly needs a new economic engine. In the health sector, research can be a powerful lever for enhanced efficiency of our own health delivery systems. As well, research can underpin an important export effort, directed to sharing our advances in both health products and services, with other nations.

All of the companies described in the previous two chapters require sustained investment in research and development simply to survive. Success will require luck, proficient marketing and skilful management. Without research the prospects are dismal. Canada is rapidly expanding a talented network of researchers, as noted in Chapter 9, this network includes a cluster of new health services or applied clinical epidemiology research organizations.

As hospital duties unbundle to the outpatient and community setting, hospital space often becomes available for other purposes. One potential use for this real estate is conversion to research. The success of a research enterprise requires it to have separate and identifiable leadership from a hospital in which it resides or is associated.

Health is a technology and knowledge based endeavour. We need to devote a greater share of our national health resources to research. Many successful companies producing knowledge intensive products or services devote 10% or more of their annual *revenues* to R & D. Canadian health care devotes only about 1–2% of total expenditures to R & D in aggregate. This is far too little.

---

5   Sir David Weatherall, Editorial, *Science and Public Affairs*, University of Oxford, Autumn, 1993, p.5.

One of the most compelling arguments for strengthening our research base is the need to retain talented young Canadians. Our education system, through the university graduate level produces bright, well-educated researchers. These people constitute our future health intelligence capacity. We need to employ, nurture and develop their skills to solve the problems we face.

There are good reasons for favouring a balanced Canadian research programme with more resources, both human and financial. Health systems and biomedical research are both vital ingredients in healing Medicare. We need vaccines against new diseases, new medicines and new surgical techniques. Science tools deployed against medical problems will give us real progress. We also need better techniques for promoting health.

Many of our successes in building health research excellence have been achieved by pioneers motivated by dreams of finding a better way to tackle health problems. Three examples are located in St. Boniface, Manitoba, on the grounds of the Sunnybrook Health Sciences Centre and on University Avenue in downtown Toronto.

St. Boniface Hospital Research Centre

Today, a modern research building, standing on the bank of the Red River which divides Winnipeg and St. Boniface, provides a home for the St. Boniface General Hospital Research Centre. A decade ago, the research centre was a dream, and a remote one at that. Realizing this vision required a remarkable voyage with a varied and talented cast of characters drawn from all over the world. One key player was the long-time Manitoba Minister of Health, Larry Desjardins. As Minister for Lotteries, Mr. Desjardins allowed the Research Foundation to sell break-open lottery tickets and to operate a major annual lottery. Mr. Desjardins boosted the Foundation's efforts. The International Award and Dinners, organized by the Foundation, have brought major world figures, from Andre Sakharov to Christian Barnard to the St. Boniface General Hospital. The Award and Dinners focused the entire enterprise of the Research Foundation and Centre on excellence in the world context. In travelling to Moscow to arrange for Dr. Sakharov to visit, St. Boniface leaders were determined to secure a visa for Dr. Sakharov and his wife Yelenna Bonner. They conquered the formidable Soviet bureaucracy to bring their guest to Canada.

The profile and stature of the Research Foundation has also been elevated by the quality and international stature of Award recipients. The late Sam Cohen, who, along with Cam MacLean was one of the key leaders of the St. Boniface Foundation. The former wagered with a wealthy member of the Bronfman family that a St. Boniface researcher would win a Nobel Prize for medical research before the Montreal Expo's won a World Series. Having left Winnipeg I lost track of the St Boniface Research Centre until I arrived back in Winnipeg for Christmas, 1993. The front page of *The Winnipeg Free Press*, prominently featuring Dr. Naranjan Dhalla, head of the cardiovascular science research team at the St. Boniface Research Centre, rapidly brought me up to date. The article noted, "In what is one of the largest medical research teams in the world — and the only one in Canada concentrating on heart research — more than 80 faculty, students and staff from 28 countries are working together to understand the causes of heart disease."[6] It also mentioned an exceptionally large grant — $5.2 million — from the Medical Research Council of Canada.

From 50 cent break open Nevada tickets and the vision of a handful of remarkable Canadians, a research endeavour now flourishes on the banks of the Red River. Whether a Nobel Prize eventually honours work at the Centre or not, Sam Cohen's bet is well won. A legacy of excellence is deeply entrenched.

Institute for Clinical Evaluative Sciences

The Institute for Clinical Evaluative Sciences, also known as ICES, was a dream of Dr. Adam Linton, an exceptional medical leader in Ontario. ICES came into being shortly after Dr. Linton's premature death in 1991. As president of the Ontario Medical Association, Dr. Linton convinced his profession that partnership with government was preferable to confrontation. He also insisted that evaluation of medical practice outcomes and development of guidelines should be insulated from government and from the profession's direct control. His vision was ICES, an independent body pursuing very practical research with dedicated and adequate financial resources.

The reality is that a well-run ICES will, on different issues, antagonize either the medical profession or government, or both. The public is the constituency that should defend ICES. Health care

---

6   *Winnipeg Free Press*, December 22, 1993, p.1.

consumers only stand to gain from improving our knowledge of what works and, how well it works.

Today, ICES is a reality. A $4.5 million per year research enterprise with bright, research and practice minds. Under the determined leadership of Dr. David Naylor, ICES has produced an impressive stream of very practical studies which will profoundly influence the way medicine is practised and health care services delivered. At Sunnybrook Health Sciences Centre, where ICES is located there is a powerful mix of excellence in delivery and in research about clinical outcomes.

With six career scientists supported by external peer reviewed awards ICES is successfully developing its core funding to expand its activities.

Reshaping University Avenue

The largest concentration of health care resources in Canada is on University Avenue in downtown Toronto. Major hospitals, such as the Hospital for Sick Children, Mt. Sinai Hospital, The Toronto Hospital and the new Princess Margaret Hospital stand cheek by jowl on the broad avenue leading from the business district to Queen's Park. Long known for health care excellence, University Avenue and the University of Toronto are changing with the times, placing greater emphasis on research.

Dr. Louis Siminovitch is the gentle but determined giant of health research on University Avenue. As the Geneticist in Chief at the Research Centre at the Hospital for Sick Children and, more recently, as Director of the Samuel Lunenfeld Research Institute at Mt. Sinai Hospital Research, Dr. Lou has been a leader, mentor and instigator of health research.

The strengthening between researchers and patients and researchers and funders are among Dr. Siminovitch's innovative contributions. At the Hospital for Sick Children, he stressed the need for researchers to meet patients and to be motivated by real medical problems, not just theory.

Dr. Tak Mak is proof that research dollars are drawn to talent. Amgen, a major U.S. biotechnology company has invested $10 million per year for ten years, a total of $100 million, in Dr. Mak's team at the Ontario Cancer Institute/Princess Margaret Hospital. With world leadership in research on the immune system, Dr. Mak is another Canadian bright light. He has received the largest investment in Canadian research ever made by a biopharmaceutical company. The Amgen Institute, dedicated to study of the immune system, will be located immediately adjacent to the new Princess Margaret Hospital on University Avenue.

The work of Dr. Siminovitch, Dr. Mak and hundreds of others is reshaping the activities on University Avenue. With luck and determination, this one street alone will continue to transform itself into a research collaboration with dynamism.

Redirecting the Medical Research Council of Canada

Improving management of health services in Canada will require a greater investment in health services research. This necessity has recently been recognized by the Medical Research Council of Canada (MRC) our major national medical research institution in its new strategic plan. Research councils in many countries including the United Kingdom, Australia and South Africa have already recognized the need to balance their overall health research agenda. Historic emphasis on biomedical research is being equalized by investments in health services research.

In 1992, the MRC and its sixty-five staff distributed some $250 million. This supports a network of 2,200 researchers, 1,500 research trainees and 4,000 technical staff. Yet total MRC spending across Canada is about the same annual amount as the budget of one large, urban teaching hospital. MRC spends less than 0.4% of our total Canadian health budget. This is too little for the challenges ahead.

Over the past two years, the Medical Research Council, undertook a sweeping reappraisal of its role. Broad consultation and development of a new strategic plan assisted the MRC in planning its future.

Three areas emerged from the planning exercise for new attention and focus by MRC:
- a broadened vision encompassing all areas of health research
- building greater excellence in existing activities
- evaluating more thoroughly the outcomes of MRC activities

Implementing this new and expanded vision will be a phenomenal challenge for the MRC. The organization will need to reach beyond its roots in the biomedical research community and embrace a broad spectrum of health research, including disciplines such as economics, political science and sociology. With a more comprehensive approach, the MRC can assist in healing Medicare by enhancing quality and affordability in health service delivery. It must not, however, abandon the essential core of biomedical research for which it will remain the key funder.

QED

Canada is a wonderful place in which to undertake research. We have a solid base of scientific talent, an excellent data base for population health studies and a diverse multicultural population. We need to expand our health research sector.

Others have forcefully stated the reasons for investing in research, include jobs and knowledge benefits. These views understate the full rationale. Consider the sentiments expressed by Professor Doolittle of Dalhousie University: "A good theory about the nature of the physical or biological world is as valuable a product of our culture as a ballet or painting. It should not, any more than art, have to justify itself only in terms of new products and job creation."[7] The stress should be on the "only." Research has many virtues and values.

Surely we want it all, within the limits of our resources. We want to dream and have our curiosity supported for its own merit. We want our ideas to translate into jobs and real progress for our fellow Canadians and, more importantly, for our fellow human beings. Balance can be struck between competing research demands. We must also find clever, creative and entertaining ways to secure necessary resources, to dramatically expand the research enterprise in Canada. National leadership from the Medical Research Council of Canada and others is paramount. So, too, is grassroots energy in the spirit of the St. Boniface Research Foundation.

Good Stuff to Read

The Next Canadian Economy by Kristin Shannon and Dian Cohen. Although nearly ten years old, it is still very relevant. It captured the main themes of the new economy early and with insight.

Shifting Gears: Thriving in the New Economy, by Nuala Beck, Harper Collins, 1992. A provocative and insightful look at the new

---

7   Professor Doolittle, *Globe and Mail*, December 15, 1993, p. 21.

economy. The strong focus on how to measure the new economy is refreshing with a key analysis of knowledge workers.

Healthy & Wealthy — A Growth Prescription for Ontario's Health Industries. The Report of the Health Industries Advisory Committee to the Ontario Minister of Health, March, 1994. Queen's Printer for Ontario, IBSN 0-7778-2558-9. This is the report of the Committee chaired by Bill Blundell. The report notes Canada's major trade deficit in health care products and proposes a strategy to create jobs, industry and exports in the health industries sector.

Investing in Canada's Health, A Strategic Plan for the Medical Research Council of Canada, Minister of Supply and Services, Ottawa. Available from the Medical Research Council of Canada, Holland Cross, Tower B, 5th Floor, 1600 Scott Street, Ottawa, Ontario, K1A OW9.

Annual Reports of the following Canadian health research organizations as well as their publication lists are well worth obtaining:
- Mt. Sinai (Samuel Lunenfeld Research Institute)
- St. Boniface Research Institute
- Hospital for Sick Children
- Medical Research Council of Canada
- Centre for Health Economic Policy Analysis (CHEPA). Although older than many of the other health policy centres, CHEPA has the wisdom and maturity of its rich history of contributing to better thinking about health policy. Located at McMaster University it retains the pioneering spirit of the McMaster Medical School.

Towards the Next Canadian Health Care System

> Learning disabilities are tragic in children, but they are fatal in organizations. Because of them, few corporations live even half as long as a person — most die before they reach the age of forty.[1]

Canadian Medicare is twenty-five years old. Will it see a fortieth birthday? Will it celebrate it in good health? Can we heal and nurture Medicare to a full and continuing vigour?

What lies ahead is a tremendous amount of difficult but crucial work in reforming Canadian health care delivery. The stakes are high, not only for Canadians, but for nations looking to Canada as a model and a guide.

A marriage of technology to the challenges of re-engineering is one clear trend. Affordability and quality are being added as the sixth and seventh principles of the Canada Health Act, in practice, if not in law. All our new ways of making choices are the result of provincial governments seeking simultaneously to improve the quality of the health care delivery system and its affordability. As well, governments are also adopting a population health, or determinants of health, perspective.

We are in the early days of Canadian health care reform. Most of the improvements, excluding Quebec, have only been underway for months or a few years, not decades. The real results will be seen through the 1990s, as Canadian governments and other stakeholders in the health care system grapple with the problems. Some early evidence is encouraging. Expenditure growth rates within the health care delivery system have shrunk dramatically from levels of 10% per annum or more through the 1970s and 1980s, to levels in the minus 3% per annum in the early 1990s. There has been no significant proof of adverse health outcomes. Nor is there evidence of

1   Senge, op. cit., p. 17.

adverse outcomes for individual political leaders and elected governments. There is an increasing sophistication in the Canadian
media with emphasis shifting from stories of financial crisis and
waiting lists, to management of the health care delivery system.
There is a profound sense of innovation at the level of individual
hospitals as they introduce utilization measurement and better information systems.

The introduction of user fees in Canada has been debated. Most
Canadians believe that an accessible health care system is one of the
most consequential achievements of the Canadian nation. Most
individuals involved in health care in Canada — managers, providers
or consumers — have confidence that with a managed re-engineering
of the delivery system and greater emphasis on the determinants of
health, Canadian health care is sustainable and affordable. Quality
improvement is a reasonable expectation. A significant minority of
Canadian physicians, and some others however, view Canadian
Medicare as financially unsustainable. They favour movement to a
two-tiered system with patient co-payments, premiums or user fees.
By the late 1990s, it should be evident whether health reform has
achieved preservation of the principles of Medicare within a restructured delivery system or whether a fundamental privatization of the
system is underway.

My conclusion is that reform is underway but must be accelerated in some parts of the country. Transforming so many aspects of
the delivery system is a huge challenge but — on the evidence to
date — we are equal to that challenge. More leadership is needed
from within health provider groups. Resistance to change is counter-
productive. It needs to be replaced by constructive advocacy for
reform which improve *both* quality and affordability.

Policies and initiatives of various Canadian provinces illustrate
the evolution of differing choice options. Saskatchewan and New
Brunswick provide evidence of the consequences of a devolution
approach. Ontario will prove an interesting area for examining
innovative negotiated outcomes with providers, as well as clinical
epidemiology research efforts. We'll look to Manitoba for both
interventionist public policy and health policy research approaches.

What will the next Canadian health care system look like? How
will it operate? Here are a few thoughts about and hopes for the
Canadian health care system in the year 2000:
- Canada's over 900 hospitals have been consolidated into about
  200 large health systems. In several provinces, these systems

are regionally-based, with an integration of health and social services at the district level. In several other provinces, health systems focus on acute care and have been brought about by merging and networking around key hospitals.

- At each academic health science centre, specific population health agreements are in place between the local health system, the academic university-linked teaching unit, and various local health delivery authorities.
- The role of ministries of health is to set a broad policy framework based on population health, with the responsibility of funding the health systems. Most funding flows on a per capita basis adjusted for local health needs. Dollars flow to real health concerns, not to the pattern of history and politics.
- From a consumer standpoint, the system is dramatically altered. All Canadian citizens now carry health cards with smart card technology. Embedded in each card is a small chip with each person's personal identification number, their entire health history, the health histories of their immediate families, parents, grandparents (where available), record of immunizations, and record of all encounters with health systems and health providers. Individuals are able to read their health records on their television screens in their homes. All providers are able to review card records at the point of service. All consumers have access by telephone, interactive television and computer networks to health advice and information.
- Health providers work in teams. Health-system based teams are either physician-led or nurse-led. The nurse-led teams operate independently of physician's direction, but often have a consulting physician. Physician-led teams are comprised of a range of health professionals. Very few conditions require a lengthy hospital stay.
- Many births take place either in out-of-hospital free standing birthing centres or in-hospital birthing centres. Home births have regained some importance. Infant mortality has been significantly reduced through the decade.
- The previous public health system has evolved into healthy community action units. These units are accountable to both local and provincial governments, and are intensively involved in community education programmes for the education system, particularly through interactive cable television programming.

- Research infrastructure in Canada, for health services research and biomedical research has been strengthened and expanded. More than $1 billion per year has been redirected from inappropriate care to research.
- Canadian health consultants are active in a number of countries designing and installing health systems — the Canadian way! Notable involvements are in Eastern Europe, China, India and parts of the emerging African continent.
- Canadian health products and services have gained a world-wide reputation for their quality and affordability.

Our ability to re-engineer care, learn new skills and take control of our own health and health care will all be critical determinants of success. We must balance our efforts to better manage the supply of health services against new challenges. We must also invest in the wider facets of health. Necessary change will not happen by itself. We must make it happen.

Will we succeed? Are we going to take the pains to struggle for the reform of Medicare, its evolution and future success? I believe so. Canadians care deeply about health and health care. Medicare is a vital barometer of our capacity as a nation. To abandon the struggle would be to abandon our values. We will succeed.

The early evidence suggests we are on the path to healthy reform. Through their leadership, their work and their compassion, tens of thousands of Canadians involved in health and health care will determine the future. Our experience with reform is rich with lessons. We are living and making our own history. Our efforts will show us the sane road forward. We shall succeed.

Afterword & Acknowledgements

On a very personal note this book has been a transition from my public sector management role as Deputy Minister of Health for Ontario to new adventures as a writer, teacher, consultant, private sector manager and continuing advocate of progressive change. It has been a joyful and painful struggle to assemble thoughts in a fashion which endeavours to assist the continuing task of managing health system change with technology and compassion.

Our struggle for Canadian Medicare will not end with any measurable victory. We will pass the torch and the obligation to continue the struggle to our children and they to theirs. We are accountable to them and to our consciences for the quality and sustainability of what we leave as a health care legacy.

There is a significant but immeasurable risk that I will write further on the subject of health and health care. The ideas and possibilities continue to haunt me. For every health policy issue addressed there were a dozen important issues left unexplored. For every good story there are a hundred stories omitted.

My obligations are significant. While not a large work, *Healing Medicare* had many helpers. My deep gratitude to all those extremely busy friends and colleagues who took time to encourage, comment, edit and critique. Thank you.

My six months as Senior Research Scholar at the Centre for Bioethics, University of Toronto, provided the window of opportunity to write. University President Rob Prichard, Dr. Fred Lowy, Director of the Centre, Professor Peggy Leatt, Head, Department of Health Administration and Dr. Carol Nash were all responsible for this sanctuary. The Centre is a remarkable coming together of disciplines and people. I wish all of them well. Dr. Peter Singer and Dr. Eric Meslin were both influential during my all too brief sojourn.

Early inspiration to write on matters of health policy and management came from Dr. Robert Maxwell of King Edward's Hospital Fund in London, England. My inclusion as a Fellow of the King's Fund International Seminar brought me in contact with leaders in health care from the United Kingdom, the United States, Australia and New Zealand as well as Canada.

Three ministers of health with whom I have worked were powerful influences on my understanding of the art of the possible in health politics. Larry Desjardins, Frances Lankin and Ruth Grier were all excellent teachers. Several deputy ministers of health have provided inspiration to me in my career. K.O. Mackenzie and Reg Edwards in Manitoba, Tom Campbell, Graham Scott and Martin Barkin in Ontario have my respect and gratitude for their wise counsel.

Six colleagues were brave enough to read the early manuscript and provide comments. The efforts of Brad Graham, Dr. Eugene Le Blanc, Dr. David Naylor, Marilyn Knox, Lisa Priest and L.A. (Tony) Quaglia were insightful and critically important.

The journey from raw ideas to a published book was only possible with the unrelenting confidence and support of my publisher and editor, Ann Decter. The manuscript also benefited significantly from the work of Angela Hryniuk as copy editor. Gwen North, as she has for many years, aided and abetted the translation into print.

My family, Lucille, Riel and Geneviève bore the brunt of absences and frustrations. They were patient and supportive throughout.

No endeavour is as humbling as the creation of a book. All of its flaws and shortcoming are my own. Where it occasionally rises to the challenge presented by its subject, the credit must accrue to my many mentors and teachers.

Index

A
ability-to-benefit 19, 24
ability-to-pay 19
academic health science centres 133
Access Health 57
Access Health Marketing Inc. 240
Act Respecting Health Services and Social Services, An 175
ADI 239
AIDS 185, 188, 189, 190
Alberta Roundtable on Health 174
Allelix Biopharmaceuticals Inc 225, 239
ambulatory surgery facilities 51
Amgen Institute 248
Andronic Devices Ltd. 240
Apotex 235, 236, 237
applied clinical epidemiology 25
Arthur Anderson & Co. 51
Ask-A-Nurse 57
Atkinson, Dr. John 48, 56
Australia 248
AUTOLAB 223, 224
AutoMed Associates 240
autonomy 137
Axworthy, Lloyd 228

B
Barkin, Dr. Martin 224
"bed" management 51
Bell-Wade Report 48
benchmarking 25, 52
benign prostatic hyperplasia 157
best practices 51
BioCapital Biotechnology Investment Fund 239, 241
blood pressure 157
Blundell, Bill 47, 230
BPH 157
breast cancer 157

C
CAE 225
Calgary 48
California Blue Cross 212
Canadian Consumers' Association 171
Canadian exports 235
Canadian Institute for Advanced Research 238
Canadian International Development Agency 225
Canadian Steel Trade and Employment Congress 120
Canadian Union of Public Employees 120
Caritas Group 56
Castonguay, Claude 26
Champy, James 31
chemotherapy 157
CHEPA decision board 155
Chief Medical Officer in Ontario 174
clinical effectiveness 39
clinical epidemiology 25

clinical guidelines 25, 173
Clinton, President 19
CLSC 57
CME 225, 239
co-generation 61
Coalition to Keep Medicare Healthy 166
Cohen, Sam 246
Columbia Health Group Inc. 240
common cold 192
Competitive Advantage of Nations 229
Comprehensive Health System Planning Commission 176
Conference of Deputy Ministers of Health 63
Connaught 193, 223, 224, 225
consumer involvement 170
Continuous Quality Improvement (CQI) 170

D
DALY 192
Dan, Leslie 237
Dartmouth Medical School 179
Desjardins, Larry 245
Dhalla, Dr. Naranjan 246
Diagnostic Chemicals Ltd 225
diagnostic testing 51
diphtheria 192
disability-adjusted life years (DALY) 192
District Health Councils 34
Disys Corporation 241
Douglas, Tommy 13, 26

E
Economic Regional Development Agreement 228
EFOS 225
emergency services 56
energy conservation 61, 182
energy management 61
environment 25
Epp, Jake 228
Ernst & Young 63
Ethical Pharmaceuticals Ltd. (U.K.) 239
Ethical Pharmaceuticals North America Inc. 239
Expanded Programme in Immunization (EPI) 192
extramural hospital 32

F
Federal Drug Administration 186
Federation of Canadian Municipalities 227
fee-for-service 131
First Nations 194
foreign-trained physicians 132
Framework Agreement 169
Frost, Merck 223
Fulton, Jane 109

Index **257**

MICHAEL B. DECTER

Michael Decter is a health care manager, consultant and now author. He served most recently as Deputy Minister of Health for the Province of Ontario. Previously, he served as Cabinet Secretary and Clerk of the Executive Council in Manitoba. Private sector positions have included Partner, Peat Marwick Consulting Group; Chair, Shawinigan Energy; and President, Vista Strategic Information Management. Mr. Decter received his training in economics at Harvard University. He has also been Senior Research Scholar at the Centre for Bioethics, University of Toronto. He is also active in consulting with clients in Canada, the United Kingdom and the United States and is Director-Canada for APM Inc., North America's leading health care consulting firm. He lives in the Beach area of Toronto with his wife Lucille and children Geneviève and Riel.

Public Religion and Urban Transformation

RELIGION, RACE, AND ETHNICITY
General Editor: Peter J. Paris

Public Religion and Urban Transformation:
Faith in the City
Edited by Lowell W. Livezey

Public Religion and Urban Transformation

Faith in the City

EDITED BY

Lowell W. Livezey

New York University Press

NEW YORK AND LONDON

NEW YORK UNIVERSITY PRESS
New York and London

Library of Congress Cataloging-in-Publication Data
Public religion and urban transformation : faith in the city / edited by
Lowell W. Livezey.
p. cm. — (Religion, race, and ethnicity)
Includes bibliographical references and index.
ISBN 0-8147-5157-1 (alk. paper) —
ISBN 0-8147-5158-X (pbk. : alk. paper)
1. Chicago (Ill.)—Religion.   I. Livezey, Lowell. II. Series.
BL2527.C48 P83 2000
200'.9773'11—dc21   99-050622

Manufactured in the United States of America

10 9 8 7 6 5 4 3 2 1

Contents

Illustrations

Maps

Photographs

Tables

Preface and Acknowledgments

The Religion in Urban America Program at the University of Illinois at Chicago has been from the beginning a collective, collegial undertaking. The authors of this book were all members of the staff during the program's first three years, 1992–1995, when we conducted most of the field research, and each author studied the congregations, organizations, and neighborhoods he or she writes about here. Several researchers participated at each site, however, because we wanted to observe our subjects "through each other's eyes," aware that we had different capacities for perception and distortion. We tried, wherever possible, to include a relative insider (for example, a Muslim observing a mosque) and an outsider (a Euro-American Catholic observing a black Protestant church). In forming the group to work at each site, we also considered the academic discipline, language skills, gender, age, and temperament of each researcher. As a result, we all have used field research conducted by other authors.

We also wish to acknowledge the contributions of research associates and assistants who are not authors of this volume but whose field research provided data and whose ideas enriched the discourse that we have drawn on for our chapters. Research associates included Julie Kaufman, Lois Gehr Livezey, Anthony Mansueto, Larry G. Murphy, William Peterman, Uma Sharma, and Ariel Zamarripa. Research assistants included Susana Angélica Bañuelos, Danit Ben Ari, Joy Bostic, Shalanda Dexter, Karen Ephraim, Jennifer Feenstra, Jeannie Lukacek, Damien McAnany, Evelyn Parker, April Payton, Reece Pendleton, Mari Philipsborn, Iraida Rodriguez, Sabri Samirah, and Authens Smith. In addition, the whole project depended heavily on the intelligent and cheerful support of undergraduate office assistants including Alex Gervacio (who made the computers work for us), Stephanie Prazak (who managed the bibliographic database and much more), Jennifer Chang, Monique Malek, Tricia Mazzone, Cynthia Suarez, and Julianna Whiteman.

Nearly everyone in the Religion in Urban America Program contributed to the research for multiple chapters and to the rich discourse that has been sustained over several years by the research team. Accordingly, as chapter authors, we acknowledge our deep sense of gratitude to one another and to the rest of the team. With rare exceptions, we do not identify each member of the team who contributed to a particular chapter, in order to avoid repetition and to emphasize the overriding importance of every person's contribution to the whole.

Academic colleagues and religious and civic leaders have been generous with advice. To launch the advisory process, we convened a meeting in October 1992 with Michael Conzen, Theo Feliciano, Sr. Mary Hennessey, Philip Nyden, Wardell Payne, George W. Pickering, Calvin Pressley, Yolanda Rios Rangel, Rabbi Herman Schaalman, Eldin Villafañe, R. Stephen Warner, and Julian Wolpert. Many of these, and others including Msgr. John Egan; Robert Franklin; Rev. Joseph Hacala, S.J.; Nancy Ammerman; and Carl Dudley, advised us intermittently throughout the project. R. Stephen Warner thoroughly reviewed our work and counseled with us insightfully at a midpoint retreat.

We also benefited greatly from comments on papers we presented between 1993 and 1997 at meetings of the American Academy of Religion, the Association for the Sociology of Religion, the Religious Research Association, the Social Ethics Seminar, and the Chicago Area Group for the Study of Religious Communities. Discussants at these meetings included (in chronological order) Msgr. Philip J. Murnion, Mark Chavez, Rima Schultz, Alan B. Anderson, Rhys H. Williams, Helen Rose Ebaugh, Preston N. Williams, Anthony Orum, Dennis McCann, Donald E. Miller, and Nancy L. Eiesland. Their public comments and continued dialogue with us have contributed substantially to this book.

Undoubtedly, the most generous and resourceful contributors to the research underlying these chapters are the congregations and other organizations, their members and leaders, their clergy and laity, who talked with us and allowed us to observe and participate in their religious activities. These people and organizations are the sources of our primary data, and we are most grateful for their considerable time and effort. Moreover, we recognize that they included us in some of their most intimate moments and entrusted us with information about themselves that could easily be misused. To protect their privacy and the confidentiality of our conversations with them, in the chapters that follow we use pseudonyms (except for clergy and chief executives of organizations, whose identity is evident from the organization itself). We know full well, however, that their trust will have been justified only by the accuracy of our description and by our insightful, appreciative use of the information they so generously shared.

We attempted to make the field research as interactive as possible, inviting our subjects to review and correct our work in progress. We are grateful for the responses of clergy and lay leaders (listed in the appendix) to interim reports and preliminary analyses of their organizations. When the field research was nearly complete in 1995, we held a conference, "Religion and Community in a Restructuring Metropolis," with workshops designed to provide for dialogue among the people of the neighborhoods and religious organizations we had studied, scholars and religious leaders, and ourselves. We wish to acknowledge all who attended, and particularly the community people and academics who spoke formally at that conference: Edwin David Aponte; Assad Basool; Warren Copeland; Larry Greenfield; Eileen Heineman; Rev. Juan J. Huitrado, M.C.C.J.; Joseph Levin; Dominic Pacyga; George W. Pickering; Ellen Skerrett; Rev. Michael J. Slattery, O.S.A.; Robert H. Stockman; and Rev. Eugene Winkler. We are also grateful to Professors Jay P. Dolan, Diana Eck, Albert Hunter, Peter J. Paris, and R. Stephen Warner for their concluding comments.

The dialogue continued during 1996 and 1997 at five "Neighborhood Forums on Religion in Chicago." Speakers and participants in these forums discussed our research with one another and with us, making a unique contribution to the thinking presented in the chapters that follow. We wish to thank Jay Caponigro, Rev. Jeffery Haynes, and Victoria Verala for participation in the "Chicago's Southwest Side" forum; Sr. Dominga Zapata, S.H., Rev. Julio Loza, and Raul Raymundo for participation in the "Pilsen's Challenge to Its Churches" forum; Rabbi Philip Lefkowitz, Robert W. Matanky, Rabbi Michael M. Remson, and Rabbi Herman Schaalman for participation in the "Jewish North Side" forum; Rev. Erwin Lutzer, Rev. Eugene Winkler, and Rev. Robert McLaughlin for participation in the "Church at the Heart of the City" forum; and Kale Williams, Imam Ahmed Rufai, Rabbi Henry Balzer, and Cathy Vates for participation in the Rogers Park forum, which was cosponsored with Loyola University.

Maps produced by UIC cartographer Raymond Brod for our 1996 research report, *Religious Organizations and Structural Change in Metropolitan Chicago,* served as a point of departure for the maps provided here. It was, however, Professor Mark Bouman and cartographer Brian Twardosz, who accepted the challenge of creating maps that would undergird the arguments and amplify the themes that appear in the text. We are also grateful to the clergy, staff, and laypeople of the congregations who provided a wide selection of photographs.

Both of our institutional sponsors, the University of Illinois at Chicago and the Lilly Endowment, have fostered the collegial character of the Religion in Urban America Program. The University of Illinois at Chicago is an excellent venue, not only because we fit the research agenda of an urban land-grant university but particularly because we have the good fortune to be situated in the Office of Social Science Research (OSSR). OSSR's director, Professor John Gardiner, is an exemplary colleague who deftly provided the optimal mix of breathing room, intellectual challenge, and support, while ensuring the proper administration of our grants and a congenial work environment. Iris Tillman, the secretary/administrator, and a series of research coordinators have cheerfully and efficiently provided logistical support. We have also benefited from interacting with other projects based at OSSR, including R. Stephen Warner's New Ethnic and Immigrant Congregations Project, Dick Simpson's research on Chicago city government, Marcia Farr's field studies of literacy among Mexican immigrants, and the Historical Encyclopedia of Chicago Women Project.

We are deeply grateful for three generous grants from the Lilly Endowment and a supplemental grant from the Lilly-funded Louisville Institute that made our work possible. But the sense of partnership with Lilly goes well beyond our funding. The initial idea for this program derived from discussions around Lilly's long-standing commitment to urban ministry and to grounding urban ministry in the best possible analysis of its urban and ecclesiastical contexts. The decision to pursue a research agenda much broader, and thus more expensive, than urban ministry alone—investigating the work of all the major religions and a wide range of religious activities—resulted from extensive discussions with Craig Dykstra, Lilly's vice president for religion, and program directors James Hudnut-Beumler, Jacqui Burton, and James P. Wind. They all, as well as a later program director, Edward Queen III, and Louisville Institute director James W. Lewis, have continued to be insightful commentators and critics. In addition, Lilly and the Louisville Institute have convened consultations with related research projects in other cities, including the Religion and Civic Order Project at University of Southern California, the Religion and Urban Culture Project at Indiana University–Purdue University at Indianapolis, and the Center for Social and Religious Research at Hartford Seminary. Thus they have fostered at the national level the collegiality we have tried to practice locally.

As editor of this volume, and as director of the program, I am deeply grateful to the other authors of this book and am even more indebted than they to our colleagues in the Religion and Urban America Program and to the many scholars and practitioners who have assisted us. I pay special tribute to three persons for their exceptional collaboration and support. William A. Simpson has followed our work closely, consistently, and thoughtfully from its conception, and his highly original thinking was ever evident in his critique of our work. Elfriede Wedam effectively combined the roles of research associate and program coordinator, rising naturally to become my partner in the leadership and serving as associate director. I shall be eternally grateful for her willingness to share overall responsibility for the program and for her intelligence, mature judgment, and grace. Finally, among the many blessings of being Lois Gehr Livezey's husband are her loyalty and her wise counsel. Both have been abundant, not only in her choosing to devote her sabbatical to participation as a theologian in the research team but in her discerning after-hours discussion of the intellectual and organizational concerns of the program. Bill, Elfriede, and Lois exemplify the larger pattern of collegiality and commitment to the whole that we were so fortunate to have in the Religion in Urban America Program, and for which I am grateful to the entire team.

Lowell W. Livezey, Director
Religion in Urban America Program

Introduction

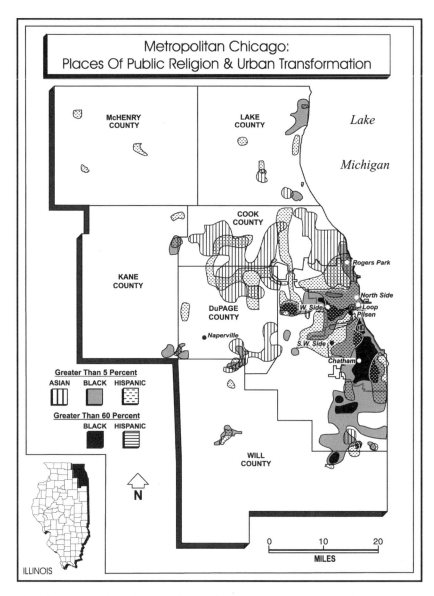

Metropolitan Chicago:
Places Of Public Religion & Urban Transformation

McHENRY
COUNTY

LAKE
COUNTY

Lake

Michigan

COOK
COUNTY

Rogers Park

KANE
COUNTY

North Side

W. Side   Loop

Pilsen

DuPAGE
COUNTY

• Naperville

S.W. Side

Chatham

Greater Than 5 Percent

ASIAN   BLACK   HISPANIC

Greater Than 60 Percent

BLACK   HISPANIC

WILL
COUNTY

N

ILLINOIS

0   10   20

MILES

The places named on this map locate the congregations discussed in chapters 2 through 9, while chapters 10 and 11 encompass much of the region. The population distribution shows that racial and ethnic diversity are important considerations for these congregations. Map by Brian Twardosz, BMT Printing and Cartographic Specialists.

The New Context of Urban Religion

Lowell W. Livezey

"Viva Mexico!" calls the youthful nun, standing in full habit at the front of the large Gothic Catholic church. "Viva Mexico! Viva Mexico!" respond a thousand voices from the crowded pews and aisles. The evening is in early December 1993, and like thousands of others in this large Midwestern American city, these Mexican families have gathered in Catholic churches to serenade La Virgen de Guadalupe, the Mother of Jesus who appeared to the peasant Juan Diego and thus to the indigenous poor of Mexico.

Thousands of red roses adorn the Virgin in a brightly lit shrine that is easily seen from anywhere in the nave. People of all ages kneel in prayer and present her with more roses, which they have purchased from young boys outside the church. The worshipers then move to the already crowded pews and join in singing love songs to the Virgin and in shouting patriotic slogans.

Only a few blocks away and a month later, a committee gathers in a Protestant church located between the city's wealthiest neighborhood and a public housing project, home to the "ghetto underclass." The committee represents the churches of the wealthy neighborhood. Laypeople and clergy, mostly white Protestants, are listening to one of their members explain the intricacies of a city policy that will gradually dismantle the adjacent public housing project, which has become notorious for its level of violence and gang warfare. What concerns the committee is the fate of the families now living in the project. The committee members have expertise and "good connections," but they don't fully agree about what to do; so they authorize some research and decide to meet again soon.

Every Sunday morning, about twenty-five African American children gather in a multipurpose room at another of the city's public housing projects. Sports equipment has been moved to the corners, and a few adults from the nearby Baptist church are putting up posters with Bible verses and pictures of black biblical characters. The adults begin singing children's choruses; the children join in. One of the church's many ministers, an African American woman, then asks for quiet and, ignoring the continuing low-level chatter, offers a passionate prayer, greets the children effusively, and directs them to adjacent rooms according to their age.

The prosperous black Baptist church also conducts Sunday school in its well-appointed educational plant, but, the ministers say, the children from the housing projects will not come to Sunday school at the church (only two blocks away). So the church takes the Sunday school to the projects.

On a Saturday morning in spring 1994, in a neighborhood sometimes called the bastion of the black middle class but now threatened by the loss of nearby employers, the Christian Men's Fellowship is cooking breakfast. Eggs and sausage, biscuits and gravy, and grits. The breakfast is for the Save Our Sons program—boys mostly from the neighborhood but not from the families of the church. The men have long been involved in the church with their wives and children, nieces, nephews, and cousins. But recently they have been hearing a new message about what it means to be a Christian man. As people of African heritage, they have been told from the pulpit, men must be fathers to all the boys of the neighborhood. The church is family to all the children and young people. So even if these men and their families have moved to other parts of the city and suburbs (following the jobs), they return to mentor the new generation of neighborhood kids. After breakfast, the boys and men will study the Bible together, recite African proverbs (in Swahili or Zulu), and go on an outing to a forest preserve or a theme park.

That same Saturday morning, in still another part of the city, the Khutbah Committee of a large mosque is meeting. The mosque, a converted theater that accommodates fifteen hundred for prayers, is alive with the voices of more than three hundred children attending Islamic school and the smell of curries being prepared for a wedding feast. The committee meets in the corner of a large room that also serves as a thoroughfare among other activities. The dozen members are all men and relatively young. Except for one African American, they are immigrants—mainly from Jordan, India, and Pakistan. There is also an Egyptian and a Nigerian. The committee chairman, Muhammad Said, is the Egyptian. His fluency in Arabic is an important qualification for the committee, which selects an Arabic-speaking *khatib* to give the *khutba* (sermon) at the *jum'ah* prayer each Friday. In this mosque, a measure of theological, political, and ethnic diversity is maintained by rotating the honor of speaking each week. This in turn gives the committee a great deal of prestige. At this meeting, the man who had been designated the *khatib* for the next Friday was called to Palestine on business for his engineering firm, and a substitute was needed. Some members objected to the fact that all the candidates were Indo-Pakistani, which, they said, had been the nationality of all the recent *khatibs.*

It is Tuesday, a few minutes after 7 A.M., and as on most weekday mornings, the rabbi is reading psalms to several other men seated in chairs on one side of the modern synagogue. Each man wears the *kippah* (skullcap), the *tallith* (prayer shawl), and the *tefillin* (the small leather box containing bits of Torah scroll that is lashed to the forehead by strips of leather). They have gathered for morning prayers, but the order of service cannot begin until a *minyan* (a minimum of ten men) is present. Two more men arrive, carefully remove the *tallith* and *tefillin* from their pouch, and put them on. Then another enters, and after a few minutes—and several more psalms interspersed with greetings—the tenth.

Most of the men know the place in the prayer book and turn to it comfortably as the rabbi indicates the page. They chant the prayers, psalms, and scriptures with ease and confidence acquired over decades of repetition. But they do not chant completely in unison, for each voices a cantillation learned in his country of origin—Turkey, Morocco, Spain, Israel, Armenia. After prayers, the men's breakfast includes baked eggs as well as lox and bagels.

Middle-class blacks appropriating African folk culture on the South Side, Indo-Pakistani immigrants planning their mosque's prayer service on the Northwest Side, Moroccan cantillations in a North Side synagogue . . . these are only glimpses of what the authors of this book have seen and heard since beginning research with the Religion in Urban America Program in 1992.[1] But they also point beyond specific people and congregations in this particular city to the larger reality of religion interacting with changing urban environments.

Studying Urban Religion in the Late Twentieth Century

Since World War II, change in American cities has been so fundamental as to be termed "urban restructuring." During the same period, organized religion has been undergoing a widespread, pervasive change that is now commonly called, following the title of Robert Wuthnow's important book, the restructuring of American religion.[2] Both structural changes are further linked to the social transformation of the 1960s and 1970s, which extended the presumption of individual autonomy and the moral legitimacy of personal choice at the expense of traditional collective authorities, including religion.

By studying more than seventy-five congregations in eight quite different neighborhoods of Chicago, Illinois, we have witnessed a complex interaction among religion, urban structure, and social change during this extraordinary episode in the history of urban America. Congregations are adapting to profound changes in context, but our interest goes beyond their strategies of survival and adaptation to consider how and to what extent they may reflect, resist, or influence the change itself.

In the 1920s, Chicago became the research site for the early members of the Chicago School of urban sociology,[3] and it has been fertile ground for urban and religious scholars ever since. In making research in this city the basis for this book, we do not claim that Chicago is typical of American cities. It is larger and more diverse than most, and unlike cities that have come of age more recently, it was structured decisively by the requirements of the industrial economy of the late nineteenth century. But it does represent many of the dimensions of late-twentieth-century urban life with which religious organizations are learning to interact. The congregations and neighborhoods we studied include people who are wealthy, middle-class, working poor, and urban underclass. They include white, black, Hispanic, Asian, African, and Middle Eastern people. They include recent immigrants and descendants of the immigrants of many generations ago. They include adherents to most of the world's religions. And they include congregations that have been organized—some recently and some generations ago—to meet the religious needs and give expression to the religious beliefs and practices of these diverse populations. Despite its differences from other cities, Chicago exemplifies the three processes of urban restructuring, religious restructuring, and social transformation with which religious organizations must interact if they are to participate effectively in urban life today.

Urban Restructuring and the Erosion of Neighborhood Ties

As an industrial city, Chicago has undergone a pattern of city-building—the phases of entrepreneurship, growth, consolidation, and decline—that is quite common in the United States, much like the building of Milwaukee, Detroit, Cleveland, and other cities that grew with the shift from a predominantly agrarian to predominantly industrial American economy.[4] And Chicago's attempt to become a successful postindustrial city, to make a transition comparable to those of Minneapolis–St. Paul and Pittsburgh, is well underway. But Chicago also exemplifies many of the challenges associated with postindustrial growth—economic polarization, spatial dislocations, and the lack of public authority at the metropolitan level to match the metropolitan reach of the economy.[5]

The congregations discussed in this book are coping with these challenges. In chapter 3, Matthew Price explores the efforts of "Gold Coast" churches to deal with problems of the notorious Cabrini Green public housing projects nearby, which were addressed at the meeting on public housing described earlier. These churches must negotiate the economic polarization between their Gold Coast neighborhood, whose people prosper with jobs in the technical and financial sectors, and Cabrini Green, whose residents do not qualify for the new jobs and are increasingly marginalized economically and victimized by violence. Similarly, the black middle-class churches discussed in David Daniels's chapter 7 recall our earlier account of male leadership responding to a situation brought on by the exodus of heavy industry, which until recently had undergirded the neighborhood's prosperity and cohesion. Many of these churches' members now live in the suburbs, where employment is more readily available. But as Daniels shows, their return to their churches not only to worship but to care for the at-risk youth is fostered by theological innovation that transcends class boundaries.

Similarly, the Baptist Sunday school we visited is in the Henry Horner public housing project on Chicago's West Side, home of what William Julius Wilson[6] has termed the "ghetto underclass," a population whose skills matched the requirements of manufacturing jobs of the previous era but do not meet the technical qualifications of the present. In chapter 4, Lowell Livezey and Isaac Laudarji explore how churches are responding to the resulting social isolation. In contrast, the Mexican Americans of Pilsen whom we saw serenading the Virgin of Guadalupe are mostly "working poor" immigrants and transmigrants, who fill the poorly paid manufacturing and service jobs that have remained in the city. In chapter 2, Janise Hurtig examines the role of churches in the "ethnicization" of these working-poor newcomers.

Other congregations throughout the city are made up of people who are financially successful but always on the move—commuting to work, taking the kids across the city to school, driving to shopping malls. The "edge-city" congregations reviewed in Paul Numrich's chapter 8 perhaps best illustrate this reality, but the recent Muslim, Hindu, and Sikh immigrants (see Numrich's chapter 10) too are highly mobile and widely distributed. Thus the local ties of the more prosperous congregations of all faiths are weakened by the centrifugal forces of people on constant reassignment and the speed of capital allocation. These cause members to spend little time in their own neighborhoods and to have few occasions to work with neighbors on problems and projects of common concern.

How did the city's deindustrialization and restructuring come about? Chicago's charter was granted in 1833, but as built space, most of Chicago dates from the Fire of 1871. Over the 125 years since the fire, most of the city's neighborhoods have been rebuilt at least twice, and some high-rises are the third buildings erected on certain sites. Before World War II, the entire design and layout of buildings, railroads, ports, streets, and highways were uniformly directed toward the expansion and consolidation of an industrial city. But since the war the city of Chicago, and more recently, industrial suburbs near the city, has suffered the loss of the manufacturing industries on which its economy primarily was based and around which the physical layout was organized. From 1947 to 1980, Chicago's employment in manufacturing dropped by more than 50 percent and in "TUC" (transportation, utilities, and communication) by 25 percent. Even with employment expansion in the government, service, and "FIRE" (finance, insurance, and real estate) sectors, the city of Chicago suffered a net loss of 189,000 jobs. In contrast, suburban employment increased dramatically (over 300 percent) during the same period. Yet despite this increase, employment in manufacturing and TUC in the Chicago Standard Metropolitan Statistical Area (SMSA) as a whole suffered a net decrease of 62,000 jobs.[7] By the 1990s, metropolitan Chicago had fundamentally changed both where and how it made its living.

Rapid and disruptive change is not new to the urban landscape. The changes that had taken place in Chicago neighborhoods and in the city as a whole since the late nineteenth century were of great interest to the founders of the Chicago School of urban sociology in the 1920s.[8] Indeed, the Chicago School was influential precisely because it provided an explanation for the dynamics of urban change associated with industrial growth.

But in the last decades of the twentieth century, Chicago and other large industrial cities were to undergo a different kind of change. A new metropolitan structure was emerging, one that was highly decentralized and multipolar, with edge cities[9] and other concentrations of employment and commerce distributed throughout the metropolitan area.[10] Moreover, although Chicago's central business area continued to prosper and grow as a focal point for employment, it had been transformed from the control center for Chicago-area enterprise into a niche in a global matrix of capital and information flows. Thus business decisions affecting the lives of Chicagoans were made not only in Chicago but in the major financial centers around the world. In turn, Chicago's economic power, represented in its thriving downtown and in its edge cities, increasingly was exercised over a global labor force and a worldwide network of productive enterprises. The city's labor force was competing in a growing global market, made possible by easier migrations of workers and technologically supported flows of capital. And major corporations now needed not brawny laborers, living near factories, ports, and railroads, but rather a highly educated workforce, which could afford to live in safe, pleasant residential areas with good schools and cultural amenities. These structural changes have complicated religious social ministries that once focused on issues of justice in an industrial economy.

The Changing Voices of Religion

Chicago's religious organizations grew up as part of the social and institutional structure characteristic of an American industrial city, representing what Daniel Bluestone calls "a parallel moral power."[11] The city's first settlers built churches and synagogues along with shops and houses near the Chicago River and its confluence with Lake Michigan. Some of these congregations, such as Old Saint Patrick's Roman Catholic Church (chapter 9) and First United Methodist Church, Chicago Temple (chapter 3), remain strong spiritual forces in the central city. But beginning before the Fire of 1871 and continuing through the 1920s, with the expansion and consolidation of the industrial infrastructure along waterways and railroads, many churches and synagogues moved from the central commercial district to the densely populated residential neighborhoods that were integral to that infrastructure. Bluestone argues that this represented a partial dissociation of religion from the commercial and public affairs of the city and a primary association of religion with morality and femininity, with the social and nurturing functions of community life.

Many of these congregations formed part of the growing denominationalism that was to be a hallmark of disestablished American religion. From 1916 to 1939, Archbishop George Mundelein led the Roman Catholic Archdiocese of Chicago to prominence as an exemplar of the "American Church," which evolved as a distinctive religious presence in a country in which Protestantism was culturally dominant but not officially established. Under his leadership, the archdiocese exercised effective institutional authority over territorially defined parishes that, in turn, established Catholic cultural hegemony in neighborhoods throughout much of Chicago, including Pilsen (chapter 2) and the Southwest Side (chapter 5). As in other American industrial cities, labor unions built supportive relationships with Catholics and their parishes. After the Second World War, the Chicago Archdiocese provided essential support for Saul Alinsky's innovative organizing in the Back of the Yards neighborhood, which launched the strategy of church-based organizing that has since been implemented in urban neighborhoods throughout the United States.

Although Chicago was home to as many Protestants as Catholics, most Protestant churches were smaller than Catholic parishes, and they were divided among so many denominations and sects that they could not hope to speak in a single public voice, as the Catholic Church could. The Protestant denominations, as H. Richard Niebuhr[12] argued, reflected not only doctrinal and organizational alternatives but the ethnic, racial, and class divisions of American society. Nevertheless, the Protestants of Chicago organized their numerous congregations in an Episcopal diocese, a presbytery, Methodist districts and a conference, synods of the various Lutheran churches, and various associations of congregations. These structures provided internal discipline, vehicles for social mission, and the capacity to speak publicly in the affairs of a burgeoning industrial city. Although fewer in number and membership, Jewish organizations served the same function.

Like Protestant churches in other major cities, soon after 1900, Chicago's churches crossed denominational lines to form clergy associations at the neighborhood level as well as citywide organizations. The Church Federation of Greater Chicago was founded in 1907 and continued until the late 1980s.[13] While it never united all Protestant churches, it was sufficiently strong to be recognized as an authoritative Protestant voice, a presence parallel to the Catholic Archdiocese of Chicago and the Chicago Board of Rabbis. Black churches, including those of black Protestant denominations, operated more autonomously, but many joined in issue-specific coalitions, especially when the civil rights movement came north in the 1960s.

Just as Chicago's ecumenical and denominational organizations were reaching the peak of their strength in the 1950s, however, they were also beginning to reflect the national process now known as religious restructuring.[14] While the people of the United States remain among the most likely in the world to believe in God, pray, and go to church, their religious institutions are being fragmented and realigned. The national and regional institutions of the mainline Protestant churches—the Church Federation of Greater Chicago and its member denominations, for example—have been disbanded or seriously weakened as local congregations have withheld support and questioned their authority and as individuals have directed support more to religious special-purpose organizations than to their own denominations and ecumenical agencies. This means not only that the mainline Protestant churches' economic base is attenuated but that increasingly each denomination cannot speak on public issues in a single, unified voice. Such has been the fate of the very institutions that most actively sought to have an impact on government and other public institutions and policies, that were the main expressions of what was generally considered "the public church."[15]

The Roman Catholic and Evangelical churches' concern with public policy has increased, however, and the "New Christian Right" has become a force to be reckoned with in electoral politics.[16] While the public prominence of the Chicago Archdiocese is hardly new, its visibility as a force in public life is accented by the retreat and fragmentation of Protestantism. Yet even these elements of increased strength in public religion appear to be only loosely related to the denominational structures that evolved before the Second World War.

The public role of religion was never limited to denominational and ecumenical bodies, of course, and restructuring has enhanced the relative stature of congregations and parishes. Their public importance is particularly impressive when one takes their cultural activity into account. This book highlights the publicly significant cultural work of congregations by examining the symbolic images and language, narrative stories, and social identities that they generate.

Since the 1960s, the rapid immigration from South and East Asia, the Middle East, Africa, and Latin America has altered the shape and character of religion in Chicago and in other large American cities, as Paul Numrich shows in chapter 10.[17] By most accounts, metropolitan Chicago is now home to at least three hundred thousand Muslims, seventy-five thousand Hindus, seventy-five thousand Buddhists, and smaller numbers of Sikhs, Jains, and Zoroastrians. All but a few thousand of these have arrived or were born here since 1960, but they have already formed well over a hundred thriving worship centers. Moreover, for the first time in U.S. history Christians have been arriving in large numbers from countries in which Christianity is not the majority religion or the religious basis of the predominant culture. Thus, for example, Methodists and Syrian Orthodox from India and Presbyterians from Korea add significantly to Chicago's cultural and religious diversity. Although these immigrants have largely been ignored in the literature, several scholars[18] have recently demonstrated their nationwide distribution and impact on American religious and cultural pluralism. Chapters 2, 5, 6, 8, and 10 in this book include studies of congregations that the recent wave of immigrants has created, and explore the new dimensions of pluralism that have resulted.

Social Transformation and the Refocus of Moral Culture

In Chicago as elsewhere, both urban and religious restructuring have been intimately linked to what some critics have called the "social revolution" of the 1960s and 1970s. The rejection of traditional values and extrication from traditional authorities during these decades are most often interpreted as a triumph of individual freedom and choice at the expense of community. Drawing on Philip Rieff's "triumph of the therapeutic," Christopher Lasch's "culture of narcissism," Robert Bellah's "expressive individualism," and Phillip Hammond's rise of "personal autonomy," scholars of culture John R. Hall and Mary Jo Neitz describe—and for the most part, decry—a fundamental shift in moral culture, from one in which authority lies with collectivities and their traditions to one that recognizes the authority of individual choice.[19] This thesis concerning the "loss of community" and the resulting amoral character of American society suggests one dimension—an ambiguous one, to be sure—of what has been happening in Chicago. Chicago is known as a "city of neighborhoods,"[20] and it is widely believed, not without reason, that these neighborhoods have had a moral character. While they never have been as homogeneous, stable, and cohesive as Chicago mythology would have it, there is little reason to doubt that in many neighborhoods a moral culture was shaped by overlapping interactions among people who were brought together by jobs, shopping, schooling, worship, and various services that were located relatively close together. Among immigrants, a common language and culture reinforced these material incentives to follow a shared path. For Catholics, the parish structure not only required them to attend church in their areas of residence but also established the sacredness of those particular spaces and thus of the relationships and cultural norms within them. Among industrial workers, the solidarity that the labor unions fostered reinforced the solidarity of workers and working-class families in their neighborhoods, which were typically not far from their places of employment.

These moral cultures, nostalgically recalled by Alan Ehrenhalt in *The Lost City,*[21] were inevitably eroded by urban restructuring, which caused people to spend less time, meet fewer of their needs, and achieve fewer of their aspirations near home. Moreover, these "natural communities" and their moral cultures were, in fact, morally ambiguous, as became increasingly apparent during the civil rights era, when many of them proved to be "defended neighborhoods."[22] Several chapters in this book—most poignantly chapter 5, on the Southwest Side parishes—offer lenses on congregations struggling with problems of boundaries and change as they attempt to preserve or reconstruct the moral cultures considered essential to social life.

But the old moral cultures and forms of social control have been challenged not only by economic and demographic change but by religion itself. In the Catholic Church, the Second Vatican Council's *Declaration on Religious Freedom* offered increased recognition of freedom of conscience. As Elfriede Wedam (chapter 9) and Peter D'Agostino (chapter 11) argue, the implementation of Vatican II in the Chicago Archdiocese has also afforded Catholics greater flexibility in associating with parishes and schools and has enhanced their authority and responsibility for the shape and direction of parish life. Mainline Protestant churches, perhaps more historically rooted in American individualism than other religious groups, train pastoral counselors in methods and settings that share many of the assumptions and principles of the therapeutic culture.[23] The mainline Protestants, along with Reform Jews, led the way in advocating removal of legal restrictions on divorce, and more recently, many have urged the same for abortion and the practice of a homosexual lifestyle, making all these increasingly a matter of individual choice and less subject to social control.

Yet the rise in personal autonomy has not been the only thrust of the social transformation. While many traditional sources of collective authority (such as neighborhoods, parishes, and unions) have been weakened, and others (churches) have chosen to support a greater degree of personal choice, there has been a simultaneous increase in the recognition of new collectivities and their moral claims. The events of the 1960s were fostered by social movements that both depended on and articulated group solidarities. The civil rights movement had as its goal increasing the individual rights of black people, but the movement presumed solidarities both among blacks and between blacks and whites that had not yet been articulated. These presumptions remain evident, newly reformulated, in the activities and cultures of the neighborhoods and congregations discussed in this book. Even though the feminist movement sought to advance the individual rights of women, sometimes at the expense of their communal ties, it also has both identified and fostered an "ethic of care"[24] in which individuals see themselves constituted by and embedded in their relationships, not as autonomous selves. And the two major 1990s community-organizing initiatives in Chicago, led by the Gamaliel Foundation and the Industrial Areas Foundation, suggest that the thrust of social change is not all in the direction of individualism and personal autonomy. In contrast to the personal growth and self-awareness movements, the prevailing idioms of these efforts are "relational power" and collective action for the "common good."

During the 1960s and 1970s, America underwent a profound discontinuity in its moral culture, and this is evident in the congregations discussed in this book. But if a new moral paradigm is emerging, it is doing so by fits and starts. Old authorities may be in disrepute and moral communities in disarray, but many individuals still repair to existing communities or attempt to build new ones in order to find their moral bearings. Some of these communities are congregations, whereas others compete with congregations for the hearts and minds of urban people.

Chicago: The Known City

Chicago has proved itself many times to be a rich resource and a fertile setting for both urban and religious research.[25] As Richard Sennett has argued, the early Chicago School sociologists distinguished themselves from their German teachers in part by examining and analyzing the gritty details of Chicago's neighborhoods and by studying its subpopulations and neighborhood organizations. By assembling these scholars' writings in *Classic Essays on the Culture of Cities,* Sennett shows that Georg Simmel (with whom Robert Park had studied at Heidelberg), Max Weber, and Oswald Spengler sought to contrast the distinctive city culture with that of farm and village and thus concerned themselves with what was common to cities, rather than with the variety and differentiation within them. In contrast, Park and his colleagues sought to discern the urban culture in its own "ecology," in the ways in which it was internally divided and operative. As Sennett puts it, Park believed that a city's "functional, tangible character would ultimately reveal the cultural and ethical possibilities for life within it."[26]

It was in Chicago, during the decades of its growth and consolidation as a great industrial city, that this central notion was developed and the city's specific physical and social realities, including religious life and organizations, were examined. Early Chicago School studies were conducted in some of the same neighborhoods that are the subjects of this book. The meeting concerning the demolition of public housing described at the beginning of this chapter took place in the LaSalle Street Church, which is located in what Chicago School sociologist Harvey Warren Zorbaugh[27] called the "area of furnished rooms," which separated what was then Little Sicily (now occupied by the Cabrini Green public housing project) from the wealthy residential area to the east, known from that day to this as the Gold Coast (see chapter 3). Nels Anderson's *The Hobo,* one of the earliest sociological studies of homeless men, achieves its insight into the homelessness of the time not only by charting the relationships (or lack of relationships) between the homeless and other people but by monitoring their interaction with their physical surroundings. Anderson spent his research time in the areas he called "Hobohemia," certain blocks on the fringes of Chicago's business district, including some in Old Saint Patrick's Parish, which is discussed in chapter 9. Louis Wirth's *The Ghetto,* a study of Chicago's Near West Side, a port of entry for Jews from Eastern Europe beginning in the late nineteenth century, showed how the attempt to understand the people of a neighborhood points beyond the neighborhood to "the natural history of an institution and the psychology of a people."[28] Since the 1920s, the people of Wirth's ghetto have migrated within Chicago, first westward to Lawndale, then north to West Rogers Park, where they comprise one of what Livezey (chapter 6) calls the "religiously based, ethnoracial enclaves" that characterize the community.

Chicago School methods were also used to study churches. Shortly after Graham Taylor arrived in Chicago in 1892 to teach at Chicago Theological Seminary, he established the Chicago Commons Association on the Near West Side as a laboratory for his students.[29] Preparation for Christian ministry required field studies, using direct observation and social survey. Samuel Kincheloe, a successor to Taylor, was particularly concerned to understand the inability of Chicago's Protestant neighborhood churches to cope with the influx of non-Protestant and nonwhite populations. Kincheloe's "The Behavior Sequence of a Dying Church,"[30] was based on data from declining congregations, including the West Side's Douglas Park Christian Church, which Kincheloe, as a young pastor, had been unable to keep alive when large numbers of Catholic immigrants replaced the Protestants of its neighborhood. Kincheloe's work anticipated the challenges to congregations from immigration and neighborhood change that this book explores. Kincheloe's research, however, reflecting the ecological approach of his Chicago School mentors, is preoccupied with the ability—or inability—of a church to adapt when the conditions that have sustained it change. His essays give little attention to the spiritual and social missions of the churches or to whether or not the churches create congregational cultures and goals distinct from the secular momentum of urban life.

After the Great Depression and World War II, research in and about Chicago continued to demonstrate and develop the use of field methods for understanding both urban and religious culture and organizations. Some of the landmark sociological studies in Chicago that undergird present research, including that presented here, are St. Clair Drake and Horace Cayton's *Black Metropolis,* Morris Janowitz's *The Community Press in an Urban Setting,* Gerald Suttles's *The Social Order of the Slum,* and Albert Hunter's *Symbolic Communities.*

Studies in social ethics, history, and politics have also demonstrated the value of direct, local observation for discerning human agency and for appraising strategies of transformation. For example, *The Edge of the*

Ghetto[31] examines the dynamics of race in Chicago's Southwest Side, providing a window on the encounter, repeated throughout the United States, of "white ethnic" communities with the assertion of African Americans' civil rights. Similarly, a detailed study of Chicago's civil rights organizations in the mid-1960s, *Confronting the Color Line,*[32] and various books on the dimension of race in Chicago politics during the campaigns and incumbency of Chicago's only elected African American mayor, Harold Washington,[33] anticipate that the problematic of race continues to pervade all aspects of life in metropolitan Chicago.

Finally, Chicago-based research is not particularly rich in studies that take the metropolitan area as a system or a unit of study. The present volume makes a modest move in that direction by attempting to show how each neighborhood is linked to a metropolitan system, and how change at the metropolitan level affects the neighborhood and its congregations. One antecedent is to be found in *Sacred Sands,* J. Ronald Engel's[34] study of voluntary associations' fight to save the Indiana Dunes and the Lake Michigan shore in the state of Indiana, southeast of Chicago. Engel shows how the movement to save the Dunes was built largely by Chicago-based organizations and movements that recognized the inextricable link between Chicago and the Dunes.

The writings discussed above focus on organizations' agency more than on their adaptive capacities. This is not to say that all the organizations studied actually made a difference; indeed, the main conclusion of *Confronting the Color Line* is that after years of civil rights struggle, the color line was left intact. But these accounts show how organizations may simultaneously adapt to change and participate in shaping outcomes. And they further illustrate how research in and about Chicago can illuminate issues of wider interest and can help explain the dynamics of large cities coping with structural change.

Since the early 1970s, "congregational studies" has emerged as an interdisciplinary field of research, signaled by the publication in 1986 of the *Handbook for Congregational Studies,* succeeded by *Studying Congregations* in 1998.[35] The Chicago-based Church and Community Ministry Project,[36] which seeks to understand the factors that sustain church activities intended to transform their communities, contributed greatly to the concepts presented in these books and to the development of this nascent field. The field has also been shaped by studies of the ecologies of congregations-in-community and of congregational adaptation to neighborhood change, most recently exemplified in Nancy Ammerman's

Congregation and Community,[37] and by studies of congregational cultures, perhaps still best represented by James Hopewell's *Congregation*.[38] Although the field as a whole is concerned mainly with Protestantism, John T. McGreevy's *Parish Boundaries*[39] examines the complex church-and-neighborhood interaction on the race issue in the Catholic parishes in Chicago and other American industrial cities. And in *Gatherings in Diaspora,* scholars convened by R. Stephen Warner present ethnographic case studies of eleven "new ethnic and immigrant" congregations.[40]

The Evolution of Method

The Religion in Urban America Program continued this history of religious and community research in Chicago with particular attention to the responses of religious organizations to postwar urban and religious restructuring and social transformation. We proceeded inductively in order to avoid privileging social services and community action, the urban ministries that were prominent when cities made their living mainly by manufacturing and shipping and when Will Herberg's *Protestant-Catholic-Jew*[41] described the extent of religious pluralism. We made ethnographic case studies of congregations the core of the investigation in order to look at urban religion as much as possible "from the native's point of view," recognizing, as Clifford Geertz[42] did, that this could only be approximated. We believe the ethnographic method helped us to be equally attentive to self-initiated mission and adaptive strategies and to analyze a full range of public actions, including cultural production as well as social service and community organizing. We selected organizations as case studies without regard to the nature or extent of their engagement in such activities but with the objective that, collectively, they would reflect the social, economic, demographic, and religious diversity of metropolitan Chicago.

Because we wanted to examine congregations in relation to their geographic and social contexts, we first selected neighborhoods that, taken together, would represent the city's range of social, economic, demographic, and religious characteristics. We then inventoried congregations and other religious organizations in each neighborhood and selected from five to eight of them for investigation as case studies. These selections mainly reflected the religious diversity of the neighborhoods, but we also sought to ensure that the selections for the study as a whole would represent the religious diversity of the metropolitan area. We selected a higher proportion of organizations representing Islam, Hinduism, Buddhism, and other religions that had not been much discussed in the literature of American religion.

Thus the Religion in Urban America Program's investigative method both continues and complements the ecological model of community research that has been developed and practiced in Chicago for nearly a century. It is the Chicago empirical method in a new phase. This book presents a ground-level view of the results.

Congregations and Urban Transformation

In the chapters that follow, we offer narratives of what we saw and heard as we studied Chicago-area religious organizations in their local settings. The essays in part 2 explore the interaction between religious congregations and the neighborhoods and social settings in which they are located. The social functions of neighborhoods are changing and often declining. Consequently, many congregations are reorganizing themselves to depend less on their immediate neighborhoods, to relate to their geographic surroundings in new ways, and to emphasize more symbolic and communicative frames of reference.

The essays in part 3, therefore, are concerned with some of the ways in which religious organizations constitute themselves and serve constituencies beyond the neighborhood. Many of these, exemplified by Old Saint Patrick's Church in chapter 9, are "niche congregations" that are surviving neighborhood change and reconstituting themselves as viable, possibly growing congregations by devising programs and communal styles that appeal to specialized constituencies. Others, such as the recently established Buddhist, Hindu, Sikh, and Muslim worship centers discussed in chapter 10, have deliberately chosen their locations to accommodate participants who are dispersed throughout the metropolitan area.

Finally, despite the erosion of denominational power, these structures still have the institutional responsibility for the entire city or metropolitan area. Peter R. D'Agostino's analysis in chapter 11 of Chicago's largest denominational structure, the Roman Catholic Archdiocese, complements the ethnographic examination of parishes presented in chapters 2, 4, 5, 6, 7, and 9, enabling the reader to see the interaction between the neighborhood and the metropolitan levels of religious organization. This is particularly important at a time of adjustment to a postindustrial economy, and D'Agostino's chapter focuses specifically on the archdiocesan response to urban restructuring under the episcopacy of the late Joseph Cardinal Bernardin, who died in 1996, shortly after our field research was completed.

The narratives of all ten chapters reveal congregations and other religious institutions responding, often creatively, to the opportunities and pressures of urban change. The congregations demonstrate a combination of internal and external concerns, delivering what organizational theorists call "member benefits" as well as "public benefits." Most of the congregations principally serve their own members, with service to the wider community and advocacy for public causes relegated to small committees and discretionary portions of annual budgets. The chapters presented in this book suggest that while social action is a significant form of religious engagement, one that makes an appreciable contribution to human welfare in the city, it is not the central dynamic of urban religion.

This finding suggests a considerable expansion, if not an outright shift in focus, for the question of the urban contribution of religious organizations. At least since the Progressive Era and the Social Gospel movement, both scholarly and ministerial interest in religion's contribution has focused on benefits to poor, marginalized, and subordinated populations, whether through the salvation of souls, the delivery of social services, or the reform of the public order. In short, religious agency has been considered important in the city mainly insofar as it directly and measurably benefited, in Elam Davies's memorable expression, "the least, the last, the lost, and the lonely."[43] In the late 1990s, this long-standing expectation of religion has been expressed as part of the trend toward the privatization of services briefly considered the proper responsibility of government.

The studies presented in this book confirm that congregations of all the major faiths are collectively engaged in good deeds to benefit the "disadvantaged other," continuing the long-standing tradition known in Christianity as social ministry. But they also conclude that programs of social service and social action account for but a fraction of the religious contribution to the quality of urban life. To understand that contribution fully, it is necessary to examine the cultural life of religious organizations and to recognize that cultural production and community formation are not necessarily inward-looking and private but are often effective forms of public action. R. Stephen Warner addresses this point in the epilogue.

The religious organizations of metropolitan Chicago are shaped by their members' experience of living in extremely kinetic conditions, in which the communities and cultures of their past appear to be defunct, inaccessible, or irrelevant. This is most obvious among recent immigrants, especially those from non-European countries that were never fully dominated by European culture, the English language, and Christianity. But it is also true for American citizens whose ties to a local community have been severed by their own relocation, or by the replacement of their former neighbors by new neighbors of different language or culture or experience, or by the daily pressures preventing their interaction and cooperation with persons whose residences are nearby. And it may also be true for some who, even though geographically settled and organizationally connected, are unable or unwilling to assent to the moral authority or share in the common culture of the institutions and groups to which they belong. In short, the institutions of urban religion are made up of people whose frames of reference have been shaken by some combination of structural and cultural change.

In response, these churches, temples, synagogues, and mosques produce the cultural material that enables their members and adherents to locate themselves with respect to the places and time in which they currently live, to identify with others, to find their moral bearings, and to achieve some measure of efficacy with respect to their own needs and aspirations. Mainly through worship, education, and social activities, these congregations appropriate symbols and generate new ones, claim and revise traditions, defend and bridge social boundaries, articulate and invent meanings and values by which to make sense of changing circumstances.

This much is not new but rather a recognized role of religion in society and an expression of the fact that, as Geertz[44] has argued, religion is— whatever else it may also be—a cultural system. The importance lies in both the process and the content of that cultural production, which are complex subjects. The process of producing religious cultural material, as Robert Wuthnow explains in *Producing the Sacred*,[45] is very similar to that of creating music, art, and entertainment. The production of new cultural material always begins with what already exists. Just as even the most original painting reflects the pigments, tools, and media that the present technology and economy supply, so the sermons, music, and liturgies of every congregation are conditioned by the particular people, artifacts, technologies, theologies, and beliefs available to it. These raw materials of cultural production are different for every congregation, and the congregations discussed in this book were selected precisely to reflect as much variety as possible. Although they are located in a single metropolitan region, the differences of neighborhood, race and ethnicity, economic resources, age, and religious heritage mean that the starting point is unique to each congregation.

Yet, as we have observed the expressions and practices of urban religion, it has been possible to discern patterns and to identify some of the ways in which the cultural activities of these congregations are important to life in the city. Culture is inherently public, so cultural production by religious organizations is one kind of religious public action. Cultural production has many dimensions, but we have been particularly impressed with the ways in which it is concerned with theology, morality, and community.

First, since congregations are specifically religious, their cultural innovation is in part theological. Their central symbols are about their god or gods, and the meanings they share and the authority they exercise almost always include some claims about their relationship with the Divine. Thus, while the chapters that follow are not explicitly theological, they examine congregations that are engaged in theological discourse, and they show how that discourse has public and political as well as private and spiritual implications. For example, the incorporation of black popular culture into the worship life of a middle-class black church evokes an understanding of the God of the entire African diaspora, and this in turn provides a basis for bridging the boundary between the black middle class and the poor. Similarly, the mandatory inclusion of multiple ethnic groups in the governing structure of a mosque not only symbolizes the theological principle of the inclusiveness of the Muslim *ummah,* or "nation," but also institutionalizes procedures to ensure that diverse cultural traditions interact and evolve. The result is that Indians, Pakistanis, Palestinians, Egyptians, and African Americans, among others, find common interests and purposes that go far beyond the conduct of the mosque.

Second, most of the congregations discussed here are engaged in cultural activities that have a prominent moral dimension. This does not mean that they or the authors writing about them view culture itself as inherently good. While many of these congregations exhibit the aesthetic refinement and intellectual achievement associated with "high culture," this is incidental to the fact that they all generate systems of meaning and value that are embodied and expressed in symbols. Cultural symbols mark both the good and the bad, the better and the worse, the acceptable and the unacceptable—whether the subject is art, food, government, or personal or group behavior. And since religion is a cultural system, our focus on religious congregations enables us to ask how and to what extent congregations may be fostering collective norms and patterns of social accountability.

The picture that emerges from the essays taken together is one of multiple religious communities in which people share a concern for speaking and acting in ways they consider proper. Virtually every subject that has a "right-and-wrong" dimension came up sooner or later in the congregations we studied. But we were particularly impressed with how frequently congregations or groups within them were concerned with questions of race or ethnicity, sometimes without even articulating the relevant choices in racial or ethnic terms. Whether or not to conduct a worship service in an additional language, whether to add or change a picture or icon, how hard to try to evangelize a neighborhood or to recruit new members from a wider region—choices such as these entail racial values and choices. And the decision of whether to articulate the racial dimension or to leave it latent beneath the surface is itself a moral choice, one that the congregations discussed in this book often made and sometimes articulated. Thus, although only a small percentage of these congregations engaged in political action on race "issues," the problem of race in our society and in their own religious groups was frequently central to their cultural work.

Finally, while different congregations and groups foster different and sometimes conflicting values, their social accountability and the authority they attribute to their respective traditions contrast markedly with the individual moral autonomy sustained by the secular culture. For all their differences, congregations are collectives—associations, groups, communities. In general, the religious communities discussed in this book tend to preserve traditional values by reinterpreting them in new contexts, rather than to reject and replace them. Thus the cultural activities of religious congregations tend more toward preserving and reclaiming traditional collective goods (neighborhoods, families) than toward promoting either new collective goods (economic equality) or individual rights and freedoms. This runs counter to the individualism and moral autonomy that were central to the social revolution of the 1970s and that many alarmed critics, such as Bellah and Hammond, claim have become the dominant features of the common culture. This line of argument is more implicit than explicit in following chapters, but the reader will find rich and multifaceted evidence to support it.

NOTES

The entire Religion in Urban America Program team contributed greatly to the knowledge and perspective reflected in this introductory chapter. I am also particularly grateful to William A. Simpson for his discerning critiques and creative suggestions.

1. The authors are all members of the Religion in Urban America Program at the University of Illinois at Chicago and conducted field research—along with our colleagues in the program—in the congregations and neighborhoods we discuss in our chapters.

2. Wuthnow, *Restructuring of American Religion.*

3. See Park, "City as a Social Laboratory."

4. Orum, *City-Building in America.*

5. Soja, *Postmodern Geographies;* Orum, *City-Building in America.*

6. Wilson, *Truly Disadvantaged.*

7. Haider, "Chicagoland 2005."

8. Park and Burgess, *The City;* Wirth, "Urbanism as a Way of Life"; Hunter, *Symbolic Communities* and "The Gold Coast and the Slum Revisited."

9. Garreau, *Edge City.*

10. Soot et al., *Analysis of Employment Hubs.*

11. Bluestone, *Constructing Chicago,* 62ff.

12. Niebuhr, *Social Sources of Denominationalism.*

13. Richesin, "Eighty Years of Ministry 1907–1987."

14. Wuthnow, *Restructuring of American Religion.*

15. Marty, *Public Church.*

16. Casanova, *Public Religions in the Modern World,* esp. 135–166.

17. Also see Numrich, "Recent Immigrant Religions."

18. Williams, *Religions of Immigrants;* Warner and Wittner, eds., *Gatherings in Diaspora;* Haddad, ed., *Muslims of America;* Eck, ed., *World Religions in Boston.*

19. Hall and Neitz, *Culture,* 20–43. Their sources include Rieff, *Triumph of the Therapeutic;* Lasch, *Culture of Narcissism;* Bellah et al., *Habits of the Heart;* and Hammond, *Religion and Personal Autonomy.*

20. Pacyga and Skerrett, *Chicago.*

21. Ehrenhalt, *Lost City.*

22. Suttles, *Social Construction of Communities,* 21–43.

23. Browning, *Fundamental Practical Theology,* 245–46.

24. Gilligan, *In a Different Voice,* esp. 62–63.

25. The title for this section comes from Richard Wright's introduction to Drake and Cayton, *Black Metropolis,* xviii.

26. Sennett, ed., *Classic Essays,* 13.

27. Zorbaugh, *Gold Coast and the Slum.*

28. Wirth, *The Ghetto,* xi.

29. Stockwell, "Graham Taylor—Urban Pioneer."

30. Kincheloe, "Behavior Sequence of a Dying Church."

31. Fish et al., *Edge of the Ghetto.*

32. Anderson and Pickering, *Confronting the Color Line.*

33. See Grimshaw, *Bitter Fruit;* Green and Holli, eds., *Restoration 1989;* Travis, *"Harold" the People's Mayor.*

34. Engel, *Sacred Sands.*

35. Carroll, Dudley, and McKinney, eds., *Handbook for Congregational Studies;* Ammerman et al., eds., *Studying Congregations.* Also see Hopewell, *Congregation;* Dudley, Caroll, and Wind, eds., *Carriers of Faith;* Wind and Lewis, eds., *American Congregations,* vols. 1 and 2; Ammerman, *Congregation and Community.*

36. Dudley and Johnson, "Congregational Self-Images."

37. Ammerman, *Congregation and Community.*

38. Hopewell, *Congregation.*

39. McGreevy, *Parish Boundaries.*

40. Warner and Wittner, eds., *Gatherings in Diaspora.*

41. Herberg, *Protestant-Catholic-Jew.*

42. Geertz, *Local Knowledge,* chap. 3.

43. Scroggs, "Making a Difference," 507.

44. Geertz, *Interpretation of Cultures,* chap. 4.

45. Wuthnow, *Producing the Sacred,* chap. 1.

Religion in a City of Neighborhoods

Map 2. Pilsen, a major port of entry for Mexicans, is a symbolic center of the Hispanic population of metropolitan Chicago. Map by Brian Twardosz, BMT Printing and Cartographic Specialists.

Hispanic Immigrant Churches and the Construction of Ethnicity

Janise D. Hurtig

Every Sunday morning Rosario and her family walk four blocks to Saint Pius V, their neighborhood parish. Saint Pius is a Roman Catholic church located in the heart of Pilsen—a poor, inner-city neighborhood that over the past forty years has come to form part of Chicago's densest and most populous Mexican American district, as well as a principal port of entry for Mexican immigrants to the Chicago area. As Rosario walks up the steps of the unimposing red-brick building, she joins hundreds of her fellow parishioners—most of whom also live nearby—to attend one of three Spanish-language masses held each Sunday; two more masses are held in English. Over the course of the day, more than twenty-five hundred people attend mass at Saint Pius, and often there is standing room only in the wood-beamed sanctuary that seats around six hundred. Most of those attending, like Rosario, are Mexican immigrants; and many of them, like Rosario, speak little or no English.

While Rosario walks to Saint Pius, Lucia drives into Pilsen, with her Salvadoran husband and their two young children, from a lower-middle-class, predominantly Hispanic[1] neighborhood several miles away, to attend services at Emmanuel Presbyterian Church. Located only blocks away from Saint Pius, Emmanuel Presbyterian is an evangelically oriented, burgeoning congregation whose two hundred Sunday worshipers consistently overflow the rather modest sanctuary. As at Saint Pius, the Sunday service is attended largely by young families—parents accompanied by their children and, at times, the grandparents. The worshipers at Emmanuel, however, tend to be slightly better off economically than Saint Pius's parishioners; and while the Presbyterian congregation is entirely Hispanic, it is nationally quite diverse.

Although many of the adults and their children are bilingual, Sunday services at Emmanuel are held in Spanish.

We[2] met Rosario and Lucia in the winter of 1994, in the course of conducting comparative research on religious organizations in Pilsen. Our objectives were, first, to learn what Pilsen's religious organizations considered to be the pressing issues for their members and communities and, second, to analyze and compare how individual organizations addressed those issues, spiritually and programmatically. We gathered information in part through the observation of religious rituals, programs, and other activities and in part through interviews with clergy, laity, and community leaders. Rosario and Lucia were among the lay leaders we interviewed at their churches.

This chapter draws on the growing research in congregational studies that looks at urban churches not as institutional mirrors of the larger secular society, nor as havens from the profane urban world, but rather as "subcultures," distinguishable from but interacting with the larger urban environment of which they are part. Each church subculture is guided by a particular logic or worldview that integrates the spiritual, social, educational, and community life of the church. It also projects certain values, identities, and social orientations that members often turn to for guidance and inspiration in their daily lives.[3]

The worldviews of immigrant churches are informed in part by their model or vision of "ethnicization"—the process by which immigrants become ethnics. Thus the orientation an immigrant church offers its members also implies a path for their incorporation into an ethnic community. Located in a Mexican American neighborhood and serving predominantly Hispanic constituencies, Pilsen's churches play an active role in the constitution and spiritual legitimation of Mexican American and Hispanic ethnicities.

By "ethnicity" I am referring to a culturally constructed category that stands for a collective identity emergent in the interaction between immigrant groups and the mainstream society. Historically, ethnicity has been represented in the popular and academic imaginations as a transcendent cultural form, thought to abide in such traits as descent, cultural heritage, and national origin and to be expressed and reproduced through shared language, customs, and traditions. Discussions of the nature of ethnicity—implicitly figured in terms of the experiences of (white) European immigrants—have been inseparable from debates regarding the likelihood and civic value of immigrant incorporation (assimilationism) on the one hand and the persistence of separate "ethnic minorities" (cultural pluralism) on the other.[4] Even the current celebration of multiculturalism and ethnic diversity, while embracing pluralism wholeheartedly, has encouraged a new wave of ethnic essentialism among scholars, cultural critics, and social activists.

In a provocative article contesting essentialist notions of ethnicity, Kathleen Conzen and her colleagues suggest instead that ethnicity be thought of as "a process of construction or invention which incorporates, adapts, and amplifies preexisting communal solidarities, cultural attributes, and historical memories."[5] Their constructivist approach to ethnicity is compelling, first, because it historicizes ethnicity as an ongoing and contested process and, second, because it emphasizes the active participation of immigrants themselves in the construction and transformation of ethnic identities and ethnic group boundaries. Ethnicity, they argue, does not inhere in immigrants; rather, it emerges through *"relationships* among specific immigrant groups and between them and the dominant ethnoculture."[6] By implication, immigrant churches would not simply offer up a preconstituted ethnic identity to their members. Rather, the invention or construction of ethnicity occurs at the intersections of the church, its members, the larger religious institutions to which it is tied, and the wider secular society with which it interacts. In the context of the urban neighborhood of Pilsen, this perspective encourages us to consider the significance and impact of each church's model of ethnicization in terms of such factors as the racialization of Hispanic ethnicity by the dominant (Anglo) society[7] and the location of Pilsen and many of its residents within a transnational, migratory circuit.

The Religious Landscape of a Transnational Neighborhood

Pilsen is a small but densely populated neighborhood bounded on the north and west by railroad tracks, on the east and south by the South Branch of the Chicago River. The boundaries signal the neighborhood's historical role as port of entry and residence for poor, laboring Eastern European immigrants, who found jobs on the rail and shipping lines and in the lumberyards, factories, and processing plants that had surrounded the area since the mid-1800s.[8]

By the turn of the century, Pilsen—named for a small town in Bohemia—had become a "tenement district": it suffered the highest concentration of poor immigrant families, the most congested and unsanitary housing, and the most militant labor force in the city.[9] Pilsen's immigrant population was also solidly Catholic, and the neighborhood was organized around national parishes—Czech, Slovak, Polish, Croatian—often built by the parishioners and run by "native" priests. For the early residents of Pilsen parish, community, faith, and national identity were of a piece.[10] It was as parish communities that Pilseners waged battles over language, ethnic discrimination, employment, housing, and education, in their efforts to assimilate into the urban U.S. mainstream while maintaining symbolic and material ties to their homelands. They also contended with the Archdiocese of Chicago for their native languages, religious practices, and clerical representation. Similar battles, both secular and spiritual, continue to be fought today by Pilsen's Mexican residents.[11]

Pilsen's population began to change from Eastern European to Mexican in the 1950s, when the coincidence of U.S. postwar prosperity and Mexican economic crisis stimulated a dramatic increase in Mexican immigration. At the same time, patterns of national and transnational migration began to shift as Mexican migrants increasingly relocated from rural agricultural to urban industrial areas on both sides of the border, under the pressures of a changing global labor market. By 1980, over 80 percent of the Mexican workforce in the United States was located in urban areas, and Chicago's Mexican population was growing dramatically: from 106,000 in 1970, to 206,000 in 1980, and to 348,000 by 1990—figures that do not take into account the tens of thousands of undocumented Mexican immigrants. The rapid influx of Hispanics into Pilsen was magnified in the 1960s by two major urban renewal projects to the north and east that displaced substantial numbers of Hispanics. At the same time, acculturated "white ethnic" residents moved to urban and suburban neighborhoods where they could buy houses and move up the socioeconomic ladder. By the 1970s, Pilsen had become a solidly Hispanic and primarily Mexican district; by the 1990s, many of the industries providing accessible, low-skill employment for immigrants had relocated elsewhere or closed.

Present-day Pilsen is a thoroughly Mexican neighborhood. The 1990 U.S. Census statistics, which tell us that over 81 percent of its nearly fifty thousand residents identify themselves as Mexican (with another 12 percent identifying themselves as Latin Americans of other national backgrounds), give us little feel for the myriad ways in which Mexican cultural and social life permeates the neighborhood. Its main streets are lined with restaurants, grocery stores, and bakeries that sell primarily Mexican food and dry goods. The sweet smell of corn tortillas wafts across every street corner. Bookstores sell Spanish-language books, magazines, and newspapers, and most street conversation and store signs are in Spanish. Mexican popular music pours out into the streets from music stores, apartment buildings, and car windows. In the spring and summer months, *paleteros* selling ice cream and *eloteros* selling corn on the cob and tropical fruit ambulate up and down the streets ringing their bells. Seven of Pilsen's nine Catholic parishes offer one or more Sunday masses in Spanish, and many church interiors include shrines to the Virgin of Guadalupe, the patron saint of Mexico and symbol of Mexican popular religious culture.

But Pilsen is not a town in Mexico. Its immigrant residents work for U.S. companies and deposit money into U.S. banks; their children attend either public or parochial schools; and the neighborhood parishes are under the jurisdiction of the Archdiocese of Chicago, which is part of the U.S. Roman Catholic Church. Pilseners face struggles common to poor, inner-city communities the United States: under- and unemployment, inadequate housing and school facilities, high rates of crime and violence, pervasive gang and drug involvement, and low levels of academic achievement among youth. These problems are exacerbated by the material and ideological barriers created by language differences, and by the gender and generational conflicts created by tensions between the cultural values and social relations of the societies of origin and of settlement.

In both the struggles Pilsen's Mexican residents face and the tendency to address those problems through their religious organizations, Pilsen's current inhabitants resemble their European predecessors. Several interrelated factors, however, distinguish the Mexican experience from that of earlier Eastern European immigrants: the neocolonial relationship of Mexico to the United States; the institutionalized, racialized discrimination against Mexican immigrants;[12] the precariousness of many immigrants' civil status, exacerbated by the current wave of anti-immigration legislation targeting Mexicans; and the circular, transnational dimension of their migration experience.

While many of Pilsen's churches address the first three of these issues spiritually and programmatically, transmigration is not on the religious agenda. And yet, Mexican migration into Chicago has become increasingly transnational in its orientation and cultural consequences. Certainly, the intention of eventual return to the homeland is not new to the immigrant experience; nor is the creation of formal and informal structures for maintaining circular flows of communication, money, and other material and cultural goods between the United States and the homelands. (Indeed, immigrant churches have often facilitated such circuits.) What distinguishes contemporary transnational communities is the rapidity, frequency, and relative ease with which family members come and go between various points of residence, so that *migration itself* becomes formative of the cultural and social life of such communities.

As ethnographers of transnational communities have suggested, transmigratory practices do not simply produce two distinct local or national cultures; rather, they create a distinct, transmigratory cultural system that sustains multiple and often conflicting social and cultural identities,[13] as well as "a powerful ideology of return migration."[14] This dream—which for many is linked to the very impetus to migrate to the United States in the first place—circulates as a force organizing many families' daily lives and thus pours out into the larger community of Pilsen as well. Moreover, transmigration supports a cultural logic in which returns to the homeland are among the strategies immigrants adopt in adjusting to life in the host society. Thus we can understand the common practice among Mexican American families in Pilsen of sending teenage children back to Mexico, for summers or during the school year, to "keep them out of trouble"—where trouble refers to gang involvement, drug use, or premarital sexual activity.[15] Notably, while most of the religious organizations we studied devoted considerable energy and programming to the needs of neighborhood youth, none of them considered sending youth back to Mexico as a strategy for avoiding gang involvement or drug use.

In their extensive study of Mexican migration, Douglas Massey and his colleagues found that while few Mexican immigrants come to the United States with the intention of staying, many find themselves slowly abandoning the dream of return to their homeland as they become increasingly caught up in and committed to life in the United States. And yet, established immigrants do not separate from but rather support other network members' transmigratory patterns.[16] In other words, transmigration is not a stage in a continuum from mobility to settlement; rather, the two migratory tendencies are intimately interconnected. Thus neighborhoods like Pilsen are not simply the point of entry to a unidirectional pathway that leads immigrants up and out of the poor inner city and into the suburban mainstream. Rather, they are incorporated economically, socially, and culturally into a larger, spatially dispersed, transmigrant culture. As Roger Rouse puts it, "In the United States as well as in Mexico, the *place* of the putative community—whether regional or national—is becoming little more than the *site* in which transnationally organized circuits of capital, labor, and communications intersect with one another and with local ways of life."[17] By extension, parishes like Saint Pius are themselves enmeshed in this transnational migratory flow. Emmanuel Presbyterian, a church with a substantial outsider membership and fewer recent immigrant members than Saint Pius, has a less direct relationship to the transnational social reality that permeates Pilsen. Nonetheless, it too engages with that reality: not only does it evangelize within and serve the local community, but many of its members maintain familial ties to the neighborhood.

Within the context of Pilsen's emergent transmigratory culture, the Catholic parishes, schools, health facilities, and community centers have maintained their centrality as a religious presence and defender of the people. Certainly, Pilsen has produced an impressive array of secular, community-based organizations that operate in the service and defense of Pilsen's Hispanic immigrants; some of these are descendents of community organizations that once served Pilsen's Eastern European residents. But the Catholic community of Pilsen has continued to play a central role in advocating for its immigrant residents. At the same time, it is engaged with its Protestant competitors in a battle over souls that dates back to the founding of Protestant-based settlement houses at the turn of the century.

Over the past thirty-five years, the neighborhood parishes have consolidated their efforts through the structure of the Pilsen Catholic Cluster—an association of parishes active for social justice. The Cluster describes itself as "a clearing house to share information and ideas and to assist on joint action among the parishes and other invited groups."[18] Cluster parishes work together on liturgy and sacramental programs, social-justice issues affecting the neighborhood and the wider Hispanic Catholic community, evangelization, educational issues, and youth programs.

One religious event that enacts and illustrates the integration of faith, popular culture, and social action characteristic of the Pilsen Cluster is its annual dramatization of the Via Crucis (Stations of the Cross), held on Good Friday of Saints' Week. In Mexico and across Latin America, Saints' Week is one of the most important moments in the annual ritual cycle, and the Via Crucis is a public performance vividly enacted with all the dramatis personae in full regalia. The Cluster's decision to enact the Stations of the Cross in the street exemplifies the incorporation and symbolic transformation of "native traditions": parishioners and clergy alike recognized that a street celebration not only would draw on a familiar Mexican religious practice but would also "represent Christ's passion publicly in relation to Pilsen people's everyday lives" and reaffirm "the immigrant community's identity as . . . a people on the move."[19]

The Pilsen Via Crucis has become renowned throughout the city as a powerful expression of Mexican popular religion and community solidarity. Thousands of people—Hispanics and Anglos alike—come from around the city to walk slowly and somberly behind the cross-bearing figure of Jesus from station to station. As Jesus carries the cross down the streets of Pilsen, accompanied by Mary, Joseph, Mary Magdalene, the disciples, and Roman soldiers, the procession stops at each of the twelve stations, located in front of parishes and at sites of social and political significance to the community. Among the stations of the cross included in the 1994 Via Crucis that I attended was the Rudy Luzano Public Library, a site of bittersweet significance. Named for a martyred community activist, the modern, well-equipped library is a source of tremendous community pride. The procession also stopped at the site of a drive-by gang shooting and, later, at the newly opened Guadalupano Family Center, located in a former Saint Vitus Parish building. This passionate, public display of popular religion consolidates the community around symbols of local struggle, which are made sacred as they become integral to Mexican American ethnicity.

Fig. 2-1. Jesus bearing his cross in the 1998 Via Crucis in Chicago's Pilsen neighborhood. Photo courtesy of Saint Pius V Roman Catholic Church.

Fig. 2-2. Father Charles Dahm, pastor of Saint Pius V Roman Catholic Church in Pilsen, memorializing a neighborhood killing as part of the 1998 Via Crucis. Photo courtesy of Saint Pius V Roman Catholic Church.

In the 1960s and 1970s the Pilsen Catholic Cluster also provided the structure and inspiration for the creation of a church-based neighborhood community organization and a development corporation, two separate entities that merged in 1994 to form the Resurrection Project. The Resurrection Project runs a neighborhood cleanup program, low-cost housing development and rental programs, and the Guadalupano Family Center. While the Resurrection Project is not directly accountable to the Cluster, its mission—"to shape the future of our community and the quality of its life by building relationships, organizing people with common goals and values and putting those values into practice through education, leadership training, and action"[20]—clearly echoes the Cluster's liberationist spirit. Its programs, directed against the twin threats of urban blight and Anglo gentrification, are aimed at empowering residents by increasing their pride in, control over, and ownership of the community. It is interesting that the unidirectional vision of immigrant incorporation implicit in Resurrection Project's efforts to empower Mexican immigrants by facilitating settlement is entirely in keeping with the long-standing policy of the Catholic leadership to promote home ownership as a strategy for building and sustaining the parish community.[21]

The Catholic presence in Pilsen extends beyond the parishes, schools, and church-based community organizations. Many secular community organizations and agencies also cooperate with the Pilsen parishes, in part because of the sizable population base the parishes represent and can mobilize. Cooperation is also fostered by the politically progressive orientation of the parishes and Cluster and by the recognition that the local parishes are advocates for the Mexican community. This is often expressed through their appeals to the middle-class, Anglo Archdiocese of Chicago, which much of the Hispanic Catholic community perceives as having only a token interest in its large but poor Hispanic constituency and as unwilling to promote Hispanic leadership.

As the Cluster struggles to gain both recognition and autonomy from the archdiocese while uniting with the regional Hispanic Catholic community, it finds itself contending with a growing, though relatively small, Protestant presence. In the mid-1990s there were three mainline Protestant congregations in Pilsen and fifteen small and often transitory evangelical, fundamentalist, or Pentecostal "storefront" churches, many of which have a significant outsider membership. Of these non-Catholic churches, only Saint Matthew Lutheran Church and the multiethnic Church of God are actively engaged in social-justice issues in the community. Ana Maria Díaz-Stevens and Anthony Stevens-Arroyo attribute the pastoralism of Pentecostal and evangelical churches to their millennial vision, which "often precludes concerns for social and political change."[22] While these organizations may implicitly construct Hispanicity through the homogeneity of their membership, they do not explicitly link spirituality and religious identity with ethnic identity.

Nonetheless, Catholic parishes and Protestant congregations are equally invested in recruiting souls into the faith, establishing a commitment to their religious community, and cultivating lay leadership among their members—all efforts that encourage a unidirectional model of ethnicization that prefigures their immigrant constituencies as moving along a path toward eventual, permanent settlement in the Chicago area.

Saint Pius Parish: An Immigrant Parish
Committed to Social Justice

Rosario had been living in Chicago for close to six months when she first walked up the steps of Saint Pius Parish. She, her husband, and their two young daughters had come to Pilsen from a small hamlet in the central state of Michoacán, Mexico. It was February, and the brutal Chicago winter matched the harsh urban landscape and the rough sounds of English that accosted Rosario's uncomprehending ears.

Just before leaving her native village, Rosario's pastor had counseled her: "Where the tree is, there the branches and the root should also be. The wife should follow the man. Wherever you may be, look for the pastor and your religion." His simple message made it profoundly clear that the continuity of and commitment to family and religious life were not only morally imperative but part of the natural order of things. Implicit in his counsel was the assumption of a certain universality to Catholicism—that it knows no cultural boundaries and transcends the materiality of national frontiers. Historically, this theological premise has existed in tension with the equally fundamental parochialism of that same religion, one that emphasizes the geographic and cultural situatedness of each parish and its parishioners.[23]

Perhaps the presumption of and commitment to a universal religious culture gave Rosario the courage to first walk into the parish sanctuary and attend mass when, six months after her arrival, her pastor's words resonated through her growing sense of isolation and estrangement. And in a sense he had been right: something spiritually and personally reassuring was indeed to be found in the mere act of attending Mass. And certainly, the comfort the act produced was enhanced by hearing the Mass conducted in Spanish. As Rosario told us the story of her entry and gradual immersion into parish life, she made it clear, however, that the inviting familiarity she encountered in many of the parish's ritual practices and religious symbols was due to their being specifically *Mexican,* not "universally" Catholic: the nine-day celebration (*novena*) dedicated to the Virgin of Guadalupe, the patron saint of Mexico, whose altar shines with particular brilliance inside the sanctuary; the dramatic Via Crucis procession; the Quinceañera program, which prepares young women turning fifteen for their important rite of passage; the Christmas *posadas*, house visits that symbolize the arrival of the infant Jesus.

This is not to say that Saint Pius offers its immigrant parishioners a replica of Mexican Catholic religious culture, although we heard several parishioners describe parish life as "like being in Mexico." To begin with, the very act of incorporating these familiar symbols and practices into the religious life of an urban U.S. immigrant parish imbues them with a distinct spiritual and cultural significance. Relocated, resacralized, and relegitimated as "native traditions," these components of religious life take on new meaning as ethnic symbols, effectively linking local cultural practices to a common *national* heritage. This use of ethnic symbols contributes to the nationalization of ethnicity, a process of social and symbolic relocation in which immigrants from different communities and cultural groups within Mexico are assimilated into the ethnic category "Mexican Americans."[24]

Historically, the process of transforming religious practices associated with the country of origin into cultural traditions that stand for and preserve a nostalgic identification with the homeland has been a fundamental dimension of immigrant-church subcultures in this country.[25] At a progressive, liberationist parish such as Saint Pius, however, these elements of Mexican religious life become more than performative symbols of Mexican American identity; they are also deployed as vehicles of community formation and empowerment. As one of the parish's religious staff commented, "We seek to empower our parishioners *through* their traditions" (my emphasis).

One way in which Saint Pius empowers its parishioners is to offer them positions as leaders of the groups organizing religious rituals and programs. Several lay leaders described at length the modifications they had made or planned to make in a particular religious festival or program, often in order to better capture the spirit and qualities of the festival as it was practiced in Mexico. Olivia, never an active parish member in Mexico, had been a volunteer in the Devotional Group to Our Lady of Guadalupe (the Guadalupano Group) for ten years when she assumed the position of coordinator, dedicating herself more to the group "in order to do more things, and do them differently." As she explained, she had found the activities at Saint Pius "poor, lacking" in comparison to the festivities for the Virgin of Guadalupe back in Mexico. Both the pastor and the Guadalupano Group have supported her in her efforts to embellish and enrich the group's activities and the festival. The support Olivia has received in taking a creative and determinative role indicates the parish's commitment to empowering and promoting leadership among its parishioners. Moreover, by encouraging lay participation in the renewal and transformation of these rituals,[26] Saint Pius also supports its immigrant parishioners in the construction of their emerging ethnic identities—even though for some parishioners it may also contribute to the construction of a national Mexican identity.

While signs of Mexican popular religious expression are ubiquitous at Saint Pius, most practices and programs at the parish combine familiar elements from Mexico with features that are quite new to its immigrant parishioners. But the newness is not necessarily disorienting. Indeed, it is precisely this juxtaposition of the familiar with the strange that imbues those native traditions with a spiritual significance that guides immigrant parishioners toward new, specifically ethnic identities and dispositions. Saint Pius enacts its incarnational theology by focusing spirituality on social-justice issues that affect the parish community, as well as the neighborhood of Pilsen more generally. Thus, as Saint Pius offers parishioners a social location, spiritual mission, and ideological orientation, it also legitimizes an ethnic identity that is based in their local struggles as immigrants and in their experiences of oppression as a racialized minority.

This ethnically infused localism—the very aspect of immigrant parish culture that exists in tension with its claims to transcendence—is a particularly important dimension of how Saint Pius offers guidance and orientation to its immigrant parishioners. It tells them who they were, who they are, who they should become, and how to do so. In other words, Saint Pius "invents" ethnicity in the process of fulfilling its mission to serve an immigrant community, by engaging its parishioners in struggles for social justice. However, Saint Pius's model of ethnicization and its concomitant social/civic orientation may not be identical to parishioners' experiences and orientations as transnational migrants who maintain familial, social, and economic commitments to two communities, in and between two distinct cultural contexts.

Saint Pius was first established as an Irish parish in 1874. It had become predominantly Polish by the 1920s and served a primarily Polish congregation until the 1950s. During the 1960s, the Spanish-speaking membership of the parish was on the rise at the same time that the parish's and neighborhood's Eastern European residents were moving out along the suburban corridor. In 1972 a shrine in honor of the Virgin of Guadalupe was installed, further testimony to the growing presence of Mexican Americans within the parish. By the end of the 1960s, Spanish masses had been integrated into the regular parish schedule, as was true at other increasingly Hispanic parishes such as Saint Vitus and Saint Procopius. Their current prevalence belies the long and fierce struggle for Spanish-language masses, a local initiative that unified the Spanish-speaking Catholic newcomers of Pilsen in opposition to the Anglo Catholic establishment.[27]

The use of Spanish not only in masses but as the predominant language of parish life has a complex cultural significance in a transnational neighborhood like Pilsen, where recent immigrants share the block with established immigrants or second-generation Mexican Americans, many of whose children, bilingual and bicultural, are ambivalent about their "mother tongue." The presumption of a shared language in Mexico here becomes a vehicle both of continuity with the homeland and of community formation in the host society.[28] At the same time, the church as a sacred institution imbues the Spanish language (and, by extension, Hispanic cultures) with a legitimacy that is continually under assault by the dominant Anglophone society. Nonetheless, several clergy members we spoke with referred to the problems parishes have reaching out to "English-speaking" youth, which suggests that the construction of a monolingual Mexican ethnicity may not be as meaningful to Pilsen's youth as to their parents.

Parishioners at Saint Pius frequently commented that their pastor speaks Spanish "as if he were one of us," using language to symbolize the pastor's commitment to, and perhaps his ability to stand for, the parish as an ethnic community. While the pastor's language is comfortingly familiar, the ritual form and liturgical content of the masses express the parish's distinct subculture. The pastor's homilies have a consistently liberatory orientation, emphasizing social justice and community empowerment. Various aspects of the masses symbolize an egalitarian, participatory theology: the priest speaking from a podium located close to the pews, the inclusion of parishioners in the service, the occasional clapping from congregants—all features that are quite different from the masses Rosario attended at her village chapel in Mexico.

The masses also offer a clear symbolism of the parish's model of ethnicization. The liberationist liturgy draws frequent analogies between the spiritual and historical role of Jesus, Mexicans as an oppressed third-world people in struggle, and Mexican immigrants as an oppressed minority in the United States. These associations have commonly been drawn through allusion to the Zapatista movement in the Mexican state of Chiapas, a reference that encourages parishioners to generalize their associations beyond their ongoing ties to specific home communities (which for most are not located in Chiapas) to the struggles of the Mexican peasantry more generally. The liturgy also links parishioners both to a national Mexican immigrant community, for example, through references to repressive immigration legislation in California (specifically Proposition 187), and to a local Hispanic community, by calling for opposition to such legislation in Illinois.

The church's pastor, Father Charles Dahm, a Dominican priest, is one of the most important Catholic leaders in Pilsen and a leading figure on the Catholic Left in Chicago. Since coming to the parish, he has contin-ued to stimulate its growth while taking it in a direction more progressive than that of his predecessors. In "Religious Rituals and Class Formation," a study of ritual life and class struggle at the now-defunct Saint Vitus Parish, Robert Stark identifies the orientation of the Pilsen parishes ac-cording to a three-part typology of participation in social and political life: service, patronage, or protest. He characterizes Saint Pius in the early 1970s as being oriented toward patronage, due to its close affiliation with Mayor Richard J. Daley. Under its subsequent pastor it became more ser-vice oriented, and Fr. Dahm has continued this trend while incorporating a strong social-action dimension. If Saint Pius is not a "protest" type of parish, this may be a sign more of the politically conservative times than of the political position of the parish leadership.

In an interview, Fr. Dahm characterized his theology as "incarnational and nondualistic," the focus being on God as incarnated in the world—a vi-sion and orientation that appear to be enthusiastically respected and shared by the parish staff. While Fr. Dahm cautioned against any facile characteri-zation of the parish's orientation as one of "liberation theology," a libera-tionist spirit does undergird Saint Pius's primary identity, mission, and pur-pose: to integrate spirituality with social justice in a way that empowers the congregation and "builds community," as Fr. Dahm put it.

Despite Fr. Dahm's reluctance to reduce the theological orientation of Saint Pius to an Americanized liberation theology, we heard parish staff make frequent reference to the Latin American theological movement, which seemed to stand as a symbol for the "this-worldly," human rights focus of the parish's spiritual discourses and practices. This association is enhanced by the significant effort Saint Pius devotes to the development of activist-oriented block groups, commonly known in the Hispanic Catholic world as CEBs, *comunidades eclesiales de base* (base Christian communities). Despite the association in the United States of CEBs with Latin American Catholicism, few of Saint Pius's parishioners were famil-iar with liberation theology or its application through CEBs before their arrival at the Pilsen parish. The centrality of CEBs to the lifework of Saint Pius was clearly conveyed by the associate pastor, who described CEBs as the model of the parish. He also characterized CEBs as "Latin American," in order to signal a contrast between the suburban (and, implicitly, non-Hispanic) block groups, which focus on scripture study, and the CEBs or-ganized by the Hispanic churches, which are geared—like their Latin American counterparts—toward social action.

The CEB program enacts the parish's model for immigrant incorporation, organizing liberationist spiritual training around local struggles in a way that locates the participants simultaneously within a neighborhood community and an ethnic community. The organizational centrality of CEBs, coupled with the discourse of liberation theology, associates local social-justice struggles with religiously inspired grassroots liberation struggles in Latin America. By implication, it legitimizes a specifically Latin American radical Catholicism as the principal source of inspiration and guidance for the parish. The emphasis on liberation theology links Saint Pius symbolically to both the radical Catholic community in Latin America and the U.S. Hispanic Catholic community. Notably, the Hispanic Catholic community has actively and vocally embraced CEBs, with their this-worldly spirituality, as a propitious structural and symbolic framework for organizing Hispanic Catholics as an oppressed minority within the United States.[29]

Thus, while only a tenth of Saint Pius's parishioners are actively involved in CEBs, the CEBs' visibility and organizational centrality have several important effects: they focus parishioners spiritually, socially, and politically on local struggles; they legitimate those struggles theologically; they generalize and abstract ties to the homeland as ties to Latin America; and they contribute to the construction of a Catholic Hispanic ethnicity, by linking Saint Pius's CEBs to a wider, regional Hispanic CEB organization. While Fr. Dahm and several clergy acknowledged that the individual block groups were moving slowly through the stages from "seeing" to "social action," they had no doubts that the CEBs were effective in promoting communication, developing trust, and thus building community among parishioners. The staff also shared the perception that the CEBs functioned *to replace* the familial and fictive kin networks from which some parishioners apparently became dissociated in their migration to Chicago. And indeed, many parishioners establish local ties of godparenthood through participation in CEBs. For those parishioners, however, who maintain their connections with transnational networks of family, fictive kin (*compadrazgo*), and friends, one wonders whether the CEBs replace or supplement preexisting social networks, commitments, and identities.

An important moment in the ritual cycle at Saint Pius, and a vivid display of the construction and sacralization of ethnicity, is the nine-day festival (*novena*) honoring the Virgin of Guadalupe. This elaborate festival, celebrated in early December, is organized annually by the Devotional Group to Our Lady of Guadalupe, who is the patron saint of Mexico. The Virgin of Guadalupe is a symbol of Mexican nationalism who asserts a specifically Mexican, mestizo[30] culture, identity, and popular religious expression. As an apparition that came to the native "Indian" Juan Diego during the time of the Spanish Conquest, the Virgin of Guadalupe serves as a potent reminder that the origins of the Mexican people lie in the brutal history of conquest and colonization. Guadalupe is thus a religious icon laden with political, ethnic, and racial symbolism.

Members of the Devotional Group participate in the monthly Mass for the Virgin of Guadalupe, taking down the Virgin's banner and carrying it around the sanctuary in a small procession for the Virgin. On those Sundays they also sell candles and food after Mass. The money the Guadalupano Group raises funds the elaborate nine-day festival for the Virgin, traditionally celebrated with a feast and a mariachi band. Through the festival the parish establishes symbolic, social, and material ties to Mexico. For instance, they commission an elaborate altar; the one we saw was prepared by a man who was on a return trip to Mexico at the time of our study. Most years the group also brings a Mexican priest to preach during the *novena*. But the Devotional Group is particularly proud of the contribution it makes to its U.S. parish through its fund-raising efforts. Olivia, the group's coordinator, boasted to us that the previous year they had donated a new air conditioner to the parish.

In a homily at a *novena* mass for the Virgin of Guadalupe, Fr. Dahm drew on the politicized symbolism associated with Guadalupe to give meaning and direction to the lives and experiences of his parishioners: "Just as Jesus Christ came to include the oppressed, the marginalized, the foreigners, and the excluded, so did his mother come to do the same thing in the sixteenth century . . . and just as Juan Diego, inspired by the apparition of the Virgin, went out to work among the poor, the victims of the conquest, so were they to follow the teachings of Jesus Christ and organize against the oppressions of modern-day conquest, such as NAFTA [the North American Free Trade Agreement]. Just as the Spanish treated indigenous people like animals, so do Mexicans in the U.S. think little of themselves, because of the oppression that prevails in our land." Then the pastor made reference to California's Proposition 187 and described recent incidents of racist violence against Mexican migrants.

Moving back and forth between an emphasis on poverty and on culture (ethnicity), weaving himself in and out of the discourse by alternating the pronouns *you* and *we,* the pastor effectively linked and legitimized class and ethnic identities, integrating class struggle with the battle for cultural recognition and ethnic equality. His analogic narrative effectively transposed Guadalupe, a symbol of Mexican national identity, into a symbol of Mexican American ethnic identity.

As we can see, when Saint Pius integrates spirituality, community-focused struggles for justice, and ethnicity, it offers its parishioners two distinct but not mutually exclusive ethnic identities: as Mexican Americans and as Hispanic Americans. Each of these is associated with functional and meaningful collectivities into which the parish facilitates its parishioners' entry. Importantly, the assimilation of a Hispanic and/or Mexican American identity becomes linked to a disposition toward *locally* based problems and struggles, although the possibilities of community-building and empowerment would seem to imply identification and collective engagement as ethnic *Americans*. In thinking beyond the parish subculture to its impact on parishioners, however, we should bear in mind that the mononational identities and localized orientations these activities assume and encourage may be in tension with the many local identities, affiliations, and commitments parishioners take on as participants in transnational migratory circuits.

Emmanuel Presbyterian Church: A Hispanic Christian Family in Faith

Emmanuel Presbyterian Church is an evangelically oriented, self-identified Hispanic church, unusual theologically for a Presbyterian congregation, and unusual among Pilsen's Protestant churches in that it has a burgeoning membership, with much of its growth due to successful evangelization within Pilsen.

The proximity of Emmanuel and Saint Pius belies a theologically and politically adversarial relationship, while their dramatically contrasting architectures convey distinct relationships to the neighborhood. The accessibility of Saint Pius's rather modest and unimposing architecture is matched by its policy of leaving its doors open "twenty-four hours a day" in order to be a home, shelter, and sanctuary to the community. Emmanuel's modern building and tall metal fence, by contrast, set it apart while implicitly indexing the dangerous nature of the neighborhood. Approached from the street by a metal gate, long sidewalk, and well-groomed lawn, the church conveys an inviting residential comfort while connoting a social class status that is strikingly distinct from the immediate neighborhood. The sanctuary, built in 1965, has a complex and free-flowing design, intended by the architect to convey "both a welcoming and protective shelter"[31]—qualities expressive of the distinction between Emmanuel's relationship to its congregation and to the neighborhood. Thus, where Saint Pius emphasizes its continuity with the larger community of Pilsen, Emmanuel constructs itself as a community of faith by serving and reaching out to Pilsen's residents while distancing itself from the geographic neighborhood.

Emmanuel's pastor, the Reverend Rolando Cuellar, a Peruvian with a Pentecostal background, is a warm, intelligent, and rather charismatic man in his mid- to late forties. Rev. Cuellar first came to Emmanuel in 1983, while a student at McCormick Theological Seminary in Chicago. At the time there were only thirty people worshiping at the church. Soon after, when the congregation's student pastor, (it had no regular pastor) graduated and went to Dallas, Rev. Cuellar was invited to serve as Emmanuel's student pastor, and later as its full-time pastor. The decisive role of the congregation with regard to its leadership signals its democratic, nonhierarchical organizational structure, a hallmark of U.S. Presbyterianism and Anglo Protestant religious culture—a quality that contrasts with the decidedly hierarchical Catholic Church and the patriarchal nature of Latin American societies.

Rev. Cuellar has revitalized the congregation: he brought the church out of debt, and under his leadership membership has grown steadily, primarily through a vigorous evangelization campaign waged in the neighborhood of Pilsen. In 1994, Emmanuel had a growing congregation of 120 members, with close to two hundred people overall attending the Sunday worship service, overflowing the sanctuary. In fact, the congregation had built up its membership to such an extent that they were actively looking for a larger building—one that would house not only an expanding congregation but also a variety of programs their current location could not contain. This effort constituted one of Emmanuel's principal ministries, known as "Pro Templo."

Although the pastor and lay leaders involved in the ministry preferred to relocate within Pilsen, they eventually chose to move to a nearby suburb, one with a substantial and growing Hispanic population who tend to be more affluent and settled than Pilsen's residents. The decision, however, appeared to have been made for financial rather than demographic reasons; in relocating, Emmanuel opted to occupy a space within an "American" Presbyterian church, as described by the pastor. In conversations about the

Fig. 2-3. Youth group of Iglesia Presbiteriana Emanuel of Pilsen, performing while on a visit to a church in suburban Wheeling, Illinois. Photo courtesy of Iglesia Presbiteriana Emanuel.

move before and after it took place, Rev. Cuellar focused on control and administration of the space but did not mention the ethnic composition of the host congregation. Nonetheless, the congregation still evangelizes in Pilsen and offers social programs to the community, and Rev. Cuellar continues to preach at the Pilsen sanctuary.

That ethnicity did not play an explicit role in the congregation's decision about location attests to its vision or worldview. As Rev. Cuellar put it, "The main focus of the church is first to proclaim the message of Christ and provide peace and hope for the people." Thus, unlike Saint Pius, Emmanuel does not link its status as an immigrant congregation explicitly to its theology or mission. Nor does it directly implicate its model of ethnicization in its statement of mission. Nonetheless, through its ritual life, social programs, ministries, and missions, Emmanuel enacts and expresses a particular Hispanic ethnicity that is intimately related to the model of ethnicization the church presumes for its actual and potential congregants. By projecting certain values, identities, and social orientations for its members, Emmanuel incorporates them into a larger Hispanic Christian "family in Christ," offering them both an ethnic community and identity within the U.S. mainstream.

Emmanuel's faithful represent a diversity of national backgrounds, including Mexicans, Central Americans, Puerto Ricans, and South Americans. The diversity of Emmanuel's congregation is a quality that Rev. Cuellar pointed out to us with apparent pride during our initial interview. This emphasis on national diversity contributes to the construction of *Hispanic* ethnicity as a collective identification that homogenizes and abstracts the varied social and political experiences of those it incorporates.[32] In distinction to nationally referential ethnic constructions such as "Mexicano" or "Mexican American," the construction of a Hispanic ethnicity focuses collective identification away from the country of origin (and thus away from nationally specific native traditions) and toward an abstract community created in the host country. As we will see, where Saint Pius constructs Hispanicity in part through a spiritual and political association with Latin America, Emmanuel constructs a thoroughly U.S. Hispanic ethnicity.

Nonetheless, the majority of Emmanuel's congregants are first-generation immigrants from Mexico. And while a significant number of Emmanuel's Mexican members commute to attend Emmanuel, many of them once lived in Pilsen and have familial ties to the neighborhood. Take Lucia, for instance. She was born and raised in Pilsen by immigrant Mexican parents who came from a town not far from Rosario's native village in Michoacán. Lucia and her Salvadoran husband moved out of Pilsen to a "better neighborhood" in 1992, one year after they'd joined Emmanuel. Nonetheless, Lucia still feels ties to Pilsen and its residents. Even though she is native to this country, Lucia explained, she feels she has a lot in common with "the Mexican community." "Sometimes I'm in the middle. I understand the position of older people who have lived here a long time, but I also understand the younger ones." She likes being in this position: "*Agarro dos mundos*" ("I take hold of two worlds,") she said. Lucia's comments convey her identification with Pilsen and with the Mexican community more generally, as well as a bicultural sensibility expressed by the notion of "taking hold of two worlds."

In a sense, Lucia's position differs from her church's disposition toward Pilsen and toward the immigrant Mexican community more generally. As a Hispanic Christian congregation, Emmanuel has an ambivalent relationship with Pilsen's Mexican residents. On the one hand, it differentiates the church from those Pilseners who, as Catholics, are "Others"; on the other hand it identifies itself with them, both as "potential

Christians" and as Hispanics. Unlike a national parish like Saint Pius, which asserts the *Mexican-ness* of its parishioners ritually and discursively, Emmanuel Presbyterian downplays its members' national identities and negates native traditions, constructing instead a Hispanic Christian identity for its congregants. Emmanuel constructs this ethnicity through both negation and affirmation. It negates a nationally based ethnicity, linking conversion (to Protestant Christianity) to a rupture with former religious beliefs and nationally specific cultural affiliations. Where Saint Pius embraces its members' native traditions, Emmanuel eschews them, precisely because of the intimate interconnection between Mexican popular culture and Catholicism. More than one lay leader at Emmanuel made the point that "they [Mexican Catholics] don't distinguish between religion and tradition." Particularly striking is the relationship congregants drew between the process of ethnicization and that of religious conversion. Not only were both figured as processes of rupture and rediscovery, but they also were causally linked. Lucia made this relationship explicit in our conversation. She said that "being here [in the United States], with time people begin to realize the connection between Hispanic culture and Catholicism. . . . With time they go through a rediscovery of what are the legitimate traditions."

At the same time, the congregational subculture of Emmanuel affirms and reinforces its congregants' Hispanicity through myriad aspects of its ritual, educational, and organizational life. To begin with, despite a substantial bilingual presence, Emmanuel conducts all its services in Spanish. As Chicana poet Gloria Anzaldúa puts it, "Language is twin-skin to identity";[33] and a congregation's choice of language is a forceful and formative symbol of its worldview. In the case of Emmanuel, it attests not only to its identification as a Hispanic congregation but also to its evangelizing orientation toward recent immigrants.

Nonetheless, as Lucia signaled in her identification of a *generational* distinction between the positions of the older and younger immigrant populations, Emmanuel faces the challenge of reconciling the differences between more settled and more recent immigrants, on the one hand, and between immigrant parents and their second-generation, bilingual, and bicultural children. In our conversations with Rev. Cuellar and lay leaders, this challenge was often expressed in terms of language. In fact, discussion of increased incorporation of English into worship services and religious education carried a certain urgency. The pastor explained that the services held by young people were bilingual because the youth preferred to speak English—although he added that "they are open because we also have young people who recently came from Mexico; they also speak in Spanish at home." While this ready embracing of English might suggest a more assimilationist perspective at Emmanuel than we encountered at Saint Pius, the difference may also reflect responses to distinct constituencies: where Saint Pius serves a constantly replenished population of recent immigrants and transmigrants, Emmanuel's membership ranges from recent immigrants to second-generation and settled first-generation immigrants who use English in their daily lives.

Many other features of Emmanuel's congregational life attest to the centrality of Hispanic ethnicity. For instance, the congregation belongs to the Hispanic Council within the Presbyterian Church, a body composed of lay and pastoral representatives who discuss the specific needs of the Hispanic community. Emmanuel devotes attention to those needs programmatically through worship services it holds on issues of discrimination and immigration. Emmanuel also participates in worship services with other Hispanic Christian churches in the metropolitan area. Finally, while Emmanuel does not emphasize explicit ties to Latin America through religious symbology and iconography, it does carry on formal interchanges with Latin American preachers. The relationship between ethnicity and spirituality at Emmanuel, however, is carefully bounded. The church's festival calendar, for instance, is distinctly not Latin American but rather (Anglo) American. In addition to the religious holidays of Christmas and Easter, the congregation celebrates Thanksgiving, Mother's Day, and New Year's Day—three thoroughly U.S. American *secular* holidays that are imbued with familial significance. Thus Emmanuel's ritual calendar expresses the congregation's model of ethnicization: the incorporation of mainstream, Anglo American traditions as integral to the construction of a Hispanic American lifestyle.

For several lay leaders we spoke with, it was not the tenets of Presbyterianism per se that attracted them to Emmanuel but rather a union of spiritual and interpersonal qualities that they had found lacking in their specific parish or in Catholicism more generally. Lucia told us that she preferred Emmanuel's more fundamentalist approach to scripture and the greater emphasis on reading and studying the Bible in its entirety. Lucia admitted to an early wariness as she described her initial response to the lively religious services, which had seemed loud and raucous compared to the more sober and restrained Catholic masses to which she was accustomed. But now, Lucia admitted timidly, she even likes the drumming, the rock music, and the pastor's bold preaching style—ritual practices that certainly produce an intense spirit of communality.

But the qualities Lucia most emphasized were interpersonal: communication among congregants and between pastor and the congregation, a spirit of caring and warmth that she had found absent at the more anonymous parish, and a sense not only of belonging but of being needed. "Here everyone has a role, a function," she commented. Notably, Lucia and other congregants we spoke with drew on the image of *family* to convey this combined sense of belonging and intimacy. This is not incidental. A leaflet passed out before Sunday services offers the following invitation to newcomers: "If you do not have a church, make Emmanuel your family in faith" (*si no tiene una iglesia, haga de la Iglesia Emanuel su familia en la fe*). And indeed Emmanuel, whose membership is made up primarily of families, forms a congregation that is essentially a network of families. Moreover, congregants seem to have a primary identity as members of that church; the church's identity as Presbyterian seems to be relatively unimportant and is certainly secondary to its identity as a Hispanic Christian evangelical church.

Indeed, family is the central theme running through the liturgy, program discourse, and ministry at Emmanuel. Church social events and celebrations tend to be organized around the family. The appeal of secular festivals such as Mother's Day and Thanksgiving can be understood in part in terms of their familial orientation. The church also assists its needy members on an individual or family basis (offering economic assistance, clothing, employment, counseling), rather than through participation in grassroots struggles that would locate church members within an oppressed community of Hispanics and/or "the poor."

Family issues and problems are the focus for many church ministries, including the women's club, the ministry for couples, the youth club, and the children's club. Of these ministries, the most extensive are the youth group and the children's club. The Club de Niños en Acción (Club for Children in Action) is a weekend program offering Bible study, educational and recreational activities, and a meal for children under thirteen years of age. As one club volunteer explained, the children's club was promoted with the needs of the community in mind, "to serve the community where the church resides." Of the sixty enrolled children, most are from the community. The program director noted that, while some parents have joined the church because of the quality of the program, its purpose is not to evangelize but rather to teach the children to "grow with a love of God, with positive goals, not thinking about things like gangs."

The youth group is essentially a continuation of the children's club, with a strong leadership-development component. The group meets weekly to talk, support one another, and plan a range of activities, including a youth worship service, field trips, Presbyterian Church youth retreats, and "spiritual campaigns" such as the annual "street festival," a worship service held each summer and intended to reach out to youth in the community. Several youth see their group as an alternative to gangs because it provides the kind of peer support and sense of family that youth who join gangs are looking for. In our conversations, youth emphasized the supportive sense of family, as well as social and spiritual growth, that group participation gives them.

While Emmanuel constitutes itself symbolically as a "family in Christ," structurally it is made up of a close-knit network of mostly nuclear families, many of whom seem to find their primary identification with the church. While several people we spoke to rejected Mexican culture out of hand as being inextricably bound to Catholicism, they commented that the primacy given to family was a positive quality found in "Hispanic culture" more generally. One lay leader associated the ability to discern between the positive values within Hispanic culture and the negative ones—such as *machismo*—with the process of spiritual rediscovery. In this sense, Emmanuel contributes to the construction of a Hispanic Christian ethnicity based on familial roles and identities that fit squarely within the U.S. mainstream.

As we can see, Emmanuel offers its members a location within an ethnically defined spiritual community that is wholly derived from shared religious practices (be they devotional or social), rather than from a shared neighborhood or shared struggles as oppressed immigrants, as is the case for Saint Pius's parishioners. However, Pilsen is hardly irrelevant to the construction of ethnicity at Emmanuel. To the extent that congregants work together to help a poor Hispanic neighborhood, their engagement with the geographic community—through the children's club, ministry to the local jail, distribution of food and clothing—further unites the congregation in common cause or mission. Yet these outreach efforts, as they are called, maintain the neighborhood at a distance, as the object of good works and evangelization. Moreover, Emmanuel's pluralistic, evangelical subculture is thoroughly at odds with the transnational subculture of Pilsen. Where Saint Pius's vision of ethnicization may unintentionally and indirectly support a transnational orientation by encouraging symbolic, political, and material ties to Mexico, Emmanuel constructs a Hispanic American ethnicity for its congregation on the basis of spiritual severance from those ties.

What does this comparison of two immigrant churches that are radically different—theologically, ideologically, politically, and culturally—suggest about their roles in the construction of ethnicity? To begin with, it highlights the distinct subcultures that can emerge at the intersection of a church's vision of ethnicity and its theological and political positions. Moreover, because the churches themselves constitute distinct subcultures, they also contribute to the construction of distinct ethnicities, despite the fact that both churches evangelize and serve Mexican immigrants and that both are tied into wider Hispanic religious networks. And while both churches assume and espouse positions of ethnic pluralism, their pluralistic visions and related models of ethnicity are ideologically quite distinct, as evidenced by the dramatically different strategies they adopt to guide and assist their members in making the social, civic, and psychic transition from immigrants to ethnics.

However, when examined in relation to the transmigratory circuit that incorporates Pilsen and its residents into its socioeconomic and cultural flows, a striking commonality emerges through the two churches' differences, namely, their *unidirectional* vision of immigration and ethnicization: both churches expect that settlement and incorporation into the host society entail a process of becoming an ethnic *American;* both churches are intent on helping their members make that transition; and both churches prefigure their members' struggles on that basis. Conversely, neither church actively supports the transmigratory lifestyle or culture of their members or the neighborhood, although either church may do so indirectly and unintentionally. It will be the task of further research to discern the ways in which these spiritually imbued visions of ethnicization are taken up by Pilsen's residents as they fashion their various collectivities and identities.

NOTES

1. Though it is often criticized as an assimilationist label, I use the term *Hispanic* rather than *Latino* because of its predominance in the spoken and written discourses of both churches. See Moore, "'Hispanic/Latino'"; Padilla, *Latino Ethnic Consciousness.*

2. Research for this chapter was conducted by Susana Angélica Bañuelos and myself.

3. Wind and Lewis, *American Congregations,* vol. 2, 6–7.

4. Omi and Winant, *Racial Formation,* 15.

5. Conzen et al., "Invention of Ethnicity," 4–5.

6. Ibid., 8.

7. Sánchez, *Becoming Mexican American,* 6–7.

8. Adelman, *Pilsen and the West Side,* 4–5; Stark, "Religious Ritual and Class Formation," 27.

9. Stark, "Religious Ritual and Class Formation," 27–31.

10. Liptak, *Immigrants and Their Church,* 117–118; Castelli and Gremillion, *Emerging Parish,* 15.

11. See D'Agostino, chapter 11 in this book.

12. Díaz-Stevens and Stevens-Arroyo, *Recognizing the Latino Resurgence.*

13. Rouse, "Questions of Identity"; Schiller, Basch, and Blanc, "From Immigrant to Transmigrant"; Oboler, *Ethnic Labels, Latino Lives,* 88; Rouse, "Mexican Migration." For the Chicago case, see Farr, "Language, Culture, and Literacy."

14. Massey et al., *Return to Aztlan,* 6.

15. From interviews with congregants and parishioners, and data from Marcia Farr's research on transmigrant family networks based in Pilsen (personal communication with Farr, Evanston, IL, May 16, 1999). See also Orellana and Thorne, "Year-Round Schools," 464.

16. Orellana and Thorne, "Year-Round Schools," 285–314.

17. Rouse, "Mexican Migration," 16.

18. From Pilsen Catholic Cluster, "Our Vision," Chicago May 1993.

19. Stark, "Religious Ritual and Class Formation," 210–211.

20. Pilsen Resurrection Development Corporation (PRDC), "Mission Statement," Chicago 1994. (The PRDC was merged into the Resurrection Project the same year.)

21. McGreevy, *Parish Boundaries,* 27.

22. Díaz-Stevens and Stevens-Arroyo, *Recognizing the Latino Resurgence,* 205–206.

23. Gilkey, "Christian Congregation"; Castelli and Gremillion, *Emerging Parish.*

24. See Conzen et al., "Invention of Ethnicity," 22–23.

25. Liptak, *Immigrants and Their Church.*

26. See Bass, "Congregations and the Bearing of Traditions," 170.

27. Stark, "Religious Ritual and Class Formation," 170–172.

28. See Hunter, *Symbolic Communities,* 67.

29. Sandoval, *On the Move.*

30. *Mestizo/a* refers to the racial mixture of indigenous and Spanish. Recognition of and pride in mestizo ancestry and culture has been an important dimension in the development of contemporary Mexican national identity.

31. Adelman, *Pilsen and the West Side,* 58.

32. Oboler, *Ethnic Labels, Latino Lives,* 3.

33. Anzaldúa, *Borderlands/ La Frontera,* 74.

Map 3. The greater Near North area includes Chicago's greatest concentration of wealth and power only a few blocks from the "ghetto poverty" of Cabrini Green public housing. Map by Brain Twardosz, BMT Printing and Cartographic Specialists.

Place, Race, and History
The Social Mission of Downtown Churches

Matthew J. Price

The prestigious downtown churches of the Loop and greater Near North Side have a unique place in the religious landscape of Chicago. They serve their immediate neighborhoods, and their congregations reflect the increasingly affluent and predominantly white population of the area. They also serve the larger metropolitan area, drawing on a religious constituency with an unprecedented willingness to travel in search of the church that serves their needs. In this they share certain characteristics with suburban megachurches outside Chicago, such as Willow Creek Community Church in suburban Barrington. But the central location of the downtown churches means that they address the city as a whole in a way that other churches do not: they are, symbolically and sometimes literally, the city's cathedrals.[1]

Like the prestigious "signature" buildings of architects that define the skyline of downtown, these churches are signature religious buildings at the heart of the city. For example, First United Methodist Church, Chicago Temple, the city's oldest congregation, is situated right across from City Hall. The building, according to church literature, "combines the grace of the French gothic with the practicality of an American skyscraper." With its Sky Chapel, spire, and twelve foot-high cross at its peak, the 568-foot structure is considered to be the world's tallest church building, "a beacon to the city." Like the European cathedrals that inspired its architecture, the Methodist temple, along with the other downtown churches, attempts by its physical presence to ordain with religious meaning the sense that the city as a whole has of itself.

Many of the churches studied in this chapter came of age at the beginning of the twentieth century with the rise of the corporation and its downtown headquarters. The civic-minded philanthropy of their members sought to create the epicenter of a "great city" that would present to the world the city's power and prestige and that of its professional-managerial class as one and the same. But philanthropists and advocates of the Social Gospel also attempted to fashion the image of the city as a single, corporate entity by reaching across the boundaries of class, race, and nationality through highly visible acts of compassion and social redemption. It is this combination of centrality, concentration of power and prestige, and acts of compassion articulating a responsibility for the city as a whole that still defines these churches of the downtown Loop and Near North Side.[2]

While many downtown churches in other cities have struggled, Chicago possesses a remarkable set of vibrant and strong center-city churches that not only show no signs of decline but are confident about their future growth and prospects. If, as Lyle E. Schaller claims with regard to downtown churches, "only a fraction are large, strong, vital, future-minded, and exciting congregations that today are able to attract new generations of church goers," then it seems that Chicago has a disproportionate number of such cases.[3] Nevertheless, the success of these churches is dependent on an unpredictable balance of the contradictory forces of center-city revitalization and urban decay. The churches need the former to maintain their affluent congregations and influential place within the city, but the latter also is a key part of their historic sense of mission and purpose. The churches are in control of neither force, and while from the mid-1960s through the late 1980s it looked as if the downtown churches might be overwhelmed by the forces of urban decay, in the late 1990s it was, ironically, the force of downtown revitalization that promised to transform the mission fields of these churches, removing the adjacent neighborhoods as objects of philanthropy.

Because the large downtown churches are predominantly affluent and white and the adjacent neighborhoods are predominantly poor and black, the issue of race is ever present in the churches, although rarely in the simple form of a dialectical opposition of two groups. A combination of sometimes contradictory desires and forces has created a complex racial dynamic. First, the churches' outreach theology is based on the possibility of societal redemption through a social transformation brought about by the ameliorative impact of church programs on the individual lives of the poor and, for some churches, by the advocacy of public policies that will help the poor in collective terms. Yet after thirty years of operation, the urban ministry programs begun in the late 1960s and early 1970s seem no nearer to achieving their goal of ending poverty. The seeming intractability of the problems of the urban poor has led to the construction of larger programs and the creation of a large pool of volunteers who have little or no relationship with the churches. Such programs have also led to the recruitment of full-time program staff, some of whom seem to have concluded that the problems of these areas might indeed be unsolvable. Second, the outreach theology of these prestige churches charges them to maintain their place as centers of civic leadership while also being servant churches to poor minority communities. In fulfilling this vision of a servant church, the churches have given autonomy to the programs and their administrators, some of whom see the wider white society in which the churches operate as having interests that are fundamentally opposed to the poor black communities the programs serve.

Thus powerful, mainly white churches are connected to their proximate poor black communities by a host of large outreach programs, but the connection is not a direct one. Standing between them are the army of volunteers from outside the church as well as the program staff, whose ideas about the programs can be radically different from those presented to the congregation from the pulpit. The mediating role of the volunteers allows the churches symbolically to construct their large programs as redemptive, transformative, and racially integrative while signifying the continued importance of the church in the city. But because most members of the congregation do not see the programs in action over a sustained period, they neither experience the doubts of the full-time workers nor discover the guiding philosophies of some of the programs.

The complex racial dynamic that characterizes these churches is a product of their history, one they share with many other predominantly white downtown churches in America. It has molded their sense of place and space, their role in civic leadership, and their vision of their mission to the poor and downtrodden, all of which have been, and are still, shaped by wider forces of urban restructuring.

An Overview of the Area and Its Congregations

Chicago's combined Loop and greater Near North area includes the Loop and the Near North Side, as well as the community area of Lincoln Park and the southern census tracts of Lakeview (See Map 3). Because of gen-trification, this area constitutes an almost unbroken block of business employment and residential affluence running from Roosevelt Road in the south, along the lakefront in the east, to Belmont Avenue in the north, with a western boundary that varies from Wells Street at its southern end to Ashland Avenue at its northern end. Alongside this sphere of affluence lies Cabrini Green, a public housing development occupying twenty blocks in the western third of the Near North community area. While Cabrini Green is racially and economically segregated from the Loop and the greater Near North, the outreach efforts of the downtown churches are a significant point of connection. These areas—the Loop, the greater Near North, Cabrini Green, and the Near West Side—taken together make up a functionally integrated system for the churches, sustaining their sense of place and purpose. The Loop sustains a large professional-managerial class, many of whom reside in the greater Near North area, providing a demographic base for the churches.[4] Cabrini Green and the Near West Side, in turn, are the mission fields for these churches, allow-ing them to sustain their claims to stand symbolically for the city as a whole.

In the Loop and Near North area, the Religion in Urban America Pro-gram conducted a comprehensive survey of all religious institutions listed in phone books and directories. We then selected six churches as sites for in-depth case studies and carried out interviews or observations at eight more.

In the mid-1990's—the time of our study—Fourth Presbyterian was a church of more than three thousand members, situated along Michigan Avenue's "Magnificent Mile." The church describes itself as "a light in the city," attempting urban ministry through large-scale programs for the residents of the Cabrini Green public housing development, with whom it sees itself as sharing the neighborhood.

Old Saint Patrick's Church (the focus of chapter 9), with a member-ship of fifteen hundred, sees itself as a "crossroads" where people from all over the city can meet in an atmosphere that exudes warm hospitality and a strong sense of Christian service. Its Community Outreach Group has five hundred members and sponsors seven ongoing sites and a half dozen periodic activities, including two Franciscan homeless shelters, an athletic program for Hispanic youth, and adult literacy programs at one Catholic and two non-Catholic locations.

The 950-member First United Methodist Church, Chicago Temple, has led a coalition of churches in a successful campaign for the construction of a single-occupancy hotel in the southern part of the downtown to ease the problems of homelessness.

LaSalle Street Church stands as a "bridging church" between the affluent Gold Coast and the public housing development of Cabrini Green. While the church has only 350 members, it was been the driving force in the creation of two affordable housing complexes near the church and has founded two high-profile ministries on the North Side, the Cabrini Legal Aid Clinic and the Community Youth Creative Learning Experience.

Moody Church, built in honor of the Chicago evangelist Dwight L. Moody, is the largest evangelical church in central Chicago, with more than fifteen hundred members. Although in the 1960s it considered a move out to the suburbs, as the area around the church was deteriorating, the church has benefited from adjacent gentrification and is once again solidly established in the city.

The Episcopal Cathedral of Saint James, seat of the Episcopal Diocese, lies just off Michigan Avenue's Magnificent Mile. This congregation of five hundred members saw its halcyon days during the Progressive Era, when it was a leader in social reform movements. It now operates a food pantry and a homeless shelter for men, contributes money and volunteers to a women's homeless shelter, and has an AIDS outreach ministry. At Saint James, a simple black cross, about eight feet high, stands in the cathedral plaza, where it was dedicated at Easter 1994. On it the cathedral inscribed the names of all the children who were murdered in Chicago in the previous year. Shoppers from Michigan Avenue frequently pause for a few moments by the cross. The cross and the outreach activities listed above show how the downtown churches challenge people to reach across the barriers of race and class as the churches seek the welfare of the city as a whole.

We also made on-site observations or conducted face-to-face interviews at Holy Name Cathedral, the center of the Chicago Catholic Archdiocese; Park Community Church, a member of the Willow Creek Association; Saint Paul's Lutheran Church; Saint Joseph's Catholic Church and School; Saint Luke's Church of God in Christ; and Saint Matthew's United Methodist Church, the last two of which are African American churches with strong outreach programs to Cabrini Green. In addition, we conducted interviews with organizations based in the Cabrini Green area that are involved in outreach projects.

An Evolving Racial Dynamic: Power, Responsibility, and Community

The downtown churches have historically been the places of worship for the powerful and influential citizens who lived on Chicago's Gold Coast. In *The Gold Coast and the Slum,* Harvey Zorbaugh saw the Gold Coast as "the only element in the city's life that sees the city as a whole, dreams dreams for it as a whole."[5] For Zorbaugh, these were the people who had built the city, whose "imaginations play with its future."[6] Unlike the residents of Little Sicily, now Cabrini Green, or the lodgers in "world of furnished rooms," whom Zorbaugh saw as "merely part of the landscape," "the Gold Coast has, as no other group, a sense of its . . . responsibility for the future of the city."[7]

The discourse of the destiny of the city and the responsibility of its leading citizens was heavily tinged with religious imagery. The Chicago Fire of 1871 was pictured as a divinely sent time of trial, which had ushered in a period of reform that would lead to Chicago achieving the destiny God had planned for it.[8] In 1893, British journalist William T. Stead posed the provocative question: "If Christ came to Chicago what would he wish me to do?"[9] The formation of the Chicago Civic Federation, which included such notables as Marshall Field, Cyrus McCormick, Albion Small, Jane Addams, and the pastor of Moody Church, was a direct response to Stead's revelations of poverty and squalor in Chicago's poorest neighborhoods.[10] His call to action was grounded in the growing turn-of-the-century interest in the social dimension of Christianity. This was also reflected in the ethos of Fourth Presbyterian Church, which Marilee Munger Scroggs sees as seeking to "provide for the welfare not only of church members but of whole cities."[11]

The 1890s saw the start of the tutoring programs at Fourth Presbyterian, with Cyrus McCormick Jr., among others, spending Saturday evenings tutoring immigrant men.[12] These programs expanded during the Progressive Era, and in 1913, *The Continent,* a Chicago religious journal, commented, "The great mission of Fourth Church will be to grapple with the conditions by which it is surrounded."[13] The underlying assumption in all such efforts was that wealthy native Protestants would remain in control of the destiny of the city. The great city that would be formed by the stewardship of Chicago's leading citizens would benefit all, regardless of race or ethnicity. But these visions of the city as a manifestation of God's Kingdom were not pluralistic; rather, they had within them an implicit Protestant triumphalism and an unquestioned leadership by the "enlightened," who were white, native, and Protestant.

While the downtown churches exhibit strong patterns of continuity with the Progressive Era, the 1960s brought about significant modifications to the churches' missions and their theological underpinnings. The demographic shift on the city's Near North and Near West Side, from a population that was predominantly made up of working-class white ethnics to one of poor unemployed African Americans, meant that the outreach efforts of the downtown churches now involved the crossing of racial as well as class boundaries. While the sense of insecurity that came with this change was new to many once-powerful churches, it also allowed them to articulate a mission that was more urgent and attractive to a younger generation of Christians, raised in the Civil Rights era. These churches also realized that meeting the needs of this population would require a much greater effort on their part.[14]

A 1967 report prepared under the direction of Pastor George Sweeting for the board of Moody Church, which had just a few years earlier considered leaving the city altogether, called for much greater involvement in Cabrini Green:

> We would strongly recommend that Moody Church make plans to minister to the nearly 20,000 Negroes . . . who live within the shadow of the church. . . . It seems inconceivable to us that a church that sends $1,000,000.00 a year to evangelize people of another color miles across the sea can ignore them on their back porch.[15]

It was also during the 1960s, under the pastorship of Elam Davies, that many of Fourth Presbyterian's current outreach programs were started, and it was during the early 1970s, under the Reverend Bill Leslie's leadership, that LaSalle's main ministries were initiated—Community Youth Creative Learning Experience, or CYCLE; the Cabrini Green Legal Aid Clinic; the Near North Counseling Center (now the Center for Life Skills); Young Life at LaSalle; and the ministry to seniors, including a senior housing development. The five ministries formed during the first fifteen years of Bill Leslie's pastorate account for all but one of the current outreach ministries of LaSalle.[16]

The 1960s brought the agenda of the Civil Rights movement, with its calls for racial inclusion, equality, and greater opportunity.[17] Churches were not simply to reach down with assistance to those in the adjacent communities but to make their congregations racially and economically inclusive, placing the task of racial integration in the forefront of the churches' social agenda. The churches were also asked to respect the integrity of those who lived in poor communities and to include those communities as neighbors and equals in the task of community renewal. Writers on urban ministry continue to stress the importance of this partnership approach, with programs envisioned as a means of creating a single community rather than a world of servers and clients, an ideal to which the churches in Chicago's downtown still adhere.[18]

In the late 1960s the rise of the community-organizing movement among the Protestant mainline churches, operating under the conviction that a maximum degree of autonomy should be given to community-based organizations, brought with it a cadre of program leaders who saw the existing church as an encumbrance to the progress of the communities they were serving.[19] Activist-scholar John McKnight warned against church people who had been "misled by the modern secular vision." He asked:

> Have they substituted the vision of service for the only thing that will make people whole—community? Are they service peddlers or community builders? Peddling services is unchristian—even if you're hellbent on helping people. Peddling services instead of building communities is the one way you can be sure not to help.[20]

Churches were asked to question their established practices, with the voices of the poor, now empowered by community organizing, acting as "a sorely needed check on the self-centeredness and sin which Christians should know infect all their most well meaning and charitable actions."[21]

In the late 1960s and the 1970s encounters between the activists, who saw themselves on the front lines of the fight for social justice, and the established church membership proved to be contentious and difficult. Those encounters rarely occur today, having been replaced by what theologian Langdon Gilkey has described as a "conspiracy of silence" about these contentious issues; and as we shall see, those working with church programs in poor communities may still have very different views from those espoused by their congregations.[22] The wall of separation between the thoughts and feelings of the congregations, on the one hand, and the attitudes of both those who run the programs and those who benefit from them, on the other, has been reinforced by the professionalization of urban ministry, with full-time staff assuming the major responsibilities, an intellectual subculture of urban ministry with its own institutes

and centers, and the bureaucratization that has come with the need to so-
licit steady sources of funds from beyond the church in order to maintain
the programs.[23]

This separation has meant that the issues and problems that each new
mission theology raises have remained largely unresolved and have rarely
surfaced at the congregational level. Instead, each stage of mission theology has overlain the previous one without the churches having to face the
potentially contradictory nature of these commitments. These complexities define the organizational cultures of many downtown churches. A
historic sense of responsibility for the city as a whole, based in a Progressive Era sense of civic leadership, is now combined with a Civil Rights era
orientation, predicated on equality, service, and inclusiveness, directed
toward the predominantly poor African American residents of adjacent
communities. The churches also try to follow some of the precepts of the
community-organizing model by giving the maximum level of autonomy
to the organizations they sponsor within the community, which leads to a
separation from the congregation.

The bounded nature of Cabrini Green as a mission field made it possible for us to gain some sense of the overall level of outreach to this area.
The churches that we studied are immensely effective practitioners of social ministry, and it is because of the "success" of their projects, as understood from the standpoint of urban ministry studies, that the findings of
our research in the Cabrini Green area point to some striking anom-
alies.[24] Our views of the Cabrini area came from interviews with the
salaried program officers, some of whom are white and some of whom
are African American. Through these interviews we noted three other
main actors: the residents of Cabrini Green, the church congregations,
and the program volunteers.

Cabrini Green: Place and Programs

The Cabrini Green public housing development lies in the western half of
the Near North community area, two blocks from LaSalle Street Church
and six to eight blocks from Fourth Presbyterian Church, Moody
Church, and the Episcopal Cathedral of Saint James. In 1992 the development had 6,935 official residents, but church workers in the area believe
this radically undercounts the number of adult men.[25] In many ways
Cabrini Green is similar to other housing developments and deep-

poverty areas in the city. Of its heads of household, 57 percent rely on Aid for Dependent Children as their primary source of income, only slightly lower than the percentage for the Robert Taylor Homes (59 percent). By certain other measures Cabrini Green compares quite favorably with other public housing developments. Despite its notoriety, in 1991 Cabrini's violent-crime rate was only eleventh highest of the nineteen major developments, at fifty-two violent crimes per one thousand persons.[26] Nevertheless, social conditions at Cabrini Green make it a different universe for those who attend the churches of the Loop and Near North Side, for whom Cabrini is defined by the enormity of its social problems.

The social-outreach effort at Cabrini Green is striking by its sheer scale. For example, we estimated that there were, at the time of our research, about fifteen hundred[27] tutors in the tutoring programs. Organizations running tutoring or mentoring programs include Fourth Presbyterian Church, LaSalle Street Church's CYCLE ministry, the Montgomery Ward Cabrini Connections program, Saint Chrysostom's Episcopal Church, Saint Luke's Church of God in Christ, Saint Joseph's Parochial School, Holy Family Lutheran Church, the Moody Bible Institute's Big Brother and Big Sister programs, Saint Matthew's United Methodist Church, and the Lower North Center.[28] In addition to the tutoring programs, we have counted at least forty agencies and organizations that work in the Cabrini area. These include Holy Name Cathedral, which has an established history of outreach missions to Cabrini Green; the imaginative Cabrini Greens, where Cabrini children grow designer vegetables for high-class North Side restaurants; and the summer filmmaking program.[29] This investment of resources in Cabrini Green is in stark contrast to the resources devoted to other deep-poverty areas in the city. For example, the South Side neighborhood of Englewood had a 1990 population five times the size of that in the Cabrini area, with, according to the U.S. Census, 11,911 school-age children, as opposed to Cabrini's 2,500. Yet, according to a comprehensive 1994 survey of Chicago tutoring/mentoring programs, Englewood had only two such programs, serving just 140 students.[30]

Despite the impressive scope of all the churches' outreach programs to Cabrini Green's residents, questions about the combined impact of the many efforts point to the striking absence of social transformation, or even a tangible process of improvement, relative to the major outlay of resources. Although none of these programs addresses the need for well-paying jobs for the residents, nevertheless the scale of the effort put forward by voluntary and government sectors in Cabrini is more than just a "drop in the ocean." What effect have these programs had on Cabrini Green? Unfortunately, the programs we looked at did not compile statistics that would have given an overall measure of success.

Perhaps one indicator of the impact of the programs is that the population of Cabrini Green dropped by two-thirds between 1970 and 1993. As those who have been helped by the educational programs have tended to move out of Cabrini, the population decline may be a sign of the programs' ability to help residents move up and then out of the housing project. Moreover, according to a youth worker in Cabrini, the very presence of so many white middle-class volunteers has had a cooling effect on gang conflict, because the gangs believe that the death of a white volunteer would almost certainly bring the National Guard into Cabrini. Thus these substantial efforts by the churches and other agencies have helped many individuals and given them opportunities that would have otherwise been unavailable, and they may well have made some small contribution to the gang truce and a more peaceful atmosphere in Cabrini.

Nevertheless, Cabrini is not significantly different from other Chicago Housing Authority projects. Hence we have to ask: Why have not fifteen hundred tutors and more than forty programs made more of a difference to the children who remain?

Church versus Community and the Dilemmas of Social Outreach

The tutoring programs of LaSalle Street Church and Fourth Presbyterian Church reflect by their size a sense of the magnitude of Cabrini's social problems. But the vast size of the programs complicates the church's relationship to them. The evolution of the programs illustrates the complications that can arise when attempting to conform to a mission theology whose goal is to answer the needs that develop out of overwhelming social problems, yet at the same time attempt to build community. Both LaSalle and Fourth Presbyterian are well aware of the need to help rather than hinder the creation of a strong community at Cabrini, but attempts to achieve this goal seem to distance the church from its ministries there and complicate the possibility of building a partnership between the congregation and the residents.

Both tutoring programs started small but, in order to meet the needs of the Cabrini community, expanded their pool of volunteers well beyond that of church members. LaSalle's program, Community Youth Creative Learning Experience, or CYCLE, is its oldest ministry, started in the church basement in the early 1960s. By 1994 more than three hundred CYCLE volunteers were giving about two hours each week to the learning center. Most of the volunteers at the time of our interview were young, white, middle-class professionals in marketing and accounting, and 60 percent were women. Yet, while the make-up of the volunteers resembles the LaSalle Street congregation in age, race, class, and sex, only four or five are members. To address more fully the problems of the Cabrini community, CYCLE's activities have expanded from simple tutoring to leadership development among community youth, college scholarship programs, job placement, and a GED (general equivalency diploma) and job-training program for adults. The need for money to support these ambitious programs, a full-time staff, and its own building has made CYCLE look well beyond the church for funds, with 75 percent coming from foundations, 20 percent from the public sector, and only 5 percent from individual contributions.

LaSalle's CYCLE program also adapted to Cabrini's overwhelming social problems by making a conscious decision to be closer to the Cabrini community through the relocation of CYCLE's activities from the church basement to 1441 North Cleveland, more than a mile away from the church and just to the north of the Cabrini itself, in an area that is still predominantly poor and African American. This impulse also came out of a criticism of the Progressive Era model, where social outreach by middle-class white churches was done *to* the community rather than *with* the community. Although the move made CYCLE more a part of the community it serves, it further distanced CYCLE from LaSalle; and while this has been an incredibly successful program, the growth of CYCLE and its relocation have meant that the material contribution of LaSalle members to CYCLE has become, in proportional terms, negligible. This became painfully clear to the congregation when a representative of CYCLE came to the church to talk on Ministry Sunday; it became obvious that she had no idea LaSalle and the program she worked for had ever been connected. In 1998, CYCLE moved back to LaSalle Street. The program is located in the new Cornerstone Center, just opposite the church, with the hope that the church will once again play a large part in its life.

Fourth Presbyterian Church also has struggled with the dilemmas of church versus community. Their program tutors 470 children, one-to-one, three nights per week. In Fourth Presbyterian's program, about 20 percent of the tutors are from the church. Although 90 percent of the children in the tutoring program are from Cabrini Green, the tutoring takes place at the church on Michigan Avenue, a "habitus" that, as James Wellman has pointed out, is much closer to that of the volunteers (who for the most part are professionals working downtown, single, white, and twenty-five to thirty-five years old) than to that of the children.[31]

To address the issue of community-building at Cabrini, Fourth Presbyterian opened the Center for Whole Life in 1993. The church located the center on the ground floor of a Cabrini high-rise that was scheduled for demolition. The center attempts to do three things. First, it is visible presence inside Cabrini Green and thus builds a much more direct relationship between the residents and the church than is possible with the tutoring program. Second, through the center the church can be part of the process of building community and may possibly serve in an advocacy capacity. Third, and most important, the center offers support and resources to young mothers and their children. Yet, while the Center for Whole Life is closer than the church itself to the Cabrini community, most of the program is carried out by paid staff members and a small number of volunteers; unlike the tutoring program, it does not bring many church members into contact with Cabrini residents.

Thus both churches find themselves in a dynamic in which the closeness of a program to the community it serves gives it more legitimacy and greater effectiveness than would be the case if it were seen as being carried out on the terms of the predominantly white and middle-class congregation. But the risk of such distancing is that the congregations themselves may become so uninvolved that the programs are only nominally tied to the churches. This problem of an ever-increasing divide between church congregations and the people who volunteer in their outreach programs is not confined to tutoring. In the case of Cabrini Alive—an organization sponsored by Fourth Presbyterian, LaSalle, and other Near North churches—that rehabilitates Cabrini Green apartments, observations and interviews indicate that, apart from a core of church volunteers, the bulk of the labor power comes from college and seminary students.

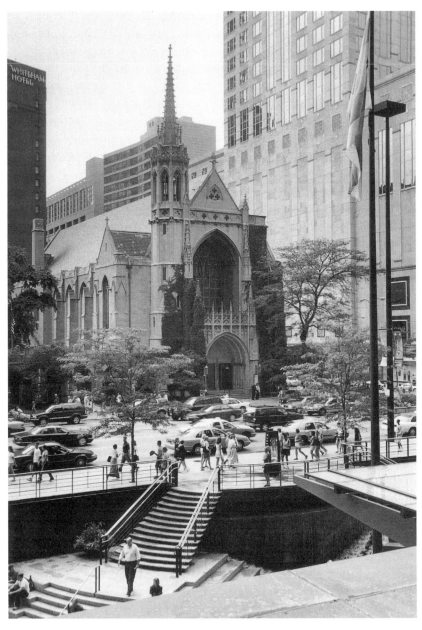

Fig. 3-1. Fourth Presbyterian Church and the "Magnificent Mile" in Chicago's Near North Side. Photo courtesy of Fourth Presbyterian Church.

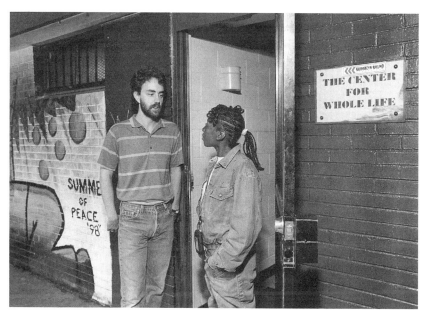

Fig. 3-2. The Center for Whole Life at the Cabrini Green public housing development, Chicago, is a project of Fourth Presbyterian Church. Photo courtesy of Fourth Presbyterian Church.

Processing the Absence of Change

In discussions with those who work for the churches in the Cabrini area we found an underlying awareness of the absence of a social transformation, even a lack of a general sense of progress, at the housing development. Some felt the lack of progress at Cabrini was due to the existence of a deeply ingrained culture of poverty, based more on the dynamics of class than of race, and saw themselves as essentially outside any possibility of change. But others identified with the community in seeing forces in society actively maintaining a system that oppresses the residents of Cabrini Green primarily on the basis of their race. This difference in the explanations of why the programs have not achieved greater success was not a simple division between white and African American program workers, although racial background made it more likely that one would adopt a particular view. African American program workers might well share Cabrini residents' experiences of police harassment, making a causal argument based on white supremacy seem more plausible to them.[32] Moreover, the middle-class position of African American program workers may, according to Jennifer Hochschild, make it more likely that they will ascribe responsibility for the problems of Cabrini Green to whites than would either whites or poor African Americans.[33] Similarly, whites might be in a difficult position if they were to identify themselves as part of the problem while having a calling to be part of the solution, although this is not unheard-of.[34] Thus, although we are not inferring hard-and-fast racial divisions, the different positions that program workers adopt in relation to the absence of success at Cabrini Green are part of the complex racial dynamic of the outreach missions.

Among those who have adopted the "culture of poverty" argument, most of whom have worked in Cabrini for many years, the mood might best be described as weary. Although these workers share a strong sense of spiritual purpose, founded on a belief that this work fulfills a religious calling, we found little faith among them that their efforts would transform Cabrini Green itself. Most of these volunteer workers focused on the possibility of helping a limited number of people. One volunteer, who has been working in Cabrini Green since the 1970s, saw himself as running the modern equivalent of the Underground Railroad in helping people to escape from Cabrini. He believed that all the families who could leave Cabrini had left, and that those who remained were trapped in overlapping and reinforcing social pathologies. Another experienced church worker said that she felt the residents of Cabrini had a fatalistic vision of life and did not see themselves as changing. While these culture-of-poverty perspectives articulate a strong sense of the intangible nature of the social problems at Cabrini, none of the program workers ever directly blamed the residents for their plight. Rather, like William Julius Wilson in *The Truly Disadvantaged,* they saw a pattern caused by structural circumstances beyond the control of individuals. In a more pessimistic vein than Wilson, they also saw a pattern of low expectations that has become ingrained because generations have lived in deep poverty, isolated from mainstream culture. Thus, although the people we interviewed work for programs and missions that present themselves as redemptive and transformative, their observations are closer to a culture-of-poverty perspective than that of a social activism and community transformation model.

Some workers associated with the ministries of the predominantly white downtown churches were uncertain about the possibility of transforming Cabrini Green through the existing programs. While issues of family and low church membership among Cabrini residents were raised, the barrier to change was also located within the larger structure of racial domination. On two occasions we were referred to Jawanza Kunjufu's *Countering the Conspiracy to Destroy Black Boys* (1985–86) as giving an explanation of the problems faced by children in Cabrini Green. Kunjufu's book offers suggestions for providing role models to young black boys, and it does so from the premise that there is a genetically driven conspiracy of whites to maintain their racial purity through dominating other races, and in particular by destroying black males. To counter this conspiracy requires a much greater involvement by older black males in the lives of young black males and creation of a curriculum that would take advantage of the learning skills of black males rather than stifling them, as a predominantly female and white teaching force tends to do. In one interview, a church worker said that the predominance of white tutors gave the children of Cabrini the idea that success was based on race and not on merit. Another worker stressed that it was a major concern of the program that there were relatively few black tutors.

The sentiments of some of the program workers who took up the viewpoint of the community as a group facing racial domination in a white society have peculiar dissonances. These programs that are addressed to a presumed white conspiracy are sponsored by white churches; they receive most of their funding from white individuals and corporate foundations; and their volunteer base is mainly white and female. The sentiments expressed by some of the African American workers and the Afrocentric philosophy of Kunjufu's *Countering the Conspiracy* seem to be at variance with the importance placed on unity within diversity in the mission statements of the churches and in the sentiments expressed in a congregational survey we administered at the LaSalle Street Church. In the survey, members stated that they valued the church because it was a place "where people from various backgrounds get together to share in Christ," because of its "diversity," because of "the variety of people at LSC [LaSalle Street Church]—different races, different socio-economic statuses." The pessimism some of the white church workers expressed and the very notion of an intractable culture of poverty also run counter to LaSalle Street Church's stated mission of fostering "Christian renewal and revitalization" in Cabrini Green.

What effect do these differing perceptions of outreach have on the programs that are at the core of these churches' identity and claim to status and influence in the city? Despite the differences between the worldviews of the program workers and the institutional culture of churches as represented by mission and vision statements, the understanding that Loop/Near North churches have of Cabrini Green as a site of redemptive activity has remained. Nevertheless, part of what sustains this image may be the separation of the congregations from the concerns and fears of those who actually work in the field. This separation is sustained by the labor of a majority of volunteers who have little relationship to the churches but who seem to move into and out of the programs through a revolving door, and so gain very little sense of how effective their efforts are in terms of the wider Cabrini community. It is a system that permits a number of mutually contradictory constructions of the interactions between middle-class white churches and a poor African American community. It is a system that aids in the continuation of the historic leadership role of the downtown churches, but it is an inherently unstable system, where a sharp fall in the number of outside volunteers or the boiling over of frustrations and disappointments by some of the full-time workers could lead to the unraveling of the delicate balance between the churches and the community they attempt to serve.

Finally, if hard questions need to be asked about the effectiveness of the programs at Cabrini Green and the subcultures of social outreach that have grown up around them, similar projects in other parts of the city also need to face these issues. On the one hand, our findings suggest that any notion that the churches can "pick up the slack" left by the curtailment of the welfare state is completely delusional; even with a limited mission and relatively substantial resources, the churches have been unable to change Cabrini Green fundamentally. On the other hand, in an era marked by increasingly hardening attitudes toward the poor, it is more important than ever that the churches formulate projects that both work and involve their members, and that there be an honest and realistic dialogue within churches about their programs' effectiveness and underlying philosophies.

New Demographics and Old Missions

Just as economic and demographic changes have challenged the churches and reshaped their mission in the past, so in the late 1990s downtown and its adjacent neighborhoods are changing again, presenting new challenges and opportunities. Although the total combined population of the

Loop and Near North Side has remained almost constant between 1970 and 1990, this seeming stability hides a massive change in the composition of the population. In 1970 roughly one-third (22,722) of the residents of this combined Loop and Near North area lived in the census tracts between Orleans Street and the Chicago River, in the area dominated by the Cabrini Green housing development—an area that was predominantly poor and African American.[35] This is the dark-shaded portion of map 3. In 1990 only one-sixth (11,142) of the population of the Loop and Near North Side lived in these tracts. Our on-site observation since 1992 indicates that even within these several tracts the composition of the population is shifting from one that is poor and predominantly black to one that is prosperous and increasingly white. This strength of the professional-managerial class can also be seen in changes in income levels. Between 1979 and 1989, the median household income of Loop residents rose by 313 percent, that of Lincoln Park residents rose by 126 percent, and that of Near North residents rose by 108 percent. Along with the contiguous neighborhood of Lakeview just to the north of Lincoln Park, these neighborhoods were the only ones in the city that had more than 100 percent increases in their median household incomes.[36]

In general, the churches have been anchor institutions in this transformation, and LaSalle Street Church with its housing program has been successful in its goal of neighborhood revitalization. By the late 1990s the area around the church had been transformed, spurred by LaSalle's Atrium Village development. In the blocks surrounding LaSalle, the percentage of workers who are managers and professionals rose from 4 percent in 1970 to 22 percent in 1990.

In the late 1990s the trend toward an enlarged presence for the professional-managerial class showed no signs of abating and, if anything, accelerated. An examination of city building permits for the greater Near North from 1991 to 1997 shows a net addition of roughly nine thousand new homes in this area, almost all by private developers and many of which consist of townhouses and condominiums.[37] It is impossible to tell if the many renovations and conversions going on in the area are adding to the total population, but they are almost certainly continuing the trend toward a more affluent population. The biggest change in the area, and the one that will transform the entire raison d'être of some of the churches that we studied, is yet to come: the comprehensive redevelopment of the Cabrini Green housing development. The city aims to redevelop the existing site into one of low-rise apartments and townhouses that will be occupied by a mixture of existing Cabrini residents, low-income tenants, and tenants paying a market rent.

The guiding philosophy behind the project is that of William Julius Wilson, as laid out in his book *The Truly Disadvantaged*. To prevent a concentrated population of the nonworking poor and a resulting a culture of poverty, the nonworking poor will be interspersed with those who work, as has been the case in the Chicago Housing Authority's Lake Shore Drive condominiums. The developer who will reshape Cabrini Green has had a number of successes already in Chicago with mixed-income housing projects, but his success has in part been based on a rigorous screening process in which roughly two-thirds of existing tenants have left the redeveloped properties.[38] This process may end up institutionalizing distinctions between the respectable and the unrespectable poor, distinctions that from the 1960s onward the churches have tried hard to shed.

Thus, in the late 1990s, with the neighborhoods around the churches undergoing a radical transformation as old railyards have been converted into more than two hundred townhouse developments for the returning middle classes, the churches have faced two main challenges, one from outside the congregation and one from within. First, if the downtown and its adjacent neighborhoods are strong, the churches have a strong demographic base for their congregations and are able to maintain their prestige place in the wider metropolitan religious world. But if the neighborhoods adjacent to the churches were to gentrify—if there were, to use Harvey Zorbaugh's terminology, only an expanded Gold Coast and no slum—the churches' sense of identity would undoubtedly change. In the late 1990s these churches have been facing the dilemma of whether they should serve what will be, after the redevelopment is complete, a very different Cabrini population working with many who are the working poor but not the desperately poor on public assistance, or whether they should look to other neighborhoods in the city to find, in Elam Davies's words, "the least, the last, the lost and the lonely."[39]

The theological self-imagery that undergirds the churches' outreach missions to the very poor is infused by the language of proximity and extremes, which brings with it both a sense of urgency to the task at hand and a certain charge that would be lacking if missions were further afield or if they were to a population that is not as desperately poor. In *Being Church, Becoming Community*, John Buchanan, pastor of Fourth Presbyterian Church, states:

The fact is that one mile from Bloomingdales and the Four Seasons is a community living in Third World squalor. Thirteen thousand people live there, mostly women and children, in high-rise apartments where most of the elevators . . . are commandeered by gang members and operated for a fee, where the smell of urine assaults everyone who walks in.[40]

While the missions of these churches and the sense of the churches' historic responsibility to the city as a whole would carry on even if the locale of their efforts were to shift to a more distant neighborhood, the sense of a shared destiny is easier to articulate when there is such a visible image of a shared space. Buchanan again cogently states the theological charge given by the proximity: "Cabrini Green represents the most dramatic contrast to the affluence of the near north side and is therefore God's clearest call to mission for the church."[41] I argue that should the proximate areas of poverty disappear, then part of the churches' identity and sense of purpose would disappear with them, a part of what makes these downtown churches so attractive to the socially conscious residents of the Near North Side. Thus the vitality of the churches depends on a contingent balance of historically volatile and unpredictable forces over which they have limited control.

The second challenge is that, with the decision of many couples with children to stay in the city, the downtown churches are finding themselves having to address new needs among their congregants that are associated with the stresses experienced by working families, something that suburban churches are used to but that has not been a major part of the downtown churches for many years. The challenge will be to meet the needs of the church members and still carry out the well-established traditions of outreach to those beyond the church door. In response to this, some of the churches have developed new mission activities that simultaneously serve the members of their congregations and aid members of the surrounding communities. This model of the church as a place where people of different socioeconomic backgrounds may have common needs fulfilled as they participate in a faith community is finding its way into the life of LaSalle Street Church and Fourth Presbyterian. Both have renovated and expanded their day-care facilities, largely at the request of their own member families, but the onset of welfare reform has provided an opportunity to share these facilities with mothers from Cabrini Green who are entering the workforce. For both the schools and the church day-care centers it is important that the scholarship parents pay some part of the cost, so the parents do not feel they are being treated as charity cases but rather all pay in accordance with their means.

This may indeed be a propitious moment to make the congregation itself a vehicle of social outreach. While the congregation's social make-up and seemingly "inward" concerns were once seen as an obstacle to the church's public mission, a new appreciation of the congregation's role gives it the potential to be more than just a bridge between public and private; indeed, it may become a moral community in and of itself.[42] Although those served by programs such as expanded day-care facilities will not be the poorest of the poor, they will still be a large population of working poor with great needs—needs that are held in common with other members of the church. Through these programs the churches may be able to achieve that as yet unfulfilled aspiration from the 1960s, namely, building an economically and racially diverse congregation.

As the churches expand services to their congregations, examples of how to build an outreach element into these services are already available to them. At Saint Joseph's Parochial School on Orleans Street, Sister Stephanie Schmidt, who runs the school's tutoring program, seems to have found a way to combine building strong institutional ties within the church with an outreach to those who live in Cabrini Green. At Saint Joseph's, a volunteer is assigned to every child. Most of the children are from Cabrini Green, and most of the volunteers live on the Near North Side or in Lincoln Park, few of them congregants at Saint Joseph's Church; this makes the program no different from those found in other area churches. But because the tutoring is centered in the school, Sister Stephanie places the tutor within a network of people that includes the student, the student's parents, the student's homeroom teacher, and Sister Stephanie herself. Moreover, although the volunteers may not be from Saint Joseph's, they are from other local Catholic parishes, and Sister Stephanie feels that she is responsible for the spiritual development of the tutors as well as the students. Thus the tutors and students are part of an organic faith community. A school as an instrument of outreach is a concept also seen at Old Saint Patrick's Church. The school is "church-sponsored" but "not parochial" and is deliberately racially, religiously, and ethnically diverse; 45 percent of the current enrollment is nonwhite. The school financially maintains 30 percent of its enrollment, with over four hundred places for "scholarship children."

Despite the promise of such an approach, this is a pattern of outreach mission that will likely benefit the working poor more than the desperately poor. In this way, the churches may start to institutionalize the same distinctions between different categories of poor people as the new developers at Cabrini Green are employing. Despite the dangers of this, such a change would, I believe, break the current dynamic of separation and subcultures that has built up between the various actors in the world of Cabrini outreach. The churches will able to bring the Cabrini community into their congregational world on the basis of common need, and the process of transforming Cabrini may well become easier if the bulk of the population is the working poor. This is a radical change for the churches. It will mean accepting the limited possibilities of "the least, the last, the lost and the lonely" as a transformative force, while still acknowledging a need to care for this part of the population, and realizing that its other goals of being in community with those of a different race and class may be more realistically realized by reaching out to a working-poor population that have not been prominent in the churches' outreach theologies.

The transformation is taking place in Cabrini Green through the workings of the market system, not through the churches. The question for the churches is: With such a transformation already occurring, what are the churches going to do? If they decide to minister to a reshaped Cabrini Green, with all their doubts about the reshaping process, they may have an opportunity to create the church as a community of diverse people living lives of mutual accountability and interdependence. In fact, because of their centrality and accessibility, it is these old downtown churches, rather than the suburban megachurches situated many miles from even the working poor, who can be on the cutting edge of creating a new type of church, while still carrying on their mission to create a better city for all its residents.

NOTES

1. These churches are similar to the "Old First" churches of Jones and Wilson, *What's Ahead;* and Bakke, *Expanded Mission,* 1–4; to "pillar churches" and "crusader churches" in Dudley and Johnson, "Congregational Self-Images for Social Ministry"; and to "Downtown Baptist" in Roozen, McKinney, and Carroll, *Varieties of Religious Presence.*

2. On the downtown Social Gospel church as the church of the whole city, see Lewis, *Protestant Experience in Gary;* and for its potential as a community of memory, see Wind and Lewis, "Memory, Amnesia, and History," 20–22.

3. See Edington, *Downtown Church,* foreword by Lyle E. Schaller, 12–13.

4. Roughly one-half of the members of churches discussed here reside within the Loop/greater Near North Side area.

5. Zorbaugh, *Gold Coast and Slum,* 274.

6. Ibid., 277.

7. Ibid., 274–275.

8. Smith, *Urban Disorder,* 37–38.

9. Stead, *If Christ Came to Chicago!* 432.

10. Smith, "When Stead Came to Chicago."

11. Scroggs, "Making a Difference," 464.

12. Ibid., 482.

13. Ibid., 484.

14. On the changing environment of downtown churches, see Jones and Wilson, *What's Ahead;* and Bakke, *Expanded Mission.*

15. "Report to the Board of Moody Church," Prepared under the direction of Pastor George Sweeting, Chicago, 1967. Copy provided by Billy Graham Center, Wheaton College Library, Wheaton, Illinois.

16. See Scroggs, "Making a Difference," 500–503; and Hefley, *Church That Takes on Trouble* (1976).

17. On the Civil Rights movement and the church, see Green, "History," 16.

18. Meyers, ed., *Envisioning the New City.*

19. See Faramelli, Rodman, and Scheibner, "Seeking to Hear and Heed," 106–108.

20. Quoted in Van Engen, "Constructing a Theology," 246.

21. From Todd, "Presbyterian Ministry," 165.

22. Gilkey, "Christian Congregation," 107.

23. See the example of Downtown Baptist in Roozen, McKinney, and Carroll, *Varieties of Religious Presence,* chap. 7.

24. Compared with the most exemplary churches cited in Dudley, *Basic Steps,* the downtown Chicago churches better understand and respond to the needs of their neighborhood.

25. From Chicago Housing Authority, *Statistical Profile,* 1991–1992 (Chicago: Chicago Housing Authority, 1993).

26. For crime statistics, see "Without Sweeps," 1 and 9.

27. *Tutor/Mentor Connection* 2 (September 1994), published by Montgomery Ward's Cabrini Connections program, puts the number of children tutored in Cabrini Green at fourteen hundred, but some children are in more than one program, which may account for our estimate of tutors being higher than Cabrini Connections' estimate of students.

28. *Tutor/Mentor Connection* 2 reported fourteen tutoring/mentoring programs in Cabrini Green.

29. See "Growth Is at the Root"; and "Cabrini Youths," 1.

30. See *Tutor/Mentor Connection* 2; and the 1990 U.S. Census.

31. Wellman, "Counter-Example"; also see Livezey, "Fourth Presbyterian Church."

32. See Cose, *Rage of a Privileged Class.*

33. Hochschild, *Facing Up to the American Dream.*

34. For example, Andrew Hacker, who is white, argues in *Two Nations* that inequalities between white and black are based on white supremacy, while William Julius Wilson, the African American author of *Truly Disadvantaged,* argues that class explains more than race.

35. This includes census tracts 804, 805, 806, 807, 808, 818, and 819. The dark-shaded portion of map 3 includes all of these except tract 818.

36. Census data published in *Chicago Sun Times* on June 3, 1992, 23.

37. This figure is a net estimation calculated by subtracting all demolition permits from new construction permits as listed by the City of Chicago. The demolitions include the destruction of a number of the tower blocks at Cabrini Green.

38. See "Developer Building a Dream."

39. Scroggs, "Making a Difference," 500.

40. Buchanan, *Being Church,* 27–28.

41. Ibid.

42. Marty, "Public and Private," 136–38 and 145–46.

Map 4. The Near West Side, with high concentrations of unemployment and poverty, suffered from the loss of manufacturing jobs in the 1960s and 1970s. Map by Brian Twardosz, BMT Printing and Cartographic Specialists.

The Churches and the Poor in a "Ghetto Underclass" Neighborhood

Isaac B. Laudarji and Lowell W. Livezey

It is 11:30 A.M., the appointed hour of Sunday worship at the Revival Center Church of God in Christ. Sunday school has just been dismissed by Brother Jerome Seavers, the secretary, after a brief report of the attendance and offering and reminders of upcoming Bible study and prayer meetings. Billy Williams is tapping rhythmically at a small set of drums under the watchful eye of Brother Benjamin, who will take over the drums when the service gets underway. Not far from the entrance, Sister Mary Perkins, the pastor's nurse and head usher, is greeting friends while she reorganizes the bags of food she and the Helping Hands Ministry plan to distribute.

Pastor Benjamin Bowman is still in the kitchen, checking the cornbread and greens that will be shared after service. But he soon exchanges his apron for a perfectly pressed dark suit coat and, with a well-worn Bible in his hand, emerges to mingle with the thirty or forty people gathering in the all-purpose basement. Making his way slowly to the pulpit area, shaking hands, hugging, and talking, he passes the drums, the Hammond B-3 electric organ, and the wooden lectern used for the Sunday school lesson and then half jumps up the three steps to the pulpit and grasps the microphone. "Let's gather round," he says in a raspy voice and a deep Mississippi dialect. "Gather round now, we gon' praise the Lord today."

He begins conversationally, noting that worship will be "right here" rather than in the sanctuary above. He shares information about members and neighborhood people he has seen during the week, about Sister

Josephine and the fact the doctors don't give her much of a chance but, with prayer, God will give her a chance. He mentions matter-of-factly that he "took the kids to Dwight" yesterday—meaning he had taken some of the children to visit their mother in the women's prison in Dwight, Illinois, some eighty miles from Chicago. He begins to pray, prayers of gratitude for the day, for the light, for the church, for health, for healing, for God's power. Gradually, people start repeating, "Thank you Jesus. Praise the Lord." The organist plays softly, then builds as more voices are lifted in thanks and praise. The drummer accents the beat; more people voice their praise; some begin moving about the floor, clapping, singing, and praying, while more worshipers come into the church. The reading from God's Holy Word, the recitation of the Statement of Faith, and selections by the choir of four adults and fourteen children prepare the congregation, now about eighty-five people, for the morning message.

Sister Katrina reads the biblical story of Jehoshaphat, the embattled king of Judah, and the prophets' assurance that however numerous and brutal the enemy tribes may be, the ensuing battle is God's to fight, not the king's, and God will win it. The pastor then spins out the analogy to his people living in the West Side. The tribes are the devil, and the devil's weapons are the "D" weapons of Doubt, Discouragement, and Despair. Just as they worked on Jehoshaphat, they work on each of us. But our God is the same God that delivered Jehoshaphat, and God will deliver us. Therefore we praise God today and every day.

As the sermon builds to its climax, the drums tap quietly, then louder, and the sweet chords of the Hammond B-3 organ complement the pastor's voice. He makes his way to floor level, and his movements evolve into the "holy dance" for which he is locally renowned. By now, half the congregation are standing, moving, singing, shouting, and a few are "slain in the spirit" (briefly fainting and falling, to be lovingly caught by a nearby worshiper). The cadence and tone of the service peak and then quiet again, and people line up for anointing with oil, laying on of hands, and prayers for healing.

At about 2 P.M. the service concludes and the pastor says a benediction, but people continue to move about, now greeting and hugging one another (including visitors), and children play in the open areas. Some are staying for greens and cornbread; a few have arrived only in time for the food. They will all take a the break in the late afternoon, some walking to their apartments in Henry Horner or driving to other neighborhoods. At least half will return for the evening service.

The Revival Center is one of twelve churches located within walking distance of the Chicago Housing Authority high-rise apartments, Henry Horner Homes, in Chicago's Near West Side neighborhood. The Near West Side is one of Chicago's poorest neighborhoods, serving as part of the empirical basis of William Julius Wilson's theory of "ghetto poverty" and the "urban underclass."[1] And, as is evident in Map 4, in the two census tracts that comprise Henry Horner (and surround the Revival Center), the 1990 Census recorded a population that is 100 percent black, with unemployment rates in the two tracts of 40 percent and 66 percent, respectively, and with an astounding 74 percent and 86 percent living in poverty. These rates had increased dramatically since 1980, caused in part by the exodus of employed and employable people as their manufacturing jobs relocated away from the city of Chicago, leaving the unemployed and unemployable even more concentrated and isolated.[2] Alex Kotlowitz brought national attention to Henry Horner in *There Are No Children Here*[3] after ten-year-old resident Lafayette Rivers told him in an interview, "If I grow up, I'd like to be a bus driver." That "if" caught Kotlowitz's attention.

Thus the vicinity of Henry Horner provides an opportunity to explore the interrelationship between churches and very poor people who live in neighborhoods of extreme poverty. For this reason, we and our colleagues in the Religion in Urban America Program surveyed all the churches in the neighborhood and conducted ethnographic studies of four that, taken together, represent the variety of its religious life. Because Henry Horner, more than the West Side in general, is characterized by "extreme" and "concentrated" poverty, we also selected churches that either include Henry Horner residents among their members or serve them through their social ministries.

Across Damen Avenue from the Revival Center is Saint Stephen African Methodist Episcopal (AME) Church, a large, well-maintained stone structure with stained-glass windows and brightly painted red doors. At Saint Stephen, the Sunday-morning worship service starts promptly at 11 A.M., with two hundred or more well-dressed people already seated. The dignified processional, the elegantly robed choir and ministers, and the beautifully appointed sanctuary and finely tuned organ all signify a prosperous congregation. Much of the service is sung, including prayers and responses, giving the service a "high church" feeling. Yet the hymns are traditional Protestant hymns, recalling biblical, often rural, imagery and anticipating a personal salvation.

It is only slightly atypical that on this particular Sunday the procession includes a bishop visiting from Africa, for the congregation is actively dedicated to benevolent activities at home and abroad, and its pastor is a leader in the AME denomination and in the local community. One of the announcements asks members to attend a "claiming and cleansing" ceremony at the property and to come dressed for work. For most, this will be a strictly charitable undertaking, caring for the neighborhood of their church, even though they have long since moved into cleaner, quieter, and safer places of residence.

Continuing west on Washington Boulevard, one sees the security screens and shabby exterior of the small grocery and liquor store, old row houses and "two-flat" buildings in various states of disrepair, and vacant lots. In the third block we arrive at Saint Malachy Roman Catholic Church, the seat of the parish that includes Henry Horner. By midday, Saint Malachy's Sunday mass has concluded, and the only people remaining are members of the parish pastoral council, a lay advisory body. The mass was inspirational to them, celebrated in the small but elegant church, its Greek-revival architecture expressing deep roots in Catholic tradition, while the tradition was made contemporary by percussion and piano performed in a manner suggestive of urban Gospel music. The cantor, like half the congregation, grew up in the church. His rich baritone voice has adapted well to the post–Vatican II hymnody, and he rarely invokes the Gregorian chants for which he was trained. Only a few of the congregation and its leaders have walked to church, but for those who did not, the drive or bus ride was short compared with the commuting time of those attending nearby Saint Stephen. Saint Malachy is their "parish," and they live in the modest West Side row houses and rented apartments (but not in Henry Horner) where they have lived for many years, some for their entire lives.

Like many Catholic parishes, Saint Malachy has an elementary school and a convent, and it is mainly through these that it has been connected to the poorest people of the neighborhood. The school was recently made part of West Side Catholic Education Ministries, which the archdiocese is forming to provide quality Catholic education in poor neighborhoods (see chapter 11). The convent is the Chicago home of Mother Teresa's

Missionaries of Charity, which operates a shelter for abused and homeless women and a soup kitchen that offers hot meals every day.

Retracing our steps, past Saint Stephen and the Revival Center, continuing along the southern boundary of Henry Horner Homes, we pass more churches and the United Center, new home of the Chicago Bulls and Black Hawks, a major example of commercial interests exploiting the opportunities that decades of disinvestment and urban blight have generated. Then, tucked inconspicuously beneath the overpass of the "El" (Chicago's elevated rapid transit), one finds the Greater Pleasant Valley Missionary Baptist Church. Its members are mainly people of modest means, both working poor and welfare recipients, who come not from the immediate neighborhood but from many parts of the city because of their relationship with the minister or to participate in the particular kind of spirituality the church affords.

A block further east, just beyond the last Henry Horner high-rise building, we come to a very large, old church of light sandstone and a bulletin board displaying the words "First Baptist Congregational Church, Rev. Arthur D. Griffin, Pastor." Turning the corner to enter from the main steps, proceeding further up a red-carpeted staircase and through a large walnut-paneled vestibule, we find the thousand-seat sanctuary comfortably full of worshipers. Ten ministers, four of them women, are seated behind the pulpit one level up from the congregation. Above them, at balcony level, the choir director is conducting a classical anthem performed by the fifty-member Celestial Choir and several soloists, arranged for accompaniment by the large pipe organ, a concert grand piano, an electric organ, and an elaborate set of drums. At the conclusion, a ripple of "Amens" can be heard, marking the transition from the solemnity of the anthem to more spontaneous participation in the rest of the service. From the anthem onward the pipe organ is silent, and the urban Gospel sound accents Pastor Griffin's message of personal salvation as the ground of public responsibility. Before the benediction, people are reminded not to miss weekday Bible study, that more volunteers are needed for the weekly soup kitchen, and to please join the "Take Back the Streets" march against drugs that the Interfaith Organizing Project (IOP) is sponsoring the next Saturday. "Even if you don't live in this neighborhood," an assistant minister exclaims, "we worship here, our church is here, our God is here, and we believe the streets can be safe and secure for the community. So working with the IOP is our ministry, and God needs us on the streets next Saturday."

The Black Church and the Urban Poor

The black church has been an anchor of the black community in the United States from the time of slavery, through Reconstruction, Jim Crow, and the migration to the segregated cities of the North, to the present enjoyment of civil rights but simultaneous creation of an enduring ghetto underclass. In their comprehensive analysis *The Black Church in the African American Experience*, C. Eric Lincoln and Lawrence H. Mamiya show that historically "the Black Church has no challenger as the cultural womb of the black community,"[4] and that the churches of the historic black denominations continue to be vital centers of religious, social, economic, and political activity. Resisting the segmenting and differentiating processes of urban society, they argue, the black churches have remained complex, multifunctional institutions that both foster inward spirituality and unite the religious with the economic, political, and cultural dimensions of African American community life. Yet Lincoln and Mamiya voice concerns about the ability of the black churches to sustain this role, in view of growing numbers of "unchurched" blacks and because of institutional limitations their research identified. They also express concern that the black church may be increasingly divided between a middle-class church and a "church of the poor . . . , consisting largely of independent, fundamentalist, and Pentecostal storefront churches."[5]

Others scholars have extended, complemented, and qualified Lincoln and Mamiya's work in ways that inform our analysis of churches in Chicago's West Side. The writings of Cheryl Sanders, David Daniels, and Robert Franklin[6] have revised the apolitical image of Pentecostal churches and established their importance as public actors and agents of resistance to the marginalization and subordination of African Americans. Peter J. Paris and others have elaborated the black churches' role in fostering a racially inclusive and racially just society, despite the exclusion that led to their creation as racially separate institutions.[7] Cheryl Townsend Gilkes, Evelyn Brooks Higgenbotham, and others have probed questions about the status and contributions of women in the church that Lincoln and Mamiya raised but did not fully explore.[8] All these scholars interpret the black church as a culturally powerful institution that transcends the boundaries of class and that integrates religious, economic, political, and social functions to an extent that contrasts markedly with the fragmentation of modern urban life in general. The Religion in Urban America Program's studies of black churches in Chicago, discussed here and in chapter 7, generally support these mainstream perspectives on the role and character of the black church.[9]

But the black church literature, despite its general agreement about the importance of the church for the poor, offers little information about how and to what extent the poor participate in the churches. While Lincoln and Mamiya confirm the "class stratification" of the black church, they recognize that little is known about the participation or nonparticipation of the "dependent poor" (what social science calls the urban underclass) and speculate that the black church may be losing its presumed capacity to bridge the boundaries of class in the inner city.[10] A number of insightful ethnographic studies show how Pentecostal, independent, and storefront churches increase "human capital" in poor urban communities,[11] but these studies provide only general socioeconomic information on the churches' members and nothing about the participation or nonparticipation of area residents. Moreover, a few observers such as Robert Franklin[12] have recently noted the widespread decline in church participation by black men and the growing emphasis on reclaiming black men as a strategy of both church growth and urban mission.

When poor people are conspicuously absent from predominantly middle-class churches near their homes, this may mean not that the poor have opted for a Pentecostal or storefront church but rather that they are absent from church altogether. But it has been widely accepted, at least since the 1987 publication of William Julius Wilson's *The Truly Disadvantaged,* that one of the major causes of the persistence of urban poverty is the extreme *concentration* of the poor in *isolation* from mainstream institutions and societal functions,[13] so it is important to know whether and how churches either reflect or reduce the isolation. Unfortunately, the literature on urban churches tells us more about church programs to benefit the poor than about their interaction with the poor, including the participation of the poor in the churches.

This chapter explores how four black churches interact with people who live near them in conditions of "extreme" and "concentrated" poverty and in "social isolation." The ethnographic case studies we conducted allowed us to explore both this interaction and the differentiation by class and place of residence of members of four quite different black churches. We consider how churches may affect or mitigate the dimensions of isolation that poor people concentrated in residential complexes like Henry Horner Homes may experience. In view of the historic role of the black church, it was to be expected that many churches would offer social services for poor people and advocate public policy for their bene-fit. But if social isolation is an important factor perpetuating poverty, then it is important to see if church ministries involve the poor as partic-ipants as well as recipients. One point to consider is whether or not poor people attend the same churches as middle-class people, and if so, whether or not they engage in the same activities and social networks as those middle-class members. There is anecdotal evidence[14] that small, in-dependent churches, including storefronts, are not necessarily neighbor-hood churches but may be constituted as networks based on factors such as family ties, friendship, history, and religious preference that are much stronger than local geography.

Although any church participation would be a way for poor people to get out of their social isolation, it is particularly important for them to build relationships in their residential neighborhood. Here they are most likely to generate interrelated social networks in which the same people know one another in multiple contexts—for example, as friends, as shop-pers at the same stores, as parents of children at the same school, and as members of the same church. These overlapping relationships enhance an individual's effectiveness more than relationships that are limited to a single function or purpose. In the language of social science, "social capi-tal" (the networks and patterns of activity that people accomplish to-gether) increases "human capital" (the capacities of individuals to be pro-ductive and effective). Moreover, these multiple layers of interrelation-ship seem to be an important ingredient of social capital. For example, James Coleman, a seminal theorist of social capital, found that children did better in school if the children's parents knew one another.[15] Simi-larly, the individual capacities of people in poor neighborhoods are af-fected not only by their individual relationships but by the networks of people in their families, their apartment buildings, and their organiza-tions (if any), including churches. By focusing on churches near Henry Horner, we can examine how the churches may be part of the networks.

The Churches in a Neighborhood of "Extreme Poverty"

Because the Henry Horner Homes had the Near West Side's greatest con-centration of the ghetto poor, we surveyed pastors of the twelve churches located within walking distance of the housing development to deter-mine the extent of Henry Horner residents' involvement in those churches. To our surprise, of the twelve churches, only the Revival Center claimed participation of Henry Horner residents as members or regular attenders, although several spoke of ministries to them, including evangelization and social services. We also conducted informal interviews on the Henry Horner grounds, asking people at random whether and where they and their friends went to church and which church they considered a resource for the community. Confirming what we learned from the pastors, with one exception, they mentioned only the Revival Center as a church they attended, and it was also described as a church one could use (for a funeral, for example) without being a member. Other churches were known for their soup kitchens, food pantries, and free clothing.

We selected the Revival Center Church of God in Christ, Saint Stephen AME, Saint Malachy Roman Catholic, and First Baptist Congregational to ensure that the case studies would include the major recognized forms of public ministry to the inner-city poor[16] and a reasonable sample of the different denominational "families." And because we were treating residence in Henry Horner as a marker of concentrated poverty and social isolation, we included churches that had different ways of connecting with this public housing complex, as well as a distribution of larger and smaller, wealthier and less prosperous churches. Saint Stephen AME Church and First Baptist Congregational Church represent the Baptist and Methodist church families, which are historically the most prominent parts of the black church. While both churches conduct active public ministries, this chapter emphasizes Saint Stephen's social service ministries and First Baptist Congregational's widely recognized leadership role in community organizing. Saint Malachy represents Roman Catholicism, a denomination whose black population is small but increasing. The Revival Center represents the rapidly growing Pentecostal newcomer (in 1907) to the list of historic black denominations.

Most churches located in the poor black neighborhood minister to a wide cross section of the black community, including the poor, and fulfill the inherited image of the vibrant, multifaceted, socially relevant institution that serves as a sorely needed anchor for both the geographic neighborhood and the black community. Yet evidence builds throughout this chapter that, however great their contributions to and on behalf of the poor, most churches—especially those with the resources to provide substantial social ministries—find it very difficult to include the socially isolated poor as participants as well as recipients. It is possible that most of the very poor do not go to church in the neighborhood and may not at-

Fig. 4-1. Revival Center Church of God in Christ and Saint Stephen AME Church, Near West Side, Chicago. Photo by Lowell W. Livezey.

tend any church, anywhere. In addition to interviewing residents and pastors, for several weeks we watched the pedestrian traffic on Sunday mornings and saw virtually no people walking to church from Henry Horner. In any event, our discussions of Saint Stephen and Saint Malachy show how both a commuter and a parish church provided social ministries to benefit the poor, and our discussion of First Baptist Congregational depicts a church that not only provided major social ministries to the poor but mobilized political and economic power to defend and transform the neighborhood. Finally, we discuss the Revival Center as a church whose social ministries were limited to mutual aid but in which persons who were not only poor but otherwise socially isolated were active participants.

Social Ministries, Social Services, and Social Isolation

Little did Saint Stephen AME Church know when it purchased the building that the 1930s depression was around the corner. Nevertheless, the church held onto the building and paid off the debt. It was a neighborhood church, where members lived around the block and looked out for one another. Sixty years later, older members would lament that the church had become primarily a commuter congregation.

Yet, despite its loss of a shared residential neighborhood and the interrelated social networks that fostered, Saint Stephen's members still find at the church a vital community. They hear and recite a common story of salvation, one that is rooted in the Bible but that extends into the present,

Fig. 4-2. Saint Malachy Roman Catholic Church and the former parish school, now part of West Side Catholic Education Ministries. Photo by Lowell W. Livezey.

in which God's saving power is manifest in human agency—including their own. As Pastor Albert Tyson III put it in an interview, they are "not just actors in a play, they are the scriptwriters." This personally empowering self-concept is nurtured through acts of mutual support. A lay ministry of care for shut-ins, a health services program led by volunteer professional nurses, and an economic development committee that matches unemployed members with jobs enable the members to take charge of their own destiny by acting collectively.

The pastor's sermons call for spiritual transformation as a source of political, social, and economic change. Politicians are recognized from the pulpit and occasionally are invited to speak from it. Ministers and church leaders call on these politicians to make good on their promises and be faithful in their stewardship.

Even though fewer than ten of the nearly seven hundred members live near enough to walk to church, Saint Stephen directs much of its social ministry to West Side residents. Its weekly food pantry and clothing closet are intended to meet immediate needs of the local residents and to bridge the social gap between them and church members. The church offers volunteers to shop for needy people, but it seldom gives out money, for fear the recipients may use it for non-essential needs. Residents walk in and out of the church facility when they come to receive material help, just as they would do in a shop. Children in the neighborhood partake of the summer afternoon lunches provided through the church but seldom join in the Sunday school or other church activities oriented to member families.

In contrast, Saint Malachy is a parish church in the Catholic tradition in which, as historian John T. McGreevy puts it, "the individual came to know God, and the community came to be church, within a particular, geographically defined space."[17] If the national pattern held in the Near West Side, we expect that the priests of Saint Malachy were still urging their members to buy homes, invest in the parish school, and put down roots in the neighborhood during the 1970s and 1980s, when Protestants were joining the "black flight" to the suburbs. Not that all the Catholics stayed; but many did, and others would return later to live with younger generations in their family bungalows and "two-flats." Thus the communal, parish values associated with white ethnic Catholics (see chapter 5) led many black Catholics to remain on the West Side.

This was not lost on the 150 families of Saint Malachy parish in the late 1990s. From the name of parish newsletter—*Believers, Neighbors, and Friends*—to requests for voluntary contributions and services, to the concerns addressed in homilies and lifted up in prayers, members and participants were reminded that "to be church" was to celebrate and care for the neighborhood and its people. The evangelization effort, initiated with the help of archdiocesan staff, began with door-to-door visitation on the block where the church building stands and fanned out from there.

Saint Malachy's social ministries also reflect the parish ideal of care for all the souls within its boundaries. Saint Malachy's school, soup kitchen, and women's shelter provide major resources for the residents of Henry Horner and for the homeless who survive on the streets. Yet the social ministries are offered with minimal contact between the recipients and the members and staff of the church.

Ironically, it was precisely to make Catholic education available to the poor, even in parishes that could not afford the costs, that Saint Malachy School was incorporated into the West Side Catholic Education Ministries. But because of its structural independence, the school no longer brings children and their families into direct contact with parishioners. Even so, the prayers, celebrations, and symbols of community life at Saint Malachy symbolically create a sacred space that includes the school, the children, and the neighborhood.

The soup kitchen operated by the Missionaries of Charity, Mother Teresa's order, is the only source of free hot meals available daily in the neighborhood, and they are offered with a minimum of moralizing or religious requirements. Each morning and afternoon, forty-five to fifty men and women (mostly men) form a line at the door of the dining room. In random interviews, only a few told us they attend church, none of them at Saint Malachy; but they knew the neighborhood churches for their feeding programs, their clothing supplies, or their shelters.

Few church members volunteer at the soup kitchen, but they take pride in it, in the shelter for homeless and abused women, and in the fact that the nuns visit the sick and shut-in and work with the children who live in Henry Horner. The mention of these ministries gives immediacy and poignancy to prayers for the poor and suffering that are included in the mass and special rituals. The "we" who have come "this far by faith" includes the food pantry, the Sisters, and the school. In short, although direct interaction between church members and the poor of the neighborhood rarely occurs, the symbolic construction of the parish identity includes not only the collective action of service to the poor but the recognition of the poor—often specifically mentioning Henry Horner residents—among the people who make up Saint Malachy Parish.

Public Ministry on Behalf of the Poor

As First Baptist Congregational Church celebrated its fiftieth anniversary in 1994, it was obvious that its history on the West Side reflected dramatic changes in the neighborhood and in its membership. The one-time community church had become a commuter church; the one-time haven for blacks of all social classes and economic levels now attracted primarily middle-class, well-educated blacks. And by the end of the 1990s, partly as a result of the church's own efforts, incipient gentrification was foreshadowing the likelihood that white folks would move in nearby, implicitly challenging the church to make good on its racially inclusive ideals. If this comes to pass, the church may benefit from its affiliation with the predominantly white American Baptist and United Church of Christ denominations, in addition to the black National Baptist Missionary Convention.

But in the 1990s, the challenge to First Baptist Congregational Church was how to include the poorest residents of the West Side. Finding that virtually no residents of Henry Horner attended the church Sunday school, the church organized a separate Sunday school at Henry Horner. During good weather, the church's ministers preach open-air sermons, and its choirs perform for residents who sit at their windows or stand on the walkways to listen. Evangelization is intentionally directed to Henry Horner.

Like Saint Stephen and Saint Malachy, First Baptist Congregational provides a feeding program, a food pantry, and clothing closet. A tutoring program enlists more than twenty church members. Information about jobs and educational opportunities is displayed on bulletin boards and provided through the church office. The Drug Ministry, led by four ministers who are themselves former drug users and dealers, offers a spiritually grounded approach to recovery and celebrates an extraordinarily low (10 to 20 percent) recidivism rate.

These social ministries are available to all, including Henry Horner residents. The Drug Ministry seems to have a metropolitan clientele reached by a word-of-mouth network of people who have been helped by it. As at Saint Stephen and Saint Malachy, the volunteer service providers do not seem to have continuing social contact with the recipients, and the recipients do not participate in the worshiping community. Yet we were told that First Baptist Congregational members offer their church as a resource to people they personally know to be in need, so to this extent the church is part of a loose social network across boundaries of neighborhood and class.

Yet it is more as a political "player" that First Baptist Congregational ministers to the West Side neighborhood, including the poor of Henry Horner. While recognition from its pulpit, as at Saint Stephen, has long been a prize coveted by politicians, the church's real clout comes from its role in creating and leading the Interfaith Organizing Project (IOP), a Saul Alinsky–style community organization that has had a formative impact on the course of events in the Near West Side from its founding in 1985. "It was right here in this room," Pastor Griffin explained in an interview, extending his arm sacramentally around the cluttered Sunday school classroom, "that Bill Wirtz and Jerry Reinsdorf came to terms with us for the United Center."

The Interfaith Organizing Project was born in 1985 out of the need to bring together "peoples of various faiths and denominations"[18] to work for community interests by linking "our congregations and neighborhoods." The new organization elected Pastor Griffin as its first president and Earnest Gates, a neighborhood resident and business owner, as its vice president. With its incorporation in 1986, IOP was faced with the challenge of mobilizing the community, empowering the people to protect their interests against the Chicago Bears' plan to build a new stadium.

The linking of congregations and neighborhoods as the focus of IOP took place through its two arms—the ministers group, comprised of pastors, which met every Saturday, and the Thursday-night group, consisting mainly of residents and business owners, not limited to church members. Guided by the professional organizers, the pastors networked with one another and mobilized their members (wherever they lived), while the Thursday-night group networked within the Near West Side area. As Thursday-night members told us later,[19] the pastors mobilized people for weekend rallies and demonstrations, but during the week it was the Thursday-night leadership who could make a show of strength from the neighborhood. Despite tensions as to who best represented neighborhood interests, the two branches maintained a close working relationship, defeated the Bears' stadium, and forced the Chicago Bulls to negotiate favorable terms with IOP in the "joint venture" to build the United Center.[20]

The taste of IOP's triumph was still palpable at First Congregational Baptist Church for several years after its successes with the Chicago athletic teams, but IOP's agenda then shifted to the daily struggle against drugs and violence on the streets. The building of housing to replace that sacrificed to the United Center was mainly "spun off" to new, specialized organizations, in which lay neighborhood residents were more prominent than clergy. And some of the clergy (including the influential Pastor Albert Tyson of Saint Stephen) withdrew in conflict over goals, constituency, and leadership styles. It became harder to raise funds for the less-dramatic projects, so staff was reduced.

Yet the IOP remained a central ministry of First Baptist Congregational Church, with the assistant pastor, the Reverend George Daniels, assuming the presidency. This sustained the congregation's identity as a public actor for the neighborhood. While the members for the most part did not know neighborhood residents personally, they knew that the neighborhood was God's concern and that their destiny as a congregation was tied up with it.

Spirit-Filled Ministries, Social Isolation, and Social Capital

The Revival Center follows the practices, disciplines, and traditions of the Church of God in Christ and has the usual components of church structure, such as the Sunday school, Sunday-morning and -evening worship, the Young People Willing Workers (youth group), and the Young Women's Christian Council. People are baptized (by immersion) and may receive Holy Communion as soon as they are saved and confess Christ as Lord and Savior. The church holds funerals and weddings when they are requested, not only for members but for anyone in the community.

The church evangelizes the neighborhood partly by praying with all who come for food, clothing, or help with their children. Elders, missionaries, and other active members also visit their neighbors in Henry Horner, those who used to be their neighbors, and those whose children are in the Sunday school or choir. Even if the recipients of services and evangelization do not come to church, they sustain enough of a relationship that the church knows when something goes wrong and the people know where to come when they are in trouble. If they come, pastor told us, "we're just so happy they've come."

Revivals are important at the Revival Center, but they are not totally distinct from other services. During revivals, church people "tarry for the Holy Ghost" and pray for healing and for spiritual renewal. It is a time to bring inactive members into the church and to reclaim the backsliders. "Everyone who comes through that door—we gon' love them, and God will deliver them."

Like other black "sanctified" churches, the Revival Center draws on the resources of African American Christianity, including rituals of shouting, healing, and holy dancing.[21] It also brings a bit of the rural South into the city, thus preserving for urban people some of what the quintessentially urban scholar Robert M. Franklin calls "the humane culture of agrarian life."[22] This is evident in the relaxed Sunday schedule, with many people staying at church most of the day and sharing a meal, which helps make the church a family-like community. The meal, open even to those who come late and miss the sermon and especially to the children who need a rare hot meal, exemplifies the communal values for which the black church, especially in its Southern roots, is renowned. The pastor's sermons, prayers, and Bible-study illustrations also draw examples from his childhood in the South and communicate the values of practical self-help over commercial or governmental services, of community and mutual care over individual choice, and of respect for nature as God made it over human technology.

The Revival Center shares in what Lincoln and Mamiya have called the "black sacred cosmos,"[23] in which all creation is sacred and is dominated by the God whose "avenging, conquering, liberating" actions in history are mostly recorded in the Old Testament but whose full revelation is in Jesus Christ. The Old Testament epics show that all of life is a great struggle between good and evil, between the power of God and the power of Satan. This cosmic power struggle is still going on in the West Side, where the power of Satan is manifest as violence, drugs, racism, despair, and illness, just as it was manifest as the Egyptian pharaohs' armies and as the tyranny of Babylonian kings.

This means, first, it is God, and not the people themselves, fighting the battles against evil; and second, God is all powerful and He will win. So, at the Revival Center, when people pray for assistance, healing, and deliverance, they mainly praise God for the *fact* that He will deliver them. This does not mean they do nothing themselves to fight off evil; indeed, returning to church or calling the pastor to help with the kids may be a major initiative. But it does mean that the core of what they do is to join in God's fight and to believe in His deliverance. In contrast with Saint Stephen's members' being told that they are not only actors in the play, but they write the script, Revival Center members learn that they are just understudies. But they also learn that the play is a great cosmic epic, and that because God is both the author and the hero, "every thin' gonna be all right!"

The Revival Center's function as an extended family is also deeply rooted in the black church. As Cheryl Townsend Gilkes[24] has shown, the common use of "Brother" and "Sister" as titles of respect and, particularly in the Church of God in Christ, the formal office of "Church Mother" reflect a pattern of social relations in which childrearing, moral education, spiritual formation, and social control have long been shared within the church. Gilkes argues that the family role of the church is especially strong in times of structural pressure on the black family—slavery, urban migration, and now deindustrialization and social isolation.

Pastor Bowman's role as father and grandfather sets the tone. Every service of worship, prayer, and praise begins with the pastor or an elder or missionary talking informally, with concern about people who are absent. His overview always presupposes that concern, and if there is any exhortation, it is about *how* to express that concern. In preparation for a funeral, for example, we observed the pastor recruiting assistance with the "repast" and then giving advice about how to talk with the bereaved— how to be available and loving, but allowing the bereaved to be alone if that is their wish.

But church-as-family was also evident in the routine behavior of adults and children. Children were constantly being trained for good behavior and adult responsibilities. The pastor estimates that about one-third of the fifty or sixty children come with parents, both married and single, and the rest are unrelated to adults in the church. Adults are expected to show the children—especially the two-thirds who come to church without their parents—how to live and to give them pride and self-respect in the process. Preschool and elementary-age children playing around the church learn standard English grammar, ways to resolve conflicts without fighting, how to address adults, and to be quiet when adults are talking. The adults interlace instruction with hugs, pick the children up, give them food, and at least one member makes a ministry of designing and sewing cloths for children who might otherwise be poorly attired. Thus the church is a loving yet disciplined environment for children, and no child is to be excluded for bad behavior. "We just love them into good behavior," Pastor Bowman says. Everyone raises all the children.

Adults also feel the Revival Center's family-like discipline, especially if the forces of evil (drink, drugs, violence, etc.) overtake them. How does the church respond? "God is married to the backslider," the pastor explained, so

> we try to find them and bring them back into church. If people are active in the church they mostly live right. So we go out and find them. The pastor goes, or the active members, elders, missionaries, they go out and say, "Pastor Bowman want to see you." If they come around, if there's a crisis, we always welcome them, never chastise them. We know it's the devil at work; these are not bad people, they were just not able to resist the devil. But God loves them and so do we.

The Revival Center is something like a "parish," which has a ministry to all the people in a given geographic area. Some members also come from further away, but most previously lived in the immediate vicinity and grew up with many of those now remaining in Henry Horner. The image of parish begins with the pastor's sense of his ministry to the people of Henry Horner and the immediate vicinity. He says that in addition to the active membership of about a hundred, there are two hundred to three hundred who occasionally come to church and call him at a points of crisis, and whose children come to church or play there during the week. He and others in the church visit the children's parents—possibly in the hospital or in prison—or the adults' parents in a nursing home.

The church is open for various programs at least five evenings each week, all day Saturday and Sunday, and much of Wednesday, so it offers an open door and a safe haven in a dangerous neighborhood. It is a social center in which friendships are fostered, visitors are welcome, and both visitors and members are helped.

Active members include a few who are paid union-scale wages or are professionals, many working poor, and a few on welfare or disability. Most of the worshipers are poor, but not desperately, chronically poor—we learned, however, about several who had been chronically poor before they joined the church. Celia, a leader of the Helping Hands Ministry, was on welfare until the pastor persuaded her to get her GED; she later became a nurse and now tithes. Alex, who came after being released from prison, has remained employed, drug free, and legal—and employed. One of the elders used to be "the project drunk" before he was saved, joined the church, then got a good job and kept it. We heard several other stories like these, all told to show that if people stay active in the church, they can help one another resist the temptations of the devil and therefore remain reliable workers. The inactive members and the nonmembers who still identify the church as "theirs" are another story—60 or 70 percent are desperately poor, are on welfare and have been for a long time, and may be addicted or in trouble with the law. But they have people reaching out to them, praying for them, trying to find them and connect.

The Revival Center is a good example of the traditional "introverted forms of black Pentecostal social intervention,"[25] with no political activity beyond the occasional circulation of the nominating petition of a Church of God in Christ member seeking public office. The members give generously, but it is a mutual aid organization, not a charitable giving program and much less a broker of government funds or secular philanthropy. It is mutual aid, however, among a group that constantly reaches beyond those who regularly give, to bring in those who constantly need.

Conclusion: A Few Children, Very Few

It was in one of the Henry Horner high-rise buildings that LaJoe Rivers gave Alex Kotlowitz the title of his best-selling book. "But you know, there are no children here," she said. "They've seen too much to be children."[26] Through the eyes of Rivers's sons Lafeyette and Pharoah, Kotlowitz saw, and enabled us to see, the violence, hunger, loneliness, and degradation experienced daily by people of all ages at Henry Horner. Through their eyes we also saw their isolation, not only from the world outside but also from one another—people too fearful to connect.

Yet, for an hour a week in First Baptist Congregational's extension Sunday school, for an hour or two when a nun from Saint Malachy visits, and for much of the week at the Revival Center, a few kids from Henry Horner can be children again. Not that they will forget what they have seen; to the contrary, they will find a way to build a social network that does not remove them from Henry Horner but helps them cope with it. Those who come to the Revival Center might be fortunate enough to find an adult who already knows a parent or grandparent or cousin; or the kids might come *with* their parents. But Kotlowitz's compelling story and most social science accounts of ghetto poverty fail to mention the communities of faith that attempt to bridge the isolation of people living in concentrated poverty.

But the bridging is meager. For individuals like Celia and Alex, the Revival Center is a blessing. But with respect to the social isolation of the neighborhood's ghetto underclass, the church activities reported here suggest an underdeveloped potential, not a major contribution. The feeding programs and clothing closets mitigate the physical impact of acute poverty and will undoubtedly become more important as part of a privatized safety net made necessary by late-1990s changes in welfare policy. But we found little evidence that these charitable activities built social networks, enabling people in concentrated poverty to interact with and participate in a wider world. Similarly, Saint Malachy School provides the children of the Near West Side not only a quality education but a safe space where they can "be children," but the restructuring by which the archdiocese has arranged to maintain the school financially also separates it from the social network of the parish membership.

The participation of Saint Stephen and Saint Malachy and the central leadership of First Baptist Congregational in the Interfaith Organizing Project demonstrated the continuing importance of the black churches as powerful public institutions that can anchor neighborhood redevelopment. But the well-being of Henry Horner residents was less central than justice for owners of the modest homes nearby in IOP's confrontations with the Bears, Bulls, and the City of Chicago. And while IOP's marches against drugs, gangs, crime, and violence have obvious relevance to the Henry Horner Homes and to other poor residents, they are more directed at the deviant residents than toward enlisting the struggling victims of isolation, like Celia and LaJoe.

Our discussion of the Revival Center has shown that a small church with meager financial resources and a modest physical plant can serve as the basis for social networks bridging the boundaries that generally divide urban underclass people from mainstream society. The church has shared food and clothing as a rural family might feed a needy neighbor or stranger by adding a potato and extra water to the soup. Moreover, the pastor and lay leaders never mentioned social isolation and did not talk of providing social services; their concern was to help people find salvation in Christ, that they might be delivered from the power of Satan. Having found salvation, they would become part of a family-like network in which the saved would provide mutual reinforcement in the Christian life; backsliders would be nurtured and reclaimed; and the backsliders' children, spouses, and parents would be prayed for and cared for in their absence.

The practice of this Christian family network was the main evidence of the church interacting with, as opposed to serving, ghetto underclass people. A major difference between Celia and LaJoe Rivers, between ex-convict Alex and LaJoe's imprisoned son, LaShawn, is that Celia and Alex found the Revival Center, and it became their extended family.

How much difference does one little church really make? How many other examples of isolation-bridging Christian community might we have missed? Members of First Baptist Congregational Church steer people they know into the Drug Ministry and the Henry Horner Sunday school, and there are undoubtedly other such connective tissues being fostered by churches on the Near West Side. Yet the Revival Center appears to be unique, not only in having Henry Horner residents as active members but also in its intense and interpersonal way of evangelizing in Henry Horner—visiting people in their apartments there and taking the initiative to maintain relationships that would otherwise atrophy. Overall on the Near West Side, we found the number of people who, through the ministries of the churches, were being woven into networks that bridged the social isolation of the poor to be exceedingly small. We hope we have only scratched the surface, and that others will further investigate the social networks of urban churches and the extent to which they bridge the social isolation of urban underclass people.

NOTES

We are particularly grateful to April Payton Bernard for exceptional assistance in field research for this chapter.

1. Wilson, *Truly Disadvantaged.*

2. Data are from the U.S. Census, 1980 and 1990, as reported in Chicago Fact Book Consortium, *Local Community Fact Book Chicago Metropolitan Area 1990.* See also Wilson, ed., *Ghetto Underclass,* 3; Kasarda, "Urban Industrial Transition."

3. Kotlowitz, *There Are No Children Here,* preface.

4. Lincoln and Mamiya, *Black Church,* 8.

5. Ibid., 384.

6. Cf. Sanders, *Saints in Exile;* Daniels, "Cultural Renewal"; and Franklin, "Safest Place on Earth."

7. Paris, *Social Teaching.*

8. Gilkes, "Storm and Light"; Higgenbotham, *Righteous Discontent.*

9. Interpretations of the black church are still contested and debated. Cf. Lincoln, *Black Church since Frazier;* and Lincoln and Mamiya, *Black Church,* on the legacy of Frazier *(Negro Church in America)* and on the "myth of the black church and politics" advanced by several black intellectuals, such as Adolph L. Reed Jr. and Gary Marx.

10. Lincoln and Mamiya, *Black Church,* 138 and 383–385.

11. Kostarelos, *Feeling the Spirit;* Paris, *Black Pentecostalism;* Sanders, *Saints in Exile.* However, Williams, *Community in a Black Pentecostal Church;* and Mukenge, *Black Church in Urban America,* provide socioeconomic profiles of members of churches studied.

12. Franklin, *Another Day's Journey.*

13. Wilson, *Truly Disadvantaged;* Wilson, ed., *Ghetto Underclass;* and Wilson, *When Work Disappears.* See also Copeland, *And the Poor Get Welfare;* and Blank, *It Takes a Nation,* which as a national, not just an inner-city, study of poverty focuses less than Wilson on concentration and social isolation. Anderson, in *Streetwise* and "Code of the Streets," focuses on the self-destructive behavior patterns adopted by those living in extreme and long-term poverty.

14. Kostarelos, *Feeling the Spirit;* and Policy Research Action Group, *Black Churches of West Humboldt Park,* also show that members of small, poor churches located in poor neighborhoods do not necessarily live in those neighborhoods.

15. Coleman, "Families and Schools," "Social Capital," and *Foundations of Social Theory.* There is a growing and increasingly popularized literature on social capital, including, for example, Putnam, "Bowling Alone." Putnam's notion of "generalized reciprocation"—the presumption that assistance rendered will be returned, but not necessarily by the direct recipient—presupposes a social network—hence reinforcing our determination to see if churches can foster such networks among the otherwise socially isolated poor.

16. Franklin, *Another Day's Journey,* 51.

17. McGreevy, *Parish Boundaries,* 4.

18. This historical information is derived from Interfaith Organizing Project, *New "West Side Story,"* and from interviews with current and former board members.

19. Earnest Gates, interview with the authors, April 12, 1995.

20. Agreements reached between the owners of the Chicago Bulls and IOP include the replacement of demolished buildings or payment of full market value of each building plus $30,000; the provision of $600,000 no-interest loan to IOP for the construction of homes for sale in the West Side; the building of a new public library in the West Side by the joint venture; provision of $75,000 to assist in reopening Mile Square Health Center; and the construction of a park in the community.

21. Sanders, *Saints in Exile;* Franklin, "My Soul Says Yes."

22. Franklin, "My Soul Says Yes."

23. Lincoln and Mamiya, *Black Church,* 2–6.

24. Gilkes, "Storm and Light," 186ff.

25. McRoberts, "Understanding the 'New' Black Pentecostal Activism," 48.

26. Kotlowitz, *There Are No Children Here,* preface.

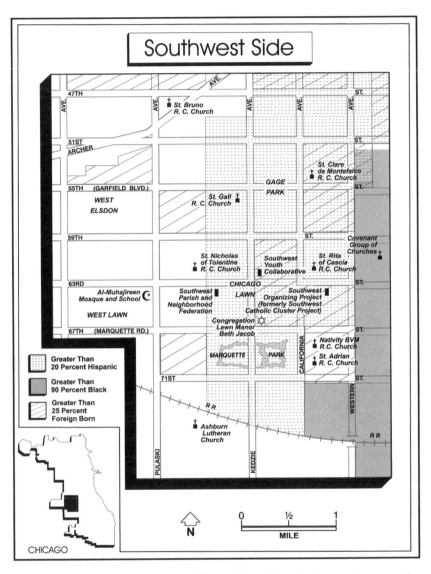

Map 5. The Southwest Side, a classic blue-collar, white-ethnic area, is now receiving Hispanic, Arab, African American, and Polish newcomers. Map by Brian Twardosz, BMT Printing and Cartographic Specialists.

"God Doesn't Ask What Language I Pray In"
Community and Culture on Chicago's Southwest Side

Elfriede Wedam

The blue-collar neighborhoods in Chicago were long known for the brightest Christmas lights in the area. Some houses had neat designs, others were gaudy. All were expressive and delightful to children's eyes, as reflected in the reactions of my siblings and me. Some blocks looked as though the neighbors had decided together what the year's style or motif would be. On others, it appeared as if there were a competition for the best, or at least the biggest, design. But however it was done, these neighborhoods distinguished themselves with the amount of light that streamed from them. Later, I wondered if the enthusiasm for Christmas decorations had to do with the Catholic propensity for material faith, since these neighborhoods were also predominantly Catholic.

Summers revealed impeccable lawns and trimmed bushes. They were curiously limited, however, in their flower gardens, at least to the eye of the passing motorist. There was just enough color to rescue the panorama from dullness, but far less of the floral vanity that stylish yards emit. There was not much space for the gardens because these small, vigorously maintained bungalows and two- and three-flat apartment buildings rested on narrow lots, arranged in soldierly rows.

The expressive quality of these homes and neighborhoods did not occur by chance. Every locale is defined by culture in the broadest sense, and these neighborhoods reflected the particular class, religious, racial, ethnic, national, and language characteristics of their residents. The outward appearance of the neighborhoods symbolized shared understandings about their meaning. It is neighborhoods like these, in five community areas on the Southwest Side of Chicago, that are the focus of this chapter. Here, residents are reexamining their self-understandings as they confront changing urban realities. I try to unravel some of these shared meanings and self-understandings. I use observations I conducted during the mid-1990s of two Catholic parishes, Saint Nicholas of Tolentine and Saint Bruno, and of a community organization, the Southwest Organizing Project, and I include data from several additional congregations, Protestant, Jewish, and Catholic, as well as other community-based groups.

The neighborhoods are located about five to seven miles southwest of the Loop, Chicago's downtown business district. I argue that these neighborhoods have been strong moral communities, not chiefly because of their high standards of behavior but because the residents act in negotiation with one another for the collective standards to which they hold each other. Historically, these neighborhoods have exemplified the "defended neighborhoods," as Gerald Suttles has described them,[1] that have responded in particular political ways to challenges by groups considered "outsiders." Defended neighborhoods contain a type of social order within which the residents can secure themselves against common apprehensions. This analysis attempts to identify the fundamental causes of those apprehensions, why the neighborhoods take the shape they do, who benefits, who loses, and how the changes in the order (or disorder) in the neighborhoods can be explained.[2] I argue that the kinds of changes that occur are related to the success or failure of new and old residents to negotiate on the basis of a shared sense of a moral order.

Community and Moral Culture in the Southwest Side

The power of community as a concept and a reality is its ability to point to a fundamental human process: the "sense of a primacy of belonging."[3] There is a "presumptive good" to community.[4] Community ties are essential for both healthy individuals and functioning civil society. For example, the strong sense of a collective identity among first-generation immigrant Poles contributed to their community mental health.[5]

The "loss of community" theme gains much of its strength from the acknowledgment that geographic mobility and changes in family life—divorce and blended families—have created certain instabilities in our expectations. Much public discourse and social criticism contrasts idealized tight-knit communities with the extreme individualism that life in modern society permits. In these critiques, moral authority is seen to have been exercised by parents, neighbors, congregations, and even politicians in customary and public ways prior to the privileging of individual rights since the 1960s. The focus on authority limited individual choices, but it also fostered lasting relationships embedded in community ties and legitimated rules that enforced social order. When authority, order, and community were rejected by the baby-boom generation, as Alan Ehrenhalt argues, they were replaced with unlimited choice, personal privacy, and free-market domination. This resulted in a loss of community accountability and an expansion of economic determinism into all areas of our lives.[6] Some of this criticism reveals an "American small town" nostalgia that overlooks the closing of ranks in the face of outsiders, often of another race or class. But it also suggests that community relationships depend on an acknowledgment of interdependence, not merely on the assertion of individual and civil rights.

Studying the culture of community is, in the largest sense, about studying "meaning" and "moral order," argues sociologist Robert Wuthnow.[7] It is studying the relations among individuals and groups in a social system that make organized, collective life possible. Meaning mostly has been analyzed as the property of individuals, but Wuthnow directs sociological inquiry toward meaning revealed in the group life of actors. In the case of the religious dimension of culture, this refers to how individuals relate in the context of their congregations and community organizations. One way to put this, then, is that culture is about how our collective life makes sense to us collectively.

Moral culture includes shared assumptions about the nature of relationships and about the norms and rules that are taught and enforced. For example, a former Southwest Side resident interpreted her neighborhood as a "village" where, when she was growing up, she and other children could roam safely. Her parents were confident that if a neighbor became a "problem," "everyone else felt the same way about it." The adherence to collective standards by members of these Euro-American ethnic neighborhoods was by no means inviolable, but widely understood norms existed by which neighbors could gauge one another's behavior. Yet norms change over time as a result of conflict, created, for example, when community members married into a different religious, ethnic, or racial group.

Interaction among residents who have different social and demographic characteristics and hold different beliefs and values creates a neighborhood community in the urban context. The Southwest Side neighborhoods were never exclusively one ethnic or cultural group,[8] but a significant degree of homogeneity distinguished certain areas—the Lithuanian neighborhood, the Polish corridor, and the like. These neighborhoods are, in the words of *Habits of the Heart*, "communities of memory."[9] They are moral communities in which the residents are connected to one another through norms of authority and stories about "who we are" and "how we do things here." These values and beliefs are taught and practiced in the schools, the neighborhood associations, and the churches.

The negative side of communal ties—the propensity to turn outsiders into enemies—has been discussed by critics of *Habits*.[10] The insider/outsider dilemma is a recalcitrant aspect of American social divisions, because recognizing and constructing others as different permits us to form identities through communal bonds that are lasting, stable, and exclusive. At the same time, tight-knit communities, including the ones of the Southwest Side, have been losing members in large numbers, partially because of economic restructuring in the latter half of the twentieth century but also because they impose restrictions on behavior and create identities that have been increasingly rejected. Participants in the churches and organizations studied here have suggested new approaches to relationships with newcomers. Where racial and ethnic diversity stimulated fears in the past, some residents are initiating discussions that search out human commonalities rather than perpetuate differences between people. Instead of simply seeing the rejection of tightly knit neighborhoods as a "decline in community," we need to examine how the new immigrants to these neighborhoods have interacted and negotiated with the current residents to re-form community cohesion and redraw the boundaries of the insider group.

The urban Catholic churches have had a long history of connecting the family with the local parish in a social and religious ecology that created a particular meaning of neighborhood. Property bought within the parish boundaries sacralized the space of the parish, argues social historian John McGreevy, and created a bond for residents with the neighborhood and with their neighbors not comparable to bonds in predominantly non-Catholic neighborhoods.[11] This interpretation was confirmed in urban historian Thomas Sugrue's account of the deindustrialization of Detroit, when he noted the ways in which neighborhoods developed an identity for their Catholic homeowners despite the fact—or perhaps because of it—that the economic foundations on which these residents made their lives was so precarious.[12] The houses "were close together on small lots. Day-to-day life was structured by countless small interactions among neighbors; little was private. Property maintenance, behavior, and attitudes seldom escaped the close scrutiny of neighbors."[13] When the residents also shared a religious identity, these bonds were reinforced.

Another norm, "to keep up the property," also expresses unity and the ability to accept community standards. In fact, individualistic standards are not well tolerated in tight-knit communities. In the Southwest Side neighborhoods I frequently heard residents unabashedly state that newcomers needed to "follow the rules" and "do the same as I do." While these rules appeared unitary in some respects, they were also reciprocal—"You treat me right and I'll treat you right," explained one resident. These were rules about civic participation and neighborly expectations. Indeed, the enforcement of these rules, another resident explained, was not about power but about "love of the neighborhood." In the words of one Catholic pastor, the meaning of neighborhood for his parishioners emerged from relationships based on and in an "emotional geography." As the ethnic, racial, and religious composition of the members in these neighborhoods has changed, the old residents have negotiated with new residents for a new local meaning based on a different emotional geography.

Two parishes and a community organization illustrate how these new relationships are being formed. The discussions among their members are about two things: first, how to create relationships between newcomers and established members, and second, how these relationships reflect the neighborhoods around the parishes and community groups and, in turn, what effect the new relationships have on those neighborhoods. In the Polish national parish of Saint Bruno, the parishioners are discussing how the Polish language and culture affect their parish. Saint Nicholas of Tolentine is a cosmopolitan parish now experiencing racial change with the steady in-migration of Hispanics and some African Americans. In the Southwest Organizing Project, initially supported by the Archdiocese of Chicago to explore the role of the church in responding to racial and ethnic changes, the members are connecting with an ever-widening array of interfaith neighborhood groups.

The Southwest Side lies several miles southwest of the Loop and includes Gage Park, Chicago Lawn (Marquette Park), West Lawn, West Elsdon (bordering Midway Airport), and Archer Heights on the northwest corner. Marquette Park and Gage Park have a mixed ethnic and racial composition, while the other three areas remain predominantly white and European. Marquette Park shifted from about 83 percent white in 1980 to 47 percent white (a small number of whom are from the Middle East), 27 percent Hispanic, and 26 percent African American in 1990. In Gage Park, the number of Hispanic residents grew from 11 percent in 1980 to almost 40 percent in 1990, and the black population increased from 1 percent to 5 percent. Archer Heights is approximately 90 percent white, with a small increase in Hispanic numbers since 1980. West Lawn and West Elsdon are about 95 percent white. The percentage of home ownership in the neighborhoods, over 70 percent, has changed little from 1960. Among the residents are six major language groups: English, Polish, Slovak, Lithuanian, Arabic, and Spanish.

The expansion of Midway Airport during the 1990s has anchored the economy of the area, which had become precarious when some of the trucking industry and light manufacturing plants left. A rapid transit line linking the airport with the Loop opened in the early 1990s. Its positive economic impact, especially as reflected in increasing real estate value, has become a symbolic and practical vehicle for connecting the neighborhoods to the outside world. Sixty-third Street, the principal east-west corridor and popular shopping district during the mid-century, still has considerable foot traffic despite the competition of nearby malls.

The Southwest Side is home to nineteen major Catholic institutions: eleven parishes, two high schools, two religious-order motherhouses, one abbey, a press headquarters, a hospital, and a home for mentally retarded children. They comprise the Southwest Cluster, designed to promote communication among geographically proximal parishes. Through the cluster, the archdiocese reinforces the spatial relationships on which parishes are based but makes each parish less insular than in the past, less a "kingdom" and more a collaboration. Alongside the Catholic institutions are approximately forty-seven Protestant churches, a Conservative Jewish synagogue, and three Sunni Muslim mosques.

Saint Bruno Parish

Surrounded by tidy brick bungalows in the middle of Archer Heights sits Saint Bruno Catholic Church, its school, and its rectory. The parish was founded in 1923 by a committee of twelve laymen, who gathered support for establishing a Polish national church by circulating petitions in the neighborhood.[14] Ground for the modern church, a cream-colored brick in a simple yet imposing design, was broken in 1955; a second school building and modern rectory were added in 1975. Saint Bruno is one of three churches in the cluster that holds Sunday masses in Polish, and one of forty-two such in the archdiocese. Our Lady of Czestochowa, a popular saint in Poland, is honored with an outdoor shrine, fittingly graced with flowers in the summer and Christmas lights in the winter.

Saint Bruno is both a national and a territorial parish, served by three full-time Polish-speaking priests; one is himself a recent immigrant. About 80 percent of the 1,850 member families live within the parish boundaries. The parish school is just shy of its capacity of three hundred children. The composition of the parish population is about half new immigrants (one-third of whom are undocumented) and half Americans of Eastern European, mostly Polish, descent. Hispanics, about 6 percent of the church's registration, play a minor but growing role in the parish. For the time being Father Joseph Grembla, the pastor, does not use his fluency in Spanish, because these Hispanics are mostly second generation and English-speaking.

Saint Bruno's extensive agenda of social, devotional, and educational activities is offered in Polish and English. The religious education program—Confraternity of Christian Doctrine, or CCD—for public school children, staffed by fifteen to twenty volunteers, serves close to four hundred children in bilingual classes. Many children from outside the parish come for instruction in Polish. The eighty-member, strong-voiced choir sings in both languages and is often a guest choir in other churches. Saint Bruno holds two out of five weekend masses in Polish. The parish elementary school has English-language tutoring for children who need help, although it offers no classes in Polish. The parish bulletin and the parish newspaper, *St. Bruno Beat,* are written in both English and Polish.

The use of both Polish and English has different meanings for different members. American Poles and new immigrant Poles share an ethnicity but not a nationality. This has opened some important opportunities for understanding how culture is both a resource to draw on and a boundary line that is negotiated daily in parish activities.

Language and Community

The annual confirmation ceremony is an important parishwide event for the young teens, their sponsors, and parents, as the young people publicly accept their adult religious responsibilities. Because of its public, ritual importance, the ceremony is held in English. When one of the parish priests included some Polish prayers, the congregation became ill at ease. Afterward, complaints flowed in to the pastor, the parish council members, and even the choir director. One parish council member suggested that no one was prepared to hear Polish, and consequently, people did not know how to respond. The sense of unpreparedness, if this was indeed the case, revealed a deeper ambivalence.

At Saint Bruno, the Polish language is a symbol of the way in which immigrants are both included in the new world and separate from their American neighbors and fellow parishioners. The multiple meanings of language permitted the congregation to make multiple interpretations, opening a debate that included ordinarily muted, negative interpretations of bilingualism. What was the *meaning* of using Polish during an English mass? Was this an attempt surreptitiously to add Polish into a formal liturgy that should represent the parish as a whole? Did the decision communicate a preference for a second language through which the parish will no longer speak as majoritarians? Was this a symbol of further ethnic encroachment, changing the identity of the parish from one that serves Poles to one that is a Polish parish? Does this mean we are no longer Americans?

The pluralist-versus-assimilationist conflict continues over the bilingual religious education classes for children of members who attend public schools. Most of the new Polish immigrant children do not attend Saint Bruno's elementary school. To fulfill the requirement for training in the faith, Polish parents send their children to the CCD program on Saturday mornings. The assimilationists in the parish wish to offer the classes only in English, whereas the pluralists see no advantages to this, only the loss of their heritage.

The conflict between pluralism and assimilation shows how divisive nonracial cultural differences can be. This conflict is about different generations of immigrants of the same national origin whose experiences are set in contrasting cultural contexts. Those contexts permit different interpretations of the meaning of the Polish language in worship and religious education and of its symbolic importance in positioning oneself in American society. Consequently, a common heritage and tradition—elements of a primordial identity—are not sufficient to create community at Saint Bruno. Rather, negotiating the *interpretations* of that heritage

Fig. 5-1. Devotion to Our Lady of Czestochowa at Saint Bruno Roman Catholic Church, Southwest Side, Chicago. Photo courtesy of Saint Bruno Roman Catholic Church.

and tradition is the cultural process through which relationships, and thus community, are formed.

Church and Neighborhood

The Archer Heights Community Organization pays special attention to housing, and it is again no accident that Saint Bruno members are active in it. One evening, the Parish Pastoral Council engaged in heated discussion on the matter of illegal housing conversions by Polish landlords who took in new immigrants. These conversions involved making additional rooms in the basements and attics of single-family houses. One of the parish leaders argued that following the housing regulations was a way of maintaining the neighborhood "as a precious asset" that must be preserved, for the good of the church and for the common good of all residents. "If the neighborhood goes down," this member asserted, "the church will go down too."

The immigrants were less appalled at the suggestion that some of their peers were trying to bend the rules for their own gain than at their perception that critics lacked sympathy for their difficulties of being uprooted and reestablished in a new world. "Immigrants have it hard," one immigrant member explained, "they have much to learn. We sacrifice a lot to try and fit in, yet, if those people [American Poles] don't have any feeling for us, you are set back." Another immigrant stated that the council should discuss such matters as the school and finances, but "they shouldn't worry about immigrants." The council should be aware of what's happening in the community but not "pick on one ethnic group."

This exchange exemplifies how the physical appearance of the neighborhood is a public and political matter, shared among long-term residents, that they scrutinize and evaluate, whereas newer residents simply feel besieged. Older residents claim that poor housing standards result in people leaving the neighborhood, and "we can't afford to lose good parishioners." Newer residents are less likely to focus on the public aspect of what is essentially—in the American definition—a private commodity, one's home. When American Poles emphasize assimilation to American rules and the values that support them, they are focusing on the muted communalist strain in American culture, rather than on the currently more pronounced individualist strain.

The economic dimension of this issue is rooted in the immigrants' continuing ties to their country of origin; for some, their "real parish" is still in Poland. Many Poles, like the Mexican immigrants discussed in chapter 2, have adopted a transnational identity, with connections to their home country continually renewed by travel, communication, and the circulation of money. These exchanges are enriching to the cultures of both the United States and the country of origin. But they are also a social and economic resource drain in each local context, because the tentativeness of commitment precludes a stable and secure involvement. The illegal conversion problem is especially irksome to some parishioners who feel that those who take advantage of American opportunities should share more of the costs. Nevertheless, the new immigrants increase parish rolls, and Fr. Grembla reported a 20 percent increase in giving as a result of a greater appeal to the newcomers. In the end, housing is highly important to long-term residents because it affects their community identity, not just their economic well-being.[15]

The matter of illegal housing conversions raised in the Parish Pastoral Council was withdrawn from discussion when the immigrant Poles on the council successfully argued in a later meeting that this was a civil issue and should not be the subject of church business. Privately, one immigrant Pole recounted to me that a number of new Polish immigrants in the neighborhood are not Catholics, or at least are not registered or practicing Catholics. (This is similar to the migration of black Protestants into heavily Catholic neighborhoods.) These people are harder for the church members to reach. But appealing to a church-state separation reduces the ability of the church to participate in the civic dialogue about what the definition of an American is and where it lies on the continuum from a whole-hearted idealism and patriotism to a crass economic opportunism.

The limitations the parishioners themselves place on the dialogue within the church also weakens its role as a moral community. In response to the push to relegate the housing issue to the civil domain, the council president argued, "Because of our ability to reach out in the Polish language, Saint Bruno Parish is in a unique position to act on this issue. We can communicate, educate, and be an agent of peace to our community. Does this sound like part of our mission as Church?" He suggested further that community issues are issues of justice on which parishioners may eventually be faced with decisions. While community issues continue to push through to become council business, they are perhaps mostly those, like community policing, on which members already agree.

For longtime residents of the Southwest Side, the neighborhood is not just a place to live but a place to which one must contribute. Several members related to me their conviction that a strong neighborhood made a strong church, not the reverse, and that because of the consequences for the church, members have a moral duty to protect the neighborhood. Maintaining control over the neighborhood was not only a response to the structural features of economic insecurity that blue-collar neighborhoods suffered but also an expression of their beliefs in community, family, and God.

Lay Leadership and Parish Planning

Saint Bruno's Parish Pastoral Council—which itself is required by the archdiocese (see chapter 11)—is using parish planning as a tool to form a more integrated parish community. The formation of the council was accompanied by different views about its role and purpose in the parish. Some members wondered, "Why get involved in this? Let the priests do it." Others were gratified that their views were being considered but worried that the council might develop its own agenda, independent of individual parish members.

In response to the statement "The toughest job of the council is to dream dreams and lay out broad visions," a member commented that as a Catholic parishioner, he had never been asked to "dream dreams." In fact, he noted that creativity was not a mark of this working-class parish. But the lay leadership at Saint Bruno is redefining the relationship between parishioners and their parish in order to reconceive their Catholic, parish, and, ultimately, community identity.

Saint Bruno's Parish Pastoral Council conducted a survey of parishioners in both Polish and English to help the council determine the administrative, spiritual, educational, and social priorities of the parish. The planning process stimulated new developments such as *St. Bruno Beat,* the parish newspaper. But it revealed many issues that affect participation and communication between ethnic groups and between generations. While steady leadership in some parish organizations provided continuity and stability, it also sometimes shut out potential leadership from younger people with new ideas. Three of Saint Bruno's council members attended archdiocesan leadership classes that included learning methods of organizing parish groups so as to overcome the tendency to form cliques. A number of parishioners requested that the parish develop a more welcoming atmosphere at church, beginning with expanding the role of the ushers beyond the taking of the collection.

The parish survey confirmed the widely shared opinion that the bilingual choir has made important strides in bridging the language communities at Saint Bruno. Before the current music director was hired, the church had two choirs, one for each language group. Through the combined choir, the members learned "not to be afraid of each other," the music director said.

The survey also confirmed a lack of inclusion of teens in parish activities, especially the liturgies. The council resolved to invite teens to become lectors and take on other lay ministerial roles, and it renewed its commitment to form a teen club that would better connect young people with the parish. Similarly, the council resolved to raise the visibility of young adults through a Parish Commission for Young Adult Ministry that would connect directly with the archdiocesan program.

Through the planning process, the council members saw how parish leadership could change their role from carrying out intraparish activities to exploring ways for the "church to be a model for the world." The pastor noted, however, that the sense of "mission" is not well understood in the parish, for example, with regard to the role of evangelization. The challenge for the council, then, becomes how to extend the envisioning process that began with the council leaders into the decisions and actions of the members.

Not all new immigrants today participate in the parish-building form of community that molded so many earlier generations of newcomers. Many of the recent Polish arrivals both seek out and are steered by well-meaning American and Polish contacts to established churches, founded generations earlier. Poles in Chicago come to churches like Saint Bruno that provide a historical ethnic mission. For immigrating Poles, Saint Bruno is one kind of "proximal host," the concept employed and adapted to religious communities by the authors of *Gatherings in Diaspora* in order to explain the relationship between new immigrants and the receiving country.[16] This relationship refers to the placement of new immigrants into proximity with Americans whom they resemble, often according to a racialized conception of their identity. Because of this particular context, these immigrants cannot shape parishes to their identities as did their predecessors, who created a refuge for themselves as they struggled with the challenges of their new, often hostile—anti-Catholic, anti-immigrant—environment. Today's Polish immigrants are given a template forged by others and shaped by their memories—which may not be recognizable to the new immigrants. Indeed, one of the parish leaders reported that many parish children remember that "grandpa never got any help." Part of the challenge facing the immigrant Poles is negotiating the fit between their newly forming identities and the templates offered by their hosts.

Neither group fully recognizes either its inclusivity or its resistance. Yet, for some members of Saint Bruno, the diversity in the parish offers alternatives not often found in a parish—it is both modern and traditional in outlook, and the dual languages offer the opportunity for expressing oneself with both an American and a European identity, tradition, and culture.

Through parish planning and the empowerment of lay members, the church has rediscovered the importance of a welcoming atmosphere and how the sharing of stories through music and writing creates opportunities to bridge cultural differences. Opening the boundaries of any in-group must include making the out-group understandable, thus "rendering the unknown into a familiar form."[17]

Saint Nicholas of Tolentine Parish

About two miles away from Saint Bruno, in the heart of the Southwest Cluster and straddling the communities of Chicago Lawn (known locally as Marquette Park, after the large and well-used city park nearby) and West Lawn, sits the parish of Saint Nicholas of Tolentine. It was founded as a mission by the Order of Saint Augustine in 1909 but organized and run as a parish by the Archdiocese of Chicago since 1916.[18] The red-brick church in an English Gothic style stands only one-half block from busy Sixty-third Street. The local public high school faces the church property on one side. There are more than twenty-six hundred registered families and almost six hundred children in the parish school, the largest in the Southwest Cluster.

The parish rolls of Saint Nicholas grew steadily during the 1990s as many first- and second-generation Latino families, mostly from Mexico, moved into this part of the city. During the year of our study, about half of the schoolchildren were Hispanic, half were white, and three African American children had recently transferred from a nearby school, which closed the year before our research visits. The church holds six masses on Sunday, one of which is in Spanish, celebrated by the pastor, Father Stanley Rataj, who recently learned Spanish in order to serve the new immigrant population. Saint Nicholas is one of 5 churches in the Southwest Cluster to offer masses in Spanish, and one of 110 in the archdiocese to do so.

Saint Nicholas has long been a large, active parish, demonstrating leadership in Vatican II liturgy and participating in community organizations. *A History of the Parishes of the Archdiocese of Chicago* calls Saint Nicholas a "cosmopolitan" parish because, despite being surrounded by ethnic parishes, it never favored any language group, having families of East European, Hispanic, Irish, and Italian descent. This is not without its special meaning. As an associate pastor phrased it, there are many boundaries to identify and respect.

The parish supports a wide variety of traditional Catholic organizations and activities, such as the Holy Thursday tour of the churches, and some nontraditional ones, such as the Passover seder and the Covenant Group of Churches, which includes several parishes in West Englewood as well as some Protestant churches. The Covenant Group emerged to work for a prayerful racial reconciliation in the aftermath of the 1992 Los Angeles riots, which erupted at the acquittal of white police officers in the beating of Rodney King. The Liturgy Committee is in high gear most of the time, and an archdiocese-mandated parish-planning effort is taking shape. In the mid-1990s, the Society of Our Lady of Guadalupe and a Latino youth group were formed, and several Latinas are members of the parish council. One Hispanic and one white couple were preparing for the deaconate.

Language and Community

Language differences reveal group boundaries within Saint Nicholas, just as they do at Saint Bruno. Saint Nicholas's strategies to address them are different, making room for a new set of members, mostly Latino, who are, in effect, building a parish in shared space. The building process has been both collaborative and segmented. The old and new members do not share a predominant ethnicity, so the parishioners have had to find ways to cross both language and racial differences.

Few priestly vocations among Hispanics means that unlike immigrants before them, the Spanish-speaking groups have few native clergy who can serve their needs. The relative poverty of Hispanics puts the financial burden of Spanish liturgies—for example, language training for priests—on the archdiocese and on the special efforts of religious orders. The previous pastor at Saint Nicholas resisted demands for a Spanish liturgy in the early 1990s, which Fr. Rataj explained later as concerning the issue of "how to do it right." Subsequently, it took over a year of committed efforts by both clergy and lay members to find and train all the liturgical ministers, altar servers, and lectors as well as ensuring a Spanish-speaking priest to say Mass regularly. While not everyone agrees that this played a role in moving the liturgy effort forward, at the time there was heavy proselytizing by Hispanic Protestants in the neighborhood around the church. One lay leader pointed out two Protestant churches nearby in which the membership changed from predominantly white to predominantly Hispanic in only a couple of years.

The Spanish mass had the unintended consequence of furthering group separation when some white members became alienated because "they didn't get a Polish mass" when they had asked for it years before. Hispanics have been able to claim ownership over language in a way that Poles at Saint Nicholas could not. The tension is not over English-speaking versus Spanish-speaking liturgy in the creation of an American as opposed to a foreign identity but over how cultural power is wielded in the parish.

Fig. 5-2. Ballet Folklorico of Mexico performing at a Cinco de Mayo celebration at Saint Nicholas of Tolentine Roman Catholic Church, Southwest Side, Chicago. Photo courtesy of Saint Nicholas of Tolentine Roman Catholic Church.

When asked why a Spanish mass is problematic—for English speakers who want English as well as for Poles who did not get their Polish mass—when there are Lithuanian, Polish, and Slovak masses in churches within a couple of miles, one elderly resident explains, "The Lithuanians built *their* church, the Spanish did not build *our* church." "Our church" signifies what historian Dominic Pacyga calls a kind of "genetic" ownership that is an important dimension of territory in Chicago ethnic parishes.[19] The sense of ownership tied to one's ethnic predecessors, who in most cases are not kin related, is part of a sense of collective identity that has some exclusionary consequences, especially for people of a different race but also for all non-Lithuanians, non-Poles, or whichever ethnic group predominates.

Yet focusing on owning overlooks the dimension of "building." Including new groups who initially are seen as outsiders requires face-to-face negotiating, addressing cultural differences, and responding to the fears these differences generate. Equally important, it is a negotiation around *perceptions* of cultural differences. As members of any social group, we need to make sense of the continuing changes that are part of ordinary life. We use our past experiences to transform new instances into forms sufficiently familiar that we can make some sense of them. If we cannot, we tend to become frightened.[20] These are often-repeated experiences. Sharing religious experiences offers the possibility of making the strange into the familiar.

Members describe one bridging event between Latinos and white parishioners as "magical" in its effect on the participants and its ability to stimulate cross-cultural understanding. A meeting between whites and Latinos was organized shortly after the forming of the Guadalupe Society to give parishioners what was hoped to be a "wide-open opportunity" to express their fears and hopes about the changing membership. Strong statements were made by both whites and Hispanics, but they came almost entirely from English-speaking participants. Despite the presence of translators, the language had been going only from English to Spanish. Finally, a seventy-eight-year-old non-English speaking Latina stood up. Through a translator, she told the story of how she recently came to live with her children in this country, despite her desire to stay in Mexico. She made a plea for a Spanish mass so that she could "talk to God, because I must talk to God." She was unable to learn English at her age and felt cut off from the liturgy by the language barrier. Her account moved many of the participants in the room. One organizer cited that event as crucial for the institution of the Spanish mass.

Yet, for other leaders in the parish, language is a barrier to the search for commonalities that community requires. I frequently heard the story from parishes with new Hispanic immigrants that "if you can't talk to your neighbors, it's a real problem." One parishioner at Saint Nicholas explained that unless you talk to people and find out how they feel, you cannot overcome stereotypes that blockade the identification of common values. She felt the emphasis on culture creates competition between nationalities. In her own Polish family, culture is unifying within the family context. But at the community level, she asserts, commitment must be to extracultural goals, such as to school, to jobs, and to God. This reflects a style of moral integration that parish life as a center for the neighborhood still contains.

Working on a common project often builds unity because it provides opportunities for interaction between groups. Saint Nicholas began this by raising over $11,000 at their first Cinco de Mayo celebration, a national holiday important to Mexicans. It was a fund-raiser for an orphanage in Mexico, where the orphans themselves came to entertain in a professionally executed performance. Many people, including the majority whites who attended, called it a success. It was important in the effort to create commonalities in order to demonstrate that a joint white-Latino event could be financially successful and equitable, with no sliding scale in the price of admission. The two gatekeepers, one Latino, one white, ensured that all paid, whether or not they were poor immigrants. But the amount of money raised was only part of the motivation. It was as important to demonstrate that parish relationships, that is, community, are not free, and that sacrifices for the collective effort are required.

Church and Neighborhood

"Where are you going to run to?"—asked the leader of Saint Nicholas's seniors group as she described the choices some white parishioners made when immigrants of color began moving into the blocks surrounding hers. In the suburbs, houses cost over $100,000, she exclaimed. Who wanted a mortgage at her age? And if you were not able to drive, you would become a prisoner in your own home. And then, there are no sidewalks in the suburbs. And crime? Her nieces told her there was all kinds of crime in their suburbs.

A few blocks away, Saint Nicholas's Parish Council held their second "block meeting" to which they invited all residents, Catholic and non-Catholic. This strategy was used to create a personal connection with residents and was an invitation for them to become acquainted, hear about the parish, and bring up their issues. One Lutheran couple attending urged their neighbors to "stay together and not move out." Rather than asking, "Why not move, if you have the chance?" they asked, "Why do it?" But the latter alternative is seldom suggested to residents who are confronting racial and ethnic population diversity. The former alternative is all too clear.

Another resident commented that although the fear days of the 1970s and 1980s were over, it nevertheless "scares people when some blacks and Hispanics move in and don't keep up the house." The history of this scenario has only reinforced people's interpretations. "It's hard to always know the reasons why people move in this context," mused one of the lay leaders. "It's hard to put my finger on why—are they running from the graffiti, or is it time to move on because they are empty-nesters, or some other reason?"

The block meetings addressed what urban planners call "tipping points." How many individual decisions have to occur before the result appears as an inexorable ecological process? One associate pastor recounted how quickly change occurs. A particular block near the church had a *Saturday Evening Post* quality to it that he would often admire as he took his evening walk. But he got word that a couple of the families were hassled by gang members, and within days, a "forest of for-sale signs" went up. Gangs are a recent visible reality among the Sixty-third street neighborhoods and present a physical and psychological threat. Graffiti is often the first sign. Saint Nicholas's mothers club sponsored a talk by the Eighth Police District gang specialist on how to recognize and respond to gang presence in the neighborhood. The sergeant's talk was so detailed that several people noted out loud that they were more afraid after the meeting than before.

When an area is perceived to be undergoing racial and ethnic change, the visibility of certain otherwise benign and casual characteristics of neighborhood housing is more salient. Houses that are not "kept up" and lawns that are not mowed take on heightened significance with regard to the neighborhood's desirability and future possibility. The nonstandard condition of even one piece of property in the hands of new in-migrants seems a harbinger of change, pointing to inevitable loss of status. Chatting after the mothers club meeting described above, one elderly resident related to me her concerns about a Hispanic family next door who didn't take care of their lawn, while another Hispanic family nearby "is very nice." Despite the approval, her hope regarding the latter was tentative; "you never know when that might change." We can see in her language that she directly links physical upkeep of the house with moral worthiness. A family that cares for its property is also interpreted to be "very nice."

This resident's apprehensions have been formed and tested by the experience of change across the South Side—in South Shore, Pullman, Englewood, and West Englewood. A leader from the synagogue recounted the climate of fear that existed in her neighborhood during the 1960s and 1970s. Many of her neighbors had moved to the Southwest Side from the Southeast not long before and felt the same kind of transition was going to take place again. She knew that "if people didn't fly, property values wouldn't go down," but many people would not believe it and left anyway. Because she and her husband moved to the Southwest Side by choice, she felt they had a different attitude about it. Since they never felt "they had to move" from a previous location, they had not experienced loss or pressure. A pastor from a neighboring parish recalled the feeling of overwhelming inevitability in the process of change in Pullman-Roseland, where he served during the 1960s: "It felt like a tidal wave coming off the lake [Michigan] and eventually will roll over everything in its path."

In the end, people also move for greed, asserted Saint Nicholas's longtime deacon Frank Sullivan. Reasons for leaving the old neighborhood include the desire for a bigger house, a bigger yard, more shopping opportunities. Decisions such as these deliberately counter the American desire for community.[21] Instead, the deacon and his family "made a decision to put down roots, to belong here." The racial and ethnic succession he observed in the Southwest Side reminded him of his growing-up experience in North Lawndale on the West Side, which is an impoverished African American neighborhood today. The neighborhood had been mostly Irish, with some Jewish areas to the south, when suddenly there was an exodus of the Irish, and into the vacuum came the Italians. The deacon remembered the first Italian-Irish wedding announcement at the local church, which proved so disruptive that the couple had to be married at Holy Name Cathedral downtown.

A narrative strategy for crossing boundaries of race, ethnicity, and cultural practices is to ask the question Saint Nicholas's deacon asked: "What's going on with others?" This opens a discussion to the discovery of other people's cultural stories. Saint Nicholas provided the setting for such storytelling, though not all people participated in it. Cultural styles also vary. Some Hispanics' reticence and preference not to intrude can easily be interpreted as resistance and unwillingness to share responsibility.

Creating culture involves the negotiation of many details of daily life at a parish. Constant discussion of issues that might not seem significant to an outsider is a sign of the cultural process at work. In describing the new model of parish they are working to form, the chair of the Parish Pastoral Council at Saint Nicholas told me, "*Doing* is what we're used to." Holding events, raising money, belonging to parish organizations, some social, others pietistic—these have been the stuff of parish life, creating solidarity and marking off the symbolic territory that parishioners identified with. As part of the archdiocesan restructuring effort, Saint Nicholas is being asked to change its focus from more grounded and insular realities—parish-focused and directed by the priests—to the creation of new visions and goals, where laity decide together with the clergy what those might be. Thus the lay members' negotiation with new residents across the language and racial barriers, essential to the formation of community in the Southwest Side, has a new place in a more open parish structure.

The Southwest Organizing Project

The Southwest Organizing Project is a values-oriented community organization that aims to create meaningful cross-racial, cross-ethnic, cross-generational, and cross-religious relationships for the purpose of creating a viable urban community. The Organizing Project was a direct outgrowth of the Southwest Catholic Cluster Project, an arm of the Catholic parishes and the archdiocesan Office of Peace and Justice.

The Southwest Catholic Cluster Project was formed in 1988 when several clergy and lay members of area churches felt that what was missing from various community efforts to address racial tolerance and neighborhood stability was an organization that "would come at the things they were dealing with in the neighborhood from Gospel values." Several pastors and lay leaders who, during the 1970s and 1980s, had been working in their Southwest Side parishes on racial and ethnic community reconciliation had become exhausted by their individual efforts. With new support from the archdiocesan Office of Peace and Justice, the leaders were able to bring most of the parishes in the Southwest Cluster into the effort and develop a collaboration among them.

The first director described the most important issue facing the neighborhood to be a "sense of powerlessness." Racial and ethnic changes were beginning to occur, and residents needed a way to overcome their feelings of isolation and to discuss these issues from a larger geographic perspective. The project developed a coordinated, areawide program to respond to problems raised by real estate interests, transportation questions, and concern over housing values. Much of the original work of the Cluster Project was to address latent problems of perception and stimulate a dialogue among the residents. Several activities, such as an ethnic parade, a banner display on which parishioners expressed their hopes for the neighborhood, and written reflections in pamphlet form about Christian perspectives on neighborhood integration, addressed residents' needs to express their concerns and come to grips with the changing reality.

In 1995, several participants in the Cluster Project decided that a larger, more aggressive agenda was needed. Mobility in the neighborhood was high; concerns about safety, both realistic and exaggerated, were accelerating. At a strategic planning meeting to decide a course of action, a Pentecost prayer was invoked. The members prayed that they might be emboldened so that they could in turn embolden the church to take necessary action on behalf of their community. They determined that an ecumenical, church-based, values-based, community-organizing model was necessary.

A community organizer trained by the Industrial Areas Foundation (IAF)—the creation of activist Saul Alinsky, whose start was in the nearby Back of the Yards neighborhood—Jerome "Jay" Caponigro had grown up in a neighboring parish. As the new director of the project, he moved quickly to restructure the organization independent of the archdiocese, so as to more easily develop an interfaith base. The Organizing Project has been able to bring several Protestant churches and one of the mosques into active participation. The ethnic balance on the steering committee is evenly divided between Euro-American and Latino, lay and clergy, and male and female.

The project's methods of engagement include a new vocabulary, one centered on "power" and "one relationship at a time." The IAF strategy involves building relationships at the public institutional level; in the Southwest Side, this means primarily the faith-based organizations. Through one-on-one meetings with members of each of the congregations, the project is working to build a community identity around public and inclusive relationships where "trust" rather than "loyalty" is fostered. These relationships form the basis of accountability to one another, that is, a relational stance that helps to refocus on the neighborhood and on one's neighbors. Caponigro regards this as essentially a Christian notion, but one that empowers all participants to become civic actors. Political activity can, he asserts, be based on values, and "relational power is one of inclusion, not exclusion."

With a (cultural) predisposition toward loyalty to and preference for one's own parish, it is but a small step toward expressing that exclusivity against outsiders who are visibly different. But the making of "otherness" cannot be simply reduced to its expression as a racial category. The question is how to help people understand the social process of difference and boundary making, and which dimensions of difference and boundary making are more and less strong in each particular context, in order to permit residents to make changes in these long-standing patterns that they have always perceived as natural. The Southwest Organizing Project has given a voice to community residents who are committed to a religiously based understanding of community in a pluralistic society.

Fig. 5-3. A Southwest Organizing Project interracial outing. In the background are a Chicago bungalow and two-flat apartment buildings characteristic of Chicago's blue-collar neighborhoods. Photo courtesty of Southwest Organizing Project.

Conclusion

This chapter has focused on ways in which Southwest Side residents are shaping the moral culture of their parishes to embrace the pluralist realities of urban life. An understanding of moral culture and its relationship to community should be connected to the economic and policy forces that affect residents. This connection has been missing.

For example, it occurred that a white couple wanted to sell their Southwest Side home and were told by an area realtor that "they would have to lower the price because minorities were moving into the area." The realtor further offered, "You had no idea this was going to happen. Ten years ago this was a good neighborhood." Was this 1967? No, it was 1997, and the incident is cited in a lawsuit claiming federal Fair Housing Act violations.[22] To construct new urban community models that cross language, ethnic, and racial boundaries, favorable economic opportunities, effective political control, and a commitment to cultural work must exist simultaneously. A different kind of culture work can then build on recognizing past mistakes as well as making visible heretofore underappreciated and underrecognized strengths.

The experience of the Southwest Side parishes demonstrates the value of two recently developed concepts in the social sciences—the social and cultural construction of ethnicity and the formation of race—fresh explanations for the changes in how Americans experience their relationships to others, especially their neighbors. This approach means we no longer have to think of race and ethnicity as immutable, biological identities. Instead, we can observe how relationships between social groups change as members come to understand their ethnic or racial heritage as partial rather than total frameworks for who they are and for what they make publicly accessible about themselves. It also means that other social categories—class, power, education, language, and religion—can be examined in order to see the more inclusive influences in the construction of racial and ethnic identities.

The Southwest Side has received notoriety in the annals of the civil rights movement. After all, this is where Martin Luther King Jr. was hit with a brick during an open housing march in 1966. But the Southwest Side is not a single entity with a single culture, despite the activities that led to such a public perception. Events of community change involve processes of symbolic boundary making and remaking that help us ask questions about what makes up the character of communities and how the formation and character of boundaries are related to communal identities in urban areas.[23] People at both parishes studied in this chapter reported in various ways how they feel closer together in their "own group" and can understand the urge to keep separate. At the same time, they acknowledged the need to overcome the primordial urge to remain with their in-group. To understand the continuing problems of racism in the United States, we need to find out about the lives of people who experience the movements of integration and/or resegregation in their neighborhoods. As one pastor asserted, these residents are looking for new urban models, just as did the members of Old Saint Patrick's Church in the Loop (see chapter 9). They are looking for ways to combine religious values and commitments with practical issues of neighborhoods.

The full story of change on the Southwest Side from the 1960s to the 1990s has not yet been told and is still unfolding in the twenty-first century. Much is at stake in those neighborhood changes, from housing equity and economic sustainability to social and cultural misunderstandings about what neighborhood viability means and how to enforce the moral norms required to achieve it.[24] In particular, a religious and moral understanding of neighborhood has not been sufficiently explored.[25] This is only a brief account, but it shows how the creation of a viable community involves both structural and cultural factors, a fair distribution of political and economic resources, and, especially, the successful negotiation of a moral order between new residents and old.

NOTES

Many thanks for helpful discussions and comments on earlier drafts are due to my Religion in Urban America Program colleagues and to Robert Aponte, Etan Diamond, Robert Lammers, Mary Mapes, Steve Warner, and Rhys Williams.

1. Suttles, *Social Construction of Communities,* 21–43.
2. Squires et al., *Chicago,* 5.
3. Cohen, *Symbolic Construction of Community,* 5.
4. Stout, "Place of Religion," 117.
5. Parot, *Polish Catholics in Chicago,* 225.
6. Ehrenhalt, *Lost City.*
7. Wuthnow, *Meaning and Moral Order.*
8. Pacyga, "Chicago's Ethnic Neighborhoods," 606.
9. Bellah et al., *Habits of the Heart,* 152–153.
10. See Wallwork, "Constructive Freudian Alternative"; and Harding, "Toward a Darkly Radiant Vision."
11. McGreevy, *Parish Boundaries.*
12. Sugrue, *Origins of the Urban Crisis.*
13. Ibid., 213.
14. Koenig, ed., *History of Parishes,* vol. 1, 153–156.
15. Sugrue, *Origins of the Urban Crisis,* 213.
16. Warner and Wittner, eds., *Gatherings in Diaspora.* See esp. McAlister, "Madonna of 115th Street Revisited," 147.
17. Cohen, *Symbolic Construction of Community,* 99.
18. Koenig, ed., *History of Parishes,* vol. 1, 659–662.
19. Dominic Pacyga. Comments at conference, "Religion and Community in a Restructuring Metropolis," University of Illinois at Chicago, June 5, 1995.
20. Cohen, *Symbolic Construction of Community,* 99.
21. Slater, *Pursuit of Loneliness,* 7–28.
22. Lydersen, "Lawsuits," 5.
23. Lamont and Fournier, eds., *Cultivating Differences.*
24. Rieder, *Canarsie;* McGreevy, *Parish Boundaries.*
25. Conzen et al., "Invention of Ethnicity"; McGreevy, *Parish Boundaries.*

Map 6. The "Rogers Parks" represent much of Chicago's ethnic and racial diversity among their 125,000 people. Map by Brian Twardosz, BMT Printing and Cartographic Specialists.

Communities and Enclaves
Where Jews, Christians, Hindus, and Muslims Share the Neighborhoods

Lowell W. Livezey

An afternoon walk along Devon Avenue on Chicago's Far North Side gives one a tangible sense of that abstract concept "social diversity." Devon offers a glimpse of the neighborhoods that make up the community areas of Rogers Park and West Ridge (known locally as West Rogers Park), which we discuss here together simply as "Rogers Parks." The area lies between Lake Michigan on the east and the North Shore Channel on the west at the northern boundary of the City of Chicago, about two and a half by two miles in size. Its total 1990 population of 125,000 showed a slight increase from ten years previous, a fact that could be claimed by very few Chicago neighborhoods. The positive population trend was due to a combination of immigration (34 percent of the residents are foreign born) and in-migration from other parts of the city (mostly blacks and Hispanics moving to a better neighborhood). The residents of these neighborhoods represent an extraordinarily wide range of the racial and ethnic groups, social and economic classes, and religious faiths of the Chicago metropolitan area. And because many small shops along Devon are operated by the local residents and cater to them, the street provides a colorful lens on the cultures of the people who live nearby.

Research by the Religion in Urban America Program from 1993 to 1998 provides the basis for my analysis of the religious dimension of local culture during that time. I argue that cultural innovation by religious organizations has encouraged the formation and maintenance of ethnoracial enclaves, which in turn characterize the diversity of Rogers Parks.

The walk eastward from Kedzie Avenue along Devon is a good way to enter the discussion. In the segment between Kedzie and California Avenues, which is officially designated Golda Meir Boulevard, Jewish residents can easily find most of the supplies needed for observance of the *halachah* (Jewish law) as interpreted by Orthodox rabbis. Here one can buy a wide variety of kosher groceries, choosing among alternatives that have been approved by different Jewish authorities determining what is kosher. And if there is any doubt about the requirements of observance, the *beth din* (rabbinic court) is nearby, not far from the *mikvah* (ritual bath) and the Kollel (a major center for adult religious study, which is visible in figure 6-1). Moreover, this part of Devon Avenue goes through an *eruv,* a geographic area constituted under Jewish law as the legal equivalent of the household—with the result that observant Jews can legally carry things on the Sabbath and on the High Holy Days.

Of the many Jewish institutions in Rogers Parks, we studied three in depth. Ezra Habonim is a Conservative congregation, the result of a merger of two German-speaking congregations. Although the older generations of its three hundred members are Germans and Austrians, it seeks to attract younger Jews of any nationality. The Sephardic Congregation is a community of about 250 Sephardic families who have come, either directly or by descent from immigrants earlier in this century, from the various Mediterranean countries in which the Spanish Jews settled. The congregation practices Orthodox observance, so most of its members live close enough to the synagogue to walk to services. Finally, we studied The Ark, a social service agency that follows *halachah* and conducts Shabbat services for staff, persons in their shelter, and many recent Jewish immigrants from Eastern Europe and the former Soviet Union.

The time was when the Jewish dominance of Devon Avenue extended much further east than the corner of California Avenue, but now the brown sign indicating the honorary street name shows the next segment to be Gandhi Marg, and the vegetarian groceries, South Asian spices, and silk saris set the tone. The religious symbolism of the community is not as obvious as on Golda Meir Boulevard, in part because Indian culture involves many different religions—Hinduism, Islam, Sikhism, Jainism, and Christianity. Moreover, the religious practices of Hinduism are not directly tied to neighborhood geography. Despite an Indian population of more than six thousand in Rogers Parks, with more in the immediately adjacent suburbs, there is only one Hindu temple here, organized and staffed by the International Society for Krishna Consciousness (widely known as Hare Krishna). In conducting our case study we learned that, although a few "new age," youthful Americans responded to Hare Krishna recruitment, the leadership and financial support for the temple come from Indian immigrants, mostly from Gujarat and Punjab, and that the temple is organized very much on the model of American congregations. Indian Christians also form American congregations, such as the First Telugu Methodist Church, which is hosted by the United Church of Rogers Park.

Continuing east on Devon, especially in the segment designated Mohammed Ali Jinnah Way, it is not uncommon to see meat markets and groceries with "Halal" signs indicating the availability of religiously approved foods for observant Muslims. Most Indian and Pakistani Muslims in Rogers Parks identify themselves as "Indo-Pakistanis," and they, along with a few Jordanians, Palestinians, Iranians, and Africans, constitute the membership of the five mosques located here. We studied one of these, the Al-Madina Islamic Center, just off Devon Avenue, where two hundred or more Muslim men of many nationalities gather for the jum'ah prayers early every Friday afternoon. But it is the Indo-Pakistanis—some speaking only Urdu, except for enough Arabic to say the prayers—who live in the rental apartments near the mosque, who support it and develop its programs and activities.

About halfway across Rogers Parks, Ridge Avenue marks a local watershed, and the terrain begins to slope gently downward toward Lake Michigan. Now the Mexican *taquerias* and restaurants become prominent and frequent, signaling the presence of Latino immigrants and transmigrants who live and work nearby. Those who participate in religious organizations mostly attend either Catholic parishes that offer the mass in Spanish or Spanish-speaking Protestant churches. We will see how Saint Jerome Roman Catholic Church organizes itself to include the Hispanic, Haitian, and white "American" Catholics living within its parish boundaries, just as in previous generations it struggled to make the Irish, German, Lithuanian, and Polish parishioners feel equally at home and spiritually nourished. We will also look at Misión Cristiana Elim, a Spanish-speaking Pentecostal church whose six hundred members have come from Mexico and Central America. And in the most economically impoverished part of Rogers Parks, "North of Howard," we find another of our case studies, the Good News Church/Iglesia Buenas Nuevas, a two hundred–member congregation of the United Church of Christ, with services in both Spanish and English.

Reaching the end of Devon Avenue, on the shore of Lake Michigan, we find the campus of Loyola, a major Jesuit university, with Saint Ignatius Roman Catholic Church not far away. These and the four other large Catholic parishes remind us that Rogers Parks is historically a "white ethnic" area, and the 1990 U.S. Census figures show that a majority still identify themselves as white.

As we can see, the diversity of Rogers Parks includes religion. By the Religion in Urban America Program's enumeration, in the years 1993–1998, the formally organized religious bodies that met regularly in a designated physical space in Rogers Parks included thirty Jewish congregations, twenty-seven Protestant churches, six mosques, five Roman Catholic parishes and the Croatian Catholic Mission, an Assyrian Catholic church, four Buddhist temples or meditation centers, a Hindu temple, a Sikh *gurdwārā,* and five or more new age meditation and worship centers. Of the Jewish congregations, twenty-one were Orthodox, three Traditional, four Conservative, one Reform, and one Lubavitcher. Of the Protestant churches, five represented mainline denominations, five were immigrant congregations associated with mainline denominations, and the remaining seventeen included Christian Science, Jehovah's Witnesses, and various Pentecostal, Evangelical, and sectarian groups—many with names indicating an ethnic or national identity.

Diversity and Controversy

Diversity is both touted evidence of American inclusiveness and a source of anxiety. At the neighborhood level, diversity often is feared as meaning that "outsiders" have arrived and will soon replace the previous population—which itself, in many cases, had replaced another population one or two generations earlier. In the first half of the twentieth century, the Chicago School of urban sociology developed theories of "invasion and succession"[1] to explain this phenomenon. Since the Second World War, the concept of "racial tipping"[2] has been used to explain and predict the point at which too much diversity will result in "white flight" and thus in the complete turnover of a neighborhood to a racially or ethnically different population. This is what David Daniels means, in chapter 7 of this book, by the "collapse of integration" in Chatham; it is how Pilsen (chapter 2) became a Mexican American neighborhood; and it is what happened in the Englewood neighborhood that so frightened the Southwest Side parishioners discussed in chapter 5. In this "city of neighborhoods,"[3] many all-white neighborhoods changed within a few years to all-black or all-Hispanic neighborhoods. And at any given time, those whose neighborhoods have recently become diverse may ask, "Will we be next?" In this respect, the Rogers Parks neighborhoods are in the same situation as those of the Southwest Side: despite significant differences (Rogers Parks does not lie next to a "color line" and a poverty ghetto), both areas exhibit a diversity that has the chance of being sustainable. In a twenty-two-city study sponsored by the U.S. Department of Housing and Urban Development, Rogers Park and the Southwest Side's Marquette Park were among the fourteen racially diverse neighborhoods selected as case studies with prospects for avoiding the pattern of tipping and white flight.[4] The study concluded that the capacity of a diverse neighborhood to be stable depends fundamentally on its quality of life, and this includes both economic and physical conditions and the values and attitudes fostered by community institutions. A study of Rogers Park conducted at Loyola University in 1993 reached similar conclusions and found that the residents valued the diversity—except that they feared the consequences of increasing poverty.[5]

Yet, for an area that was 99.5 percent white in 1960, the change has been substantial. By 1990 the population had changed from 0 to 14 percent Hispanic, from 0 to 13 percent Asian, from 0 to 15 percent black. Many of the 83,364 whites are foreign born—not only Jews and others coming from the former Soviet Union and Eastern Europe but also Arabs and nonblack Hispanics.[6] So, in light of the experience of other neighborhoods, the possibility of tipping and white flight cannot be easily dismissed.

Diversity is also controversial for more philosophical reasons. While the diversity of a neighborhood may be the consequence of market forces, attitudes toward it may result from beliefs about what it takes to have a good community and a good society. And the diversity of a particular neighborhood may result from the active creation of enclaves and boundaries, the articulation of rationales for separation, and competition for social benefits—what Iris Marion Young calls "the politics of difference."[7] Indeed, many of the religious organizations discussed in this chapter not only locate themselves in ethnoracial enclaves but help to shape them and to give them character.

The term *ethnoracial* is borrowed from David Hollinger's *Postethnic America*[8] in order to bridge the distinction between ethnicity and race, which, as socially constructed categories, are distinguishable but not separable in a fluid context such as Rogers Parks. In the late-twentieth-century American urban context, the metaphor *enclave* draws on its geopolitical roots but connotes a concentration of a subpopulation in an identifiable locale rather than a completely homogeneous population within fixed physical boundaries. While Rogers Parks is diverse, many of the microneighborhoods that make it up are much more ethnoracially concentrated, and that concentration is often fostered and defined by religious groups.

This tendency of diversity to be expressed as group self-identification and difference, often labeled "multiculturalism," is welcomed by many who perceive that the more homogeneous American culture of previous eras imposed itself on minority groups in ways that not only were unjust but that also erased the cultural enrichment of the whole society. From this perspective, some kind of politically self-conscious development of groups defined by separate identities would be necessary to prevent the conformist requirements of "coercive pluralism"—in Lawrence Fuchs's apt phrase[9]—imposed on blacks, Latinos, and immigrants as the price for participation in the wider society.

In opposition to this positive view of multiculturalism, public intellectuals such as Arthur Schlesinger Jr. were warning of "the disuniting of America," and Todd Gitlin could write nostalgically about the "twilight of common dreams,"[10] meaning that even the leftist aspirations were being fragmented by the conflicting claims of ethnic and racial groups. The American ideal of *e pluribus unum* is in danger, they said, because "the many" were identifying too much with their separate groups, rather than with the "one."

Historian David Hollinger, who agrees with the multiculturalist claims that racial and ethnic minorities have been subordinated and muscled into conformity with the norms of the dominant classes, nevertheless worries that the affirmation of separate subcultures actually undermines the social justice it seeks to promote. In *Postethnic America* he argues that the self-identification as separate groups common in the 1990s will ultimately contribute to further marginalization and loss of status of their members. There are many conflicting perspectives on multiculturalism. Minority groups' self-assertion in terms of their group identity will be viewed—positively by some and negatively by others—as fragmenting a presumably common, American culture.

Religious Congregations and Ethnoracial Enclaves

Religious organizations of all faiths produce and reproduce cultural forms that both incorporate and influence the ethnic and racial identities of their people.[11] This process defines and enforces both geographical and symbolic boundaries that distinguish the insider from the outsider, ethnically and racially as well as religiously. At the same time, these religious cultures express values and attitudes about the people, communities, and society beyond their boundaries.

Religiously defined ethnoracial enclaves are as old as the Jewish ghetto and the Catholic national parish, and many Protestant neighborhoods—such as the heavily Lutheran Swedish "Andersonville"[12] in Chicago—have had similar characteristics. But to have such enclaves within an extraordinarily diverse setting such as Rogers Parks, and in an era of highly contested multiculturalism, raises the question of whether and how they contribute to the livability and sustainability of the wider community. Of the nine congregations we examined as religious case studies in the Rogers Parks neighborhoods, seven function either as ethnoracial enclaves or as loose constellations of two or more such enclaves. Moreover, although one congregation, the United Church of Rogers Park, succeeds in its effort to be inclusive and diverse, even it is the host to the First Telugu Methodist Church, which functions as a Telugu-speaking, South Asian enclave. In this chapter we examine the internal dynamics of these enclaves and their relations with their neighborhoods.

The Jewish Community and the Neighborhood

Undoubtedly, the purest example of an ethnoracial enclave in Rogers Parks is the Jewish community. Like all ethnoracial enclaves in Rogers Parks, it shares space with many other ethnoracial and religious groups. But while the geographic space is not homogeneous or exclusive, the Jewish population is highly concentrated, and the cultural infrastructure is very dense. In a 1990 survey, more than twenty-six thousand people in 10,960 households in West Rogers Park identified themselves as Jewish. Included in these households were more than six thousand Jewish children and more than two thousand Jewish teenagers, 97 percent of whom lived with both parents. Levels of synagogue affiliation (56 percent), religious observance, and communal and civic involvement were far higher among West Rogers Park Jewish residents than among the overall Jewish population of metropolitan Chicago.[13] West Rogers Park is also the home of an extraordinary concentration of Jewish religious and cultural organizations, including a growing number of *shuls* (more than twenty-five), day schools, and social service agencies operated by and for Jews according to Jewish law and custom.[14]

The Jewish population's migration within the city is reflected in the founding of Congregation Ezra Habonim, created when Congregation Habonim moved from the South Side to join Congregation Ezra in the early 1970s. The Sephardic Congregation moved from the West Side and built its present synagogue in 1970; The Ark moved to West Rogers Park from the Albany Park neighborhood soon thereafter.

Congregation Ezra Habonim, affiliated with the Conservative branch of American Judaism, is a "Holocaust congregation" founded by refugees from Nazi Germany. As required in Ezra Habonim's bylaws, Kristallnacht, the day in 1938 when synagogues and Jewish-owned businesses were vandalized and destroyed en masse by Nazis and their supporters in Germany and Austria, is memorialized in a very moving service each year.

The intermingling of German identity with the refugee status of members has created a distinct character for this synagogue. These immigrants brought a frugal fiscal style that served them well as they struggled to start a new life in a foreign country without the benefit of public support. They bonded with one another as refugees, and the synagogue became their main social center as well as their place of worship.[15]

By the 1980s the congregation was experiencing fundamental changes, such as the aging of its founding generation; the migration of a large portion of the Jewish population, including some of its members, to the suburbs; the "social revolution" of the 1970s, with its appeal for greater equality and individual rights; and the somewhat countervailing trend within Conservative Judaism toward the reclaiming of deeper roots in Jewish tradition. Since the skills and interests of the younger generation were not the same as those of their forebears, the 1980s was inevitably a time of transition. The question of staying in West Rogers Park remained an underlying issue, but the immediate concerns were how to maintain a viable synagogue home for diverse members—no longer united by the German language and direct experience of the Holocaust—and how to educate their children in Judaism, the meaning and observance of which were being renegotiated.

Responses to these concerns reflect a combination of the immigrant/refugee experience and the urban situation in which the members live. The congregation had been a "community of memory," whose "constitutive narrative" consisted decisively in retelling the Holocaust experience. As Robert Bellah notes, "A genuine community of memory will . . . tell painful stories of shared suffering that sometimes creates deeper identities than success."[16] Indeed, the Holocaust narrative was constitutive for Ezra Habonim during the very decades, prior to Israel's 1967 Six-Day War, about which Nathan Glazer wrote that he "could see no major impact of the Holocaust . . . on the internal life of American Jews."[17] So, just as the wider Jewish community was beginning to find Holocaust history to be a source of communal identity (the national Holocaust Museum being a concrete result), Ezra Habonim's members who actually experienced the Holocaust began to retire, move to retirement homes, and die. Thus the memory could be sustained only by deliberate measures such as the Kristallnacht services and the content of religious education programs.

During the 1990s, young families with children formed a strong element in the membership of Ezra Habonim. The school, run by a professional staff and a volunteer board, provides a comprehensive education in Jewish life and customs, law and liturgy, theology and ethics, and history and language. Classes begin for prekindergarten children and continue through the high school youth group, which meets with other youth groups from the city and suburbs. In addition to classes, attendance at Shabbat services is mandatory. Both the rabbi and the *hazzan* (cantor) teach regularly in the school in addition to tutoring bar and bat mitzvahs preparing for initiation into religious adulthood. Three youth groups complement and extend the work of the school.

The progressive cultural innovation within Judaism and the wider culture was reflected in the congregation's decision to become "egalitarian," calling women to the Torah and counting them in the *minyan* (the traditional minimum of ten adult males needed for communal prayers)—the first Conservative synagogue in the Chicago area to do so. A decade later, a female *hazzan* was hired. Women can, and some do, wear the *kippah*, the same head covering as men, and they wear the *tallith* (prayer shawl). These changes identified the congregation with the liberal side of the Conservative movement, yet the general trend toward traditional observance in Judaism[18] was present here as well. The congregation hired an Orthodox rabbi, who was a good fit with the services, with most prayers in Hebrew and much interactional and joint praying. The rabbi tolerated, while seeking to correct, the members' limitations in observance of the law and their lack of Jewish "literacy."

The congregation's philanthropy is directed both to members and to nonmember Jews. The first is through a specially constituted fund for persons in need called the Gemiluth Chesed, meaning "acts of loving kindness." The anonymity of this activity is in keeping with the Jewish injunction to conduct charity privately. Second, Ezra Habonim has been active in supporting Russian Jewish immigrants by providing space for English classes, free tuition at the Hebrew school, and free initial memberships to the synagogue. Most of the Russian families, however, drop their participation as soon as the free tuition and memberships run out.

By the mid-1990s, the major concern for Ezra Habonim was to decide about the congregation's location in the heart of the only remaining Jewish neighborhood in Chicago. With most Chicago-area Jews, especially the non-Orthodox, now living in suburbs, the congregation could have increased membership by moving to a suburban location, but it decided to remain on Touhy Avenue. They thought their distinct historical identity would contribute to a viable urban Jewish life, one in which Conservative Jews who value the tough cosmopolitanism and diversity of the city could find a religious community. And the congregation itself would benefit from the dense Jewish infrastructure without giving up the broader diversity of the city. They were proactive, deciding both to strengthen their internal programs, particularly in religious education, and to market their presence to the unaffiliated Jews, especially young people, who live in the Loop, Near North, and Far North Sides of the city. Although the congregation later divided, the part of the congregation that remained in Rogers Parks are the younger families who tend toward increasing religious observance. This strong Conservative congregation, rooted in but transcending the Holocaust identity, is committed to maintaining the current Jewish enclave in an urban rather than suburban setting.

The Sephardic Congregation's members are, by constitution, all Sephardic, though multinational and multilingual by custom and practice. Sephardim[19] are descendants of the Jews of Spain, who developed a distinct subculture as a suppressed minority before the Expulsion in 1492. Elements of that subculture are evident in the Sephardic Congregation, including special rituals and customs, variations in the prayers, the use of the Ladino language (parallel to the Askenazim's use of Yiddish) in conversation and Aramaic (as well as Hebrew) in scripture study, and certain foods (such as baked eggs and Mediterranean delicacies). Because the Sephardim dispersed widely after the Expulsion, they have come to Chicago from many countries—Italy, Greece, Turkey, Iran, Israel, Egypt, Yemen, Morocco, among others. Moreover, since some came to the Western Hemisphere with the early European explorers and colonists, they are now "natives," welcoming the new immigrants from Mediterranean countries. No single group predominates in this synagogue, so the religious services reflect an amalgam of several religious and cultural traditions.

All public activities follow the norms of Sephardic Orthodox practice as interpreted by the rabbi. Services are conducted daily, with the morning prayers (described in the introduction to this book) attended by a few men and the principal Shabbat service on Saturday morning by 150 or more men and women, including the very pious who live in the immediate neighborhood or walk a considerable distance in conformity with *halachah*. The three-hour Shabbat service is conducted entirely in Hebrew except for a short sermon and announcements and involves much participation in prayers and scripture readings. The men ceremoniously remove a Torah scroll from the ark and carry it around the sanctuary for worshipers to touch with their prayer shawls before it is placed on the *bimah* and read. Women, seated behind the *mehitza*, a half-height partition, reach through to touch the Torah scroll with their prayer books.

The education of families has two substantive dimensions: what it means to be Jewish and what it means to be Sephardic. Children's programs are conducted during Shabbat service and on Sundays, teaching Bible stories, Jewish ways of living, and the Hebrew language at an early age. But the main role of the synagogue is to urge families to study together at home so that children learn, through their parents' efforts, what it means to be both Jewish and Sephardic.

The congregation's charitable activities include its Special Fund, based in contributions at daily prayers. The fund is given to persons in need, but only those who have been vetted by Agudas Israel, a recognized organization of the Orthodox Jewish community. The congregation and its rabbi are strong supporters of The Ark (discussed below), which provides a full range of social services in accordance with Orthodox interpretation of Jewish law. Congregational support for the Chicago Jewish Federation/United Jewish Appeal promotes the well-being of the Jewish community in general and, to some extent, the wider public good.

The congregation is deeply involved with the American Sephardic Federation, a secular organization that has been a significant force in the assertion of Sephardic identity in America since World War II. Leaders of the congregation are also leaders of the federation at the regional and national levels. The federation holds meetings and programs at the synagogue, which are promoted by the congregation and function, in effect, as part of the congregation's educational program. One partnership between the two organizations was the "Shabboton," a weekend conference held in December 1993, which incorporated elements of spiritual retreat, ethnic education, and social outing. The prayers, rituals, and educational programs provide a kind of social glue that holds the people together as Jews and as Sephardim, despite tremendous differences among members in language and custom. Thus, this congregation represents both the Sephardic subpopulation within Judaism and religiously observant Jews who identify as Sephardim. It is a vibrant Jewish assembly that contributes to the vitality of the Jewish community, especially in West Rogers Park. But it also creates a distinct cultural niche within the Jewish Community that fosters the development of Sephardic identity and religious practice.

The Ark, occupying the large, beautifully renovated Seymour Persky Center only a few blocks from Ezra Habonim and Sephardic Congregation, offers itself as "the Torah's vehicle for sustaining individuals in time of crisis." It is a professional social service center, but one in which Jewish volunteers can both fulfill the Torah's *mitzvot* (commandments) and do *tzedakah* (charitable deeds). The boundaries and distinctions between the many constituencies and population groups that make up The Ark are intentionally and successfully blurred. It is like the biblical Noah's ark—Noah built the ark (providing both religious leadership and skilled labor), but he also needed it as much as anyone else. While staff are well-qualified professionals and most volunteers are securely situated people, The Ark recognizes that no one is completely secure from a "sea of troubles" and thus fosters an attitude of being in this "ark" together. At The

Ark, many of the people being assisted also serve as volunteers—some of them regularly, year after year—and it is believed that their acts of charity and service may be healing for them as well as for those they assist. Staff and volunteers often serve in the same or overlapping roles, and both interact with clients without obvious signs of status.

Staff, volunteers, and clients all embody the fabric of interrelationships between The Ark and the Jewish neighborhood of West Rogers Park. Clients can be referred for religious counseling to neighborhood rabbis, many of whom interact regularly with The Ark's staff members. The Kollel, the Chicago Rabbinical Council, the Jewish Council for Elderly, the Associated Talmud Torah, and many other Jewish agencies located within easy walking distance serve as a network of organizations, professionals, and volunteers who share responsibility with The Ark for the care and nurture of people in need. Thus, The Ark is one of the pillars of neighborhood life.

The Ark's name also recalls the Ark of the Covenant, and the agency is devoted to enabling Jews to live as observant Jews, individually and collectively, regardless of their means. All food distributed through the food pantry is kosher and is available not only to the hungry but also to those who might otherwise not have kosher food. This makes The Ark's program more expensive and resources harder to obtain than they would otherwise be. But the observance is connected with a holistic support system, including a synagogue on the premises, religious services conducted both at The Ark and at secular and Christian agencies that serve Jewish people, and schedules built around observance of *halachah* by staff, volunteers, and those assisted.

Congregation Ezra Habonim, the Sephardic Congregation, and The Ark all enact both their religious and their ethnic traditions in their collective practices, and they transmit the traditions to their children and to newcomers to the neighborhood. But these are not merely acts of transmittal; they are acts of cultural adaptation and innovation, informed by the experience and practice of current adult members' parents but adapted to the requirements and competing values of their present situations.

The collective activities of these organizations are intensely local, both presupposing and promoting a high concentration of Jewish residents and an intricate infrastructure of Jewish institutions in the central part of West Rogers Park. Insofar as the three organizations look beyond

Fig. 6-1. The Ark and the Chicago Community Kollel, an adult study center, are essential to the Jewish infrastructure of West Rogers Park, Chicago. Photo by Lowell W. Livezey.

themselves, it is to the wider Jewish community, not to the non-Jewish people of Rogers Parks or to the rest of the city. While their individual members may be quite worldly in other contexts, this was not evident in organizational practice. These Jewish organizations foster an enclave within West Rogers Park and smaller enclaves within that one, but they are defined by the concentration of the Jewish population and institutions, not by exclusion of or hostility toward others. The three organizations do not explicitly espouse "common dreams" (beyond the Jewish community), but neither do they "disunite America." Moreover, we witnessed three solid and solvent institutions, with well-maintained buildings, that actively encouraged residence in the neighborhood and offered tangible support for those who choose to live there. The two synagogues made deliberate decisions not to move out of the neighborhood, not only because of the benefits they received from being in this unique concentration of Jews but also because they would contribute to a stronger Jewish neighborhood, thus helping the city remain attractive to Jewish residents and, in turn, countering the suburban migration that is often part of white flight.

A Catholic Parish and Its Ethnoracial Enclaves

Saint Jerome is a large, hundred-year old Catholic church in the northeast portion of Rogers Parks. The church has six hundred registered families, mostly older and middle-aged white people who have lived in the parish for most of their lives. In addition, by the pastor's estimate, at least four hundred Spanish-speaking families attend mass regularly and participate in various parish activities but are not formally registered as members. Given the larger size of these families, Hispanics comprise a majority of the parish population. In addition, there are about one hundred Haitian families and a few African Americans, Filipinos, and Indians. The six Sunday masses draw more than two thousand worshipers, of whom two-thirds are Hispanic. The church operated a parish school until 1994, when it became a participant in the newly created North Side Catholic Academy, with campuses at other parishes.

Saint Jerome thus exemplifies the traditional territorial parish, which ministers to all baptized Catholics—and informally, to many others—living within its boundaries.[20] Like Saint Nicholas of Tolentine, discussed in chapter 5, its territorial constitution determines that it cannot be a single ethnoracial enclave, since multiple ethnic groups live within its boundaries. It continues to be a social center, as it was for Euro-American ethnic groups in the past, but it is a center that different ethnic groups "use" for their distinct social as well as spiritual purposes. In practice, in the late 1990s, Saint Jerome has formed three differentiated social groups, distinguished by both language and race, each constructing its distinctive culture. The fact that the pastor is trilingual enhances his efforts to provide pastoral leadership to the whole parish, but both the Spanish- and French-speaking groups have their own ordained staff (a priest and a deacon).

Saint Jerome addresses a few programs to the entire church and to the entire neighborhood. A special Easter Mass is conducted in English and Spanish, and the Centennial Mass was celebrated in 1994 in English, French, and Spanish. Each year, the parish attempts other bilingual and trilingual rituals. The annual Via Crucis, a ritual strongly associated with Mexican Catholicism, which Saint Jerome celebrates in response to advocacy by Mexicans, is conducted in English and French as well as Spanish in an effort to symbolize the unity of the diverse parish. This ritually realistic reenactment of Jesus carrying the cross to his own crucifixion helps build community solidarity. By their participation, neighbors of many ethnicities and races acknowledge the status of Saint Jerome Church in the community. As they collectively move through their neighborhood, ceremonially visiting local sites where serious crimes were committed, they call attention to the problem of community violence and their common stake in ending it.

The three Sunday masses in Spanish account for the majority of the attendance, and it is in these that the preponderance of worshipful energy is evident. The Spanish-language choir, singing to the accompaniment of stringed instruments, both expresses cultural themes familiar to the worshipers and enlists their participation in the mass and in the church. Some Hispanics have been parishioners as long as twenty years, and they help organize liturgies and celebrations in Mexican traditions—including the *posadas* during the season of Advent and the *mañanitas* for the Virgin of Guadalupe. The latter, a service of love songs to the Virgin, is devoid of the Mexican nationalism we observed at *mañanitas* in other Chicago communities (perhaps because the population here includes Cubans, Central Americans, and Puerto Ricans), but it is a spirited, energetic affair, and the church is packed with families having a wonderful time.

The Hispanic youth group, Esperanza Latina, attracts fifty or more young people (twelve to thirty years of age) to its weekly meetings, which offer a combination of education in Catholic teaching (the meaning of prayer, of sexuality, of obedience); planning of youth-initiated activities (a Palm Sunday drama to be performed during Mass); and socializing among themselves (a Valentine's Day party). Throughout the many activities youth are asked to think about alternatives, and to deliberate about differences among themselves. Their differences often represent degrees of assimilation to U.S. culture and varying levels of acceptance of Catholic teaching. Saint Jerome fosters the exploration of alternatives, to the extent, for example, of inviting a Mexican American couple who had lived together before their marriage to speak to the group about sexuality, marriage, and family. All discussions are in Spanish (even though most youth speak English well), thus both selecting and encouraging those who are inclined to preserve the cultural heritage of Mexico or of the other Spanish-speaking countries from which they or their parents have come. But young people unable or unwilling to speak Spanish simply do not have a youth program to participate in.

Hispanic Pentecostals

Spanish-speaking youth, and people of all ages, will also find warm welcome and a rich array of programs at the nearby Iglesia de Cristo–Misión Cristiana Elim, a growing Pentecostal church that acquired its large auditorium and educational plant from a Korean congregation in about 1990. Elim, as the church is locally known, is part of a network of Pentecostal churches that was founded in Guatemala and expanded through Central America and Mexico. Some of the six hundred members of Elim were part of the church in Guatemala or Mexico, but most have joined the church since their arrival in Chicago. By 1995 this congregation had started four mission churches, two in Illinois and two in Mexico, forming something of a transnational circuit.

Elim shares many characteristics of "Anglo" and black Pentecostal churches and of Catholic charismatics, including expressive worship styles, rock-style music, physical and emotional healing, speaking in tongues, and many "gifts of the Spirit." Like many such churches, it devotes a great deal of preaching, teaching, and counseling to the promotion and support of nuclear families. While the church has a conservative model of the "good" family, it helps its members find an approach to family life that will work for them in a new and strange environment—urban, North American, and culturally diverse. For example, a marriage retreat promotes negotiation and accommodation between spouses, qualifying the strict patriarchal principle of deference to the husband's authority characteristic of conservative Christian teachings. Similarly, while the Youth Discipleship program includes rather strict moral teaching about chastity until marriage, it also lovingly accepts the unmarried member who becomes pregnant, and it celebrates the birth with a baby shower.

Like Saint Jerome's Hispanic parishioners, Elim's members are living on a number of cultural boundaries—between Mexico and the United States, between traditional and modern, between Christian and secular. These churches offer their members some of the tools for dealing with life on these boundaries. By using the Spanish language only, each church creates a cultural enclave within which its members have a limited protection from the pressures of the new, the urban, the secular. But while each church offers its traditional teaching as moral armor to withstand these pressures, it also offers space within which people can selectively negotiate these boundaries for themselves.

Thus the enclaves are exclusive (of non-Spanish-speakers), but within them people prepare for resilient participation in the multicultural urban world. In contrast to residents of all-Hispanic neighborhoods (for example, Pilsen, discussed in chapter 2), the participants in these churches in Rogers Parks may have no other Hispanic cultural space—unless they join a Latino gang. Both churches know that, as far as youth are concerned, the gangs are their main competitors.

South Asian Muslims

The Al-Madina Islamic Center occupies the entire basement of a large apartment building on Wallen Avenue, not far from the corner of Devon and Clark. The entrance is visible only from the alley, but at the appointed hour for *jum'ah* prayers on Friday afternoons, as many as 250 men and boys can be found there, praying, listening to a short *khutbah* (sermon) in Arabic and to other speeches in Urdu, and then socializing among themselves. Many live or work nearby, but others have chosen this mosque as the place to fulfill their obligation to pray simply because they were in this vicinity at the time. Most of the men are Indo-Pakistanis, some dressed as American laborers and professionals, others in the tunics and hats worn in India and Pakistan. Others appear to be Arabs, Africans, African Americans, Caucasians.[21]

While the *jum'ah* prayer is the central liturgical event of the week—comparable to the Sunday mass or the Shabbat service—it provides only a glimpse of the mosque and its role in Rogers Parks. All the prescribed prayers are conducted—five times every day, according to the officially established lunar timetable. At 4 P.M. Monday through Thursday, neighborhood Muslim boys and girls, often rushing back by public transportation from selective magnet schools around the city, with an Urdu-speaking instructor for lessons in Arabic, the *Qur'an,* and the moral principles of Islam. During the summer, the children spend their days studying the same subjects under the direction of professional teachers whose first language is Arabic. The children's mothers and fathers come in and out, interacting with the teachers and with one another, helping to build a community devoted to making the Islamic way of life meaningful for the next generation of Indo-Pakistani immigrants. Teachers and parents alike encourage students to seize certain opportunities the city presents—to go to the best schools, get the best jobs, advance as far as possible. But a moral discipline must also be preserved: a conservative practice with respect to sexuality and family structure and a recognition of the mosque and the Islamic community as the appropriate source of moral authority.

Participation by parents, teachers, and the mosque's leadership in educational activities, as well as family gatherings for fast-breaking and other community meals, help constitute the mosque as a neighborhood social center for Indo-Pakistani Muslims. Thus, when the men gather to make the decisions about hiring part-time teachers and *imams* or about repairing the drains, they are shaping communal life in a small corner of Rogers Parks, not only the religious practices of those who come to study and pray.

Asian Indian Hindus

The Hare Krishna Temple on Lunt Avenue is the Chicago congregation of the International Society for Krishna Consciousness (ISKCON), which came to the United States from India in 1965.[22] ISKCON was a proselytizing Hindu movement that Westerners saw as a "new religious movement." However, during the 1980s, according to Raymond Williams,[23] and by our own observation in the mid-1990s, while the religious leaders were still primarily Western converts, the regular participants and reliable supporters were mainly Indian immigrants living in Rogers Parks or nearby suburbs.

The temple conducts the prescribed traditional Hindu worship services, offering food and saying prayers to the gods five times each day. The daily practice includes the 4:30 A.M. service, which is omitted by many of the other Hindu temples in the Chicago area, including some whose priests, unlike Hare Krishna's, are Indians. On weekends the temple adds services for the convenience of persons whose work week prevents their daily attendance. The largest of these is the Sunday evening service, which is followed by a meal that not only is strictly vegetarian but is technically what is left over from what the priests have prepared for the gods. Thus the meal has been made with meticulous attention to both cleanliness and taste. Several hundred people, mostly Indians, attend this service and the meal each week.

The temple's education program inculcates Krishna consciousness in the younger members and recent converts, with an emphasis on vegetarianism, nonviolence, avoidance of intoxication and illicit sex, and the regular chanting of the Hare Krishna mantra. The "Straight Talk" program addresses issues of concern to adolescents, including dating and sexual relations. Thus the temple assists Indian parents by conveying moral norms of Hindu and Indian culture. These norms are quite conservative, but since Hare Krishna is a proselytizing sect and interested Westerners often attend the meetings, the presenters attempt to be realistic about the opportunities and pressures of adolescent life in America.

This temple serves as both a cultural and a physical space in which Indian immigrants collectively invent their ethnoracial identities as Indian Americans. The Hindu rituals and the Vedic epics they dramatize identify the participants with India and with the moral values and communal customs of their origins. The predominance of the northern Indian Gujarati and Punjabi languages and customs tends to foster ethnic differentiation from other Indian Americans. For major festivals, these Indians may travel to a larger temple, perhaps a more ecumenical one such as the Hindu Temple of Greater Chicago (see chapter 10); but Hare Krishna on Lunt Avenue is a place they can conveniently gather weekly or even more often. These Indians are dispersed throughout much of Rogers Parks and the adjacent suburbs of Skokie and Evanston but are sufficiently concentrated to make use of a local house of worship. As a result, the temple reinforces the solidarity of Indians as neighbors, as north Indians, and as Hindus.

A Protestant "Parish"

United Church of Rogers Parks is a United Methodist congregation of about 250 members, occupying a large, aging building not far from Saint Jerome, Elim, and Hare Krishna. The regular attenders (no one seems to care much about membership) include English-speaking members of many of the ethnoracial groups of the area—white, African American, and Caribbean. While most of the attenders are middle-income professionals, many are poor, and some suffer from mental problems, alcoholism, and other dysfunctions. In addition, the Indians of the First Telugu Methodist Church, which uses separate space at United Church for its weekly services, participate occasionally in Sunday worship and other programs.

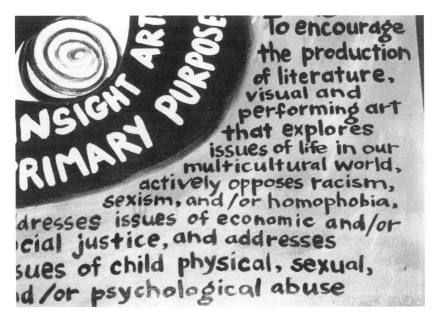

Fig. 6-2. The InSight Arts program for youth provides physically and culturally safe space at United Church of Rogers Park, Chicago. Photo courtesy of United Church of Rogers Park.

United Church is an exception to the pattern developed so far, because rather than building social solidarity on the basis of shared ethnic or racial identity, it attempts, with some success, to make inclusiveness itself a constitutive principle. The church identifies itself as a "safe space" for all, and this metaphor has several meanings. First, the Sunday morning worship service is multicultural, with a rather formal order of service holding together diverse rituals and with music drawn from various (Anglo) American, African American, African, and Caribbean traditions. Prayers and announcements invite concern for fellow human beings throughout the city, suburbs, and the world, often referring explicitly to the many ways in which they are different from the people of United Church and from one another. Worshipers who have trouble relating to the service or to other worshipers—those with mental disorders, for example—are assisted by others who have been trained and authorized to do so.

The InSight Arts program teaches performing and visual arts, but its "ministerial" purpose is to provide community youth a space that is safe from the streets (gang violence), from their homes (domestic violence),

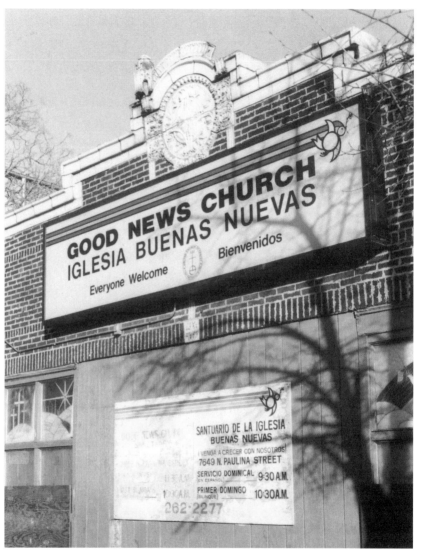

Fig. 6-3. The Good News Church/Iglesia Buenas Nuevas is one church with two congregations—English- and Spanish-speaking—in the North of Howard community, Rogers Park, Chicago. Photo by Paul D. Numrich.

and from social control (artistic censorship). The Children's Learning Center (preschool and after school), the Community House (drop-in center), the Community Feast (a weekly soup kitchen), and the Mountain Moving Coffee House (a lesbian organization) all provide security not only from physical harm but from social degradation and personal disrespect. Access to some of these groups is restricted—one must be obey the rules of respect to stay in InSight Arts, and one must be a lesbian or a lesbian's daughter to go to the Coffee House–but they are deliberately inclusive with respect to race and ethnicity.

United Church is widely known to teach a distinct sense of moral responsibility—to respect, include, and care for others—and also to teach that this respect means permitting others to make their own moral choices. In contrast to most of the immigrant congregations we have discussed, the moral culture of United Church fosters conscientious individual choice more than the moral discipline of the community. It is a decidedly liberal congregation that even in its internal life affirms only enough rules to ensure that individuals are safe and that groups can run their own affairs without interference. Thus, while the church prides itself on being inclusive and on sharing and caring among different groups, it is successful in these objectives in part by ensuring the inviolability of separate cultural, and usually physical, spaces. Except for the Telugu congregation, these spaces are not ethnoracial enclaves, but they are groups in which persons, both individually and socially, define their identities for themselves.

A Church in Mission

The Good News Church/Iglesia Buenas Nuevas began as a "house church" and then a storefront church in North of Howard, a very poor section of Rogers Parks. It was a creation of socially and spiritually committed individuals from educational institutions in the adjacent suburb of Evanston. In 1991 it merged with a Hispanic storefront church, and the joint congregation began worshiping together monthly while maintaining separate weekly worship services and prayer and Bible-study meetings. The joint congregation also sponsors a soup kitchen that serves more than one hundred people from the immediate neighborhood every day, with the assistance of suburban congregations that supply food, funds, and volunteers.

Like United Church, Good News is a "mainline Protestant" church (a congregation of the United Church of Christ), and it shares the commitment of service to the people of the neighborhood. Although it has both Spanish-speaking and English-speaking ministers, it works to hold worshipers together in a single congregation through joint activities, a single governing board, and, most important, a common commitment to community service. In some ways this approach may be compared with the distinct services of the three language groups at Saint Jerome; but Good News Church is much smaller than the Catholic parish, and the two language groups have less to do apart from the whole, so that it seems to function much more as a single spiritual community. And while the comparison with United Church is evident in its service orientation and its inclusiveness, Good News has no single, inclusive worship service to project a symbolic unity.

But there is a unity that is both symbolic and practical, and it is to be found in the service to the North of Howard section of Rogers Parks—a section that is almost entirely black and Hispanic and that is the most economically impoverished in the Rogers Parks area. Although a few members come from outside North of Howard, and although suburban churches provide volunteers and financial support, North of Howard defines the congregation as a community.

Religion and Rogers Parks' Ethnoracial Enclaves

Our walk along Devon Avenue showed the ethnoracial diversity of Rogers Parks, but as soon as we left Devon and focused on religious congregations, we found most of them to be much more homogeneous than the neighborhood as a whole, and those that were not homogeneous created distinctive subgroups that were. This looked like a multifaith variant on the aphorism that "eleven o'clock Sunday morning is the most segregated hour of the week," as the new immigrant religions repeated the ethnoracial clustering long characteristic of Protestants, Catholics, and Jews. Moreover, with the exception of United Church, the rituals and activities of each congregation gave symbolic expression to a "we" that was defined not only religiously but ethnoracially. And even United Church, like two of the other four mainline Protestant churches in Rogers Parks, hosted a congregation (Telugu Methodist) that is constituted on an ethnoracial basis.

At a time when the cultural melting pot is being replaced by a mosaic, and when Nathan Glazer confirms that "we are all multiculturalists now,"[24] the simple fact that an apparent majority of congregations actively contribute to the construction of ethnoracial identities is unremarkable. But the content of those identities, the cultural and moral values they embody, may affect how they interface with the neighborhood, the city, and the wider society. As the research on diverse neighborhoods cited earlier makes clear, the sustainability of such neighborhoods depends in part on the ways in which their diversity is interpreted by the residents and on the investment of residents' organizations and local institutions.

With the nonwhite population of Rogers Parks increasing to more than one-third in 1990, and with some census tracts as high as 40 percent Hispanic, 35 percent black, and 27 percent Asian, the area qualifies as a candidate for racial tipping and white flight.[25] Moreover, we found no congregations publicly promoting or defending the racial integration of the area, although United Church, Good News, and Saint Jerome are inclusive organizations. For these congregations of Rogers Parks, diversity is simply a fact of life.

Yet all the congregations have made commitments that add incentives for their members to remain as residents in Rogers Parks. The synagogues and The Ark help maintain a religious and ethnic infrastructure that would be hard to duplicate elsewhere (because it presupposes a geographic concentration of Jews) and thus provide a compelling reason for twenty-six thousand Jews to remain in the neighborhood. Saint Jerome, United Church, and Good News, which represent predominantly white Christian denominations, not only maintain facilities in the neighborhood and offer services to all but also involve their white members in providing those services. The youth programs, which were offered by all the organizations we studied, stabilize the community in two ways. First, parents who might otherwise move to the suburbs to find the support they need for the religious education of their youth have a Jewish, Catholic, Pentecostal, liberal Protestant, Hindu, or Muslim youth group where they now live. Second, the religious groups provide alternatives to illegal youth activities, especially gangs, possibly reducing the danger of tipping by reducing the fear of crime.

These modest positives may be either magnified or eclipsed, however, by the cultural construction of the "we" of these religious groups, the "they" who are not included, and the boundaries between the two. Far from having negative attitudes toward outsiders, these groups are primarily concerned with themselves, apparently feeling it unnecessary to actively distinguish themselves from other ethnoracial groups. Sephardic Jews might take note of their differences from Ashkenazim; German and Austrian Jews might be concerned about Russian immigrants' lack of religious literacy; and Muslims from India might define themselves as Indo-Pakistanis, thus distinguishing themselves from "Indians" and their presumably Hindu culture. Both Pentecostal and Catholic Hispanic youth defined terms of solidarity that excluded the violence, drugs, illicit sex, and *machismo* of the (Latino) gangs. But these are all boundaries within ethnoracial groups, not between them.

But do these organizations do anything positive to promote what they have in common, to build one neighborhood, one community, one American society? They clearly express a kind of American multiculturalism, each ensuring through rituals and education that its particular group will know and value what it means, *within* American society, to be, for example, Jewish, Sephardic Jewish, and Moroccan Sephardic Jewish; to be Muslim and Indo-Pakistani Muslim; to be Catholic, Hispanic, and Mexican Catholic; and so on. But do these congregations dream "common dreams," that is, American dreams? Or, by failing to do so, do they "disunite" America? David Hollinger's distinction between a pluralist and a cosmopolitan multiculturalism[26] is helpful at this point. Whereas both forms share the idea that America should be hospitable to a diversity of ethnoracially specific cultures, pluralist multiculturalism tends to "depict society as an expanse of internally homogeneous and analogically structured units, each possessed of a comparable myth of diaspora." In contrast, the cosmopolitan form shows greater consciousness of the voluntariness of individuals' affiliation with the group and of each group's dynamic interrelationships with more embracing communities, including the neighborhood, city, and America as a whole.

In Hollinger's terms, the organizations described in this chapter are more pluralist than cosmopolitan. Their programs and discourse include relatively little about "America as a whole," about American public life and culture, or about Chicago and the neighborhoods of Rogers Parks. Even the fact that these neighborhoods, because of their diversity and tolerance, include all these groups, without any of them appearing conspicuous, is taken for granted. Our research revealed no programs of education about the other religions and ethnoracial groups in the neighborhood, no intergroup visits or exchanges of musicians or instructors. An interfaith Thanksgiving service—a holdover from a period of much less diversity—was the only joint project during the time of our research. (Since then, an interfaith antihunger project has been developed, and an interfaith agency, the Council for a Parliament of the World's Religions, has organized interfaith dialogues.) United Church, and to a lesser extent, Good News and Saint Jerome, embody a cosmopolitan vision by including multiple ethnoracial groups in the same congregation and by symbolically expressing the unity of different groups through worship, education, and, in the case of Saint Jerome, through the doctrine of the inclusive territorial parish. But as we have seen, even the most cosmopolitan groups achieve their unity by creating separate enclaves in which groups differentiate themselves by race, ethnicity, language, ideology, and sexual orientation.

Yet within the religiously based ethnoracial enclaves we have seen cultural formation that, however differentiated from the wider society, is what much of the wider society claims to want. These groups are building their capacities of moral discourse, forming themselves as morally self-conscious and mutually accountable communities. More ethnically differentiated groups may be, or are trying to be, "communities of memory," constructing shared narratives based on common experiences and using inherited cultural material that they select and adapt according to the criteria of their religious traditions. The United Church, Good News, and Saint Jerome (when it acts as a whole) are ethnically diverse and thus depend more on theological and ideological principles than on shared narrative as a basis for moral formation. Nevertheless, we found all the congregations calling their members to accountability for their relationships and participation in community. If these groups did not, for the most part, define or "socially construct" the wider communities, neither did they allow the individual members to think they were sufficient unto themselves.

Rogers Parks has a variety of enclaves for the variety of people who live there. It appeals to people looking for cosmopolitan urbanity, a dense street life, but not the sort that is conceded to toughs. The area is accessible to families as well as singles. It is attractive to people who want more independence and personal freedom than a family neighborhood in the suburbs or some other parts of the city offer. Its enclaves are real, but they are not ghettos. And while the religious organizations help create and perpetuate the enclaves, they also help ensure that they are defined by the concentration and cultural self-identification of similar people, not by the exclusion or subordination of others.

NOTES

1. Park and Burgess, *The City.*

2. Taub, Taylor, and Dunham, *Paths of Neighborhood Change,* especially chap. 7.

3. Pacyga and Skerritt, *Chicago.*

4. "Racially and Ethnically Diverse Urban Neighborhoods," 23–24 and 131–160.

5. Gronbjerg et al., *Rogers Park.*

6. Chicago Fact Book Consortium, *Local Community Fact Book,* 1980 and 1990, which report U.S. Census data.

7. Young, *Justice and the Politics of Difference.*

8. Hollinger, *Postethnic America.*

9. Fuchs, *American Kaleidoscope,* 77–79.

10. Schlesinger, *Disuniting of America;* Gitlin, *Twilight of Common Dreams.*

11. For discussion of the cultural production of religion, see Wuthnow, *Producing the Sacred;* on cultural production of race and ethnicity, see Omi and Winant, *Racial Formation.*

12. Pacyga and Skerrett, *Chicago,* 146–47.

13. Jewish Federation of Metropolitan Chicago, "Fact Sheet" based on the federation's 1990 study, Chicago, 1992.

14. For the historical context and description, see Cutler, *Jews of Chicago,* esp. 249–254.

15. Sklare, "Conservative Movement," points out that the Conservative movement pioneered the "synagogue center," which offered social and recreational activities.

16. Bellah et al., *Habits of the Heart,* 152–153.

17. Glazer, *American Judaism,* 172; see also 183–186.

18. Danzger, *Returning to Tradition;* Glazer, *American Judaism,* introduction, offers a more qualified view.

19. Cohen and Peck, *Sephardim in the Americas,* especially part 3. On the Sephardim in Chicago, see Cutler, *Jews of Chicago,* 90, 196; and Zenner, "Chicago's Sephardim."

20. On the traditional parish in racially changing contexts, see McGreevy, *Parish Boundaries.*

21. For an enumeration of mosques and their ethnic concentrations in the

Chicago area, see Numrich, "Facing Northeast"; on Muslim immigrants generally, see Haddad, ed., *Muslims of America.*

22. Williams, *Religions of Immigrants,* 129–137 and 234.

23. Ibid., 234.

24. Glazer, *We Are All Multiculturalists Now.*

25. Taub, Taylor, and Durham, *Paths of Neighborhood Change,* 142.

26. Hollinger, *Postethnic America,* introduction and chap. 4. Following quote from p. 12.

Chatham & Neighboring Communities

First Census
Greater Than
90 % Black

1940
1950
1960
1970
1980
1990

67TH (MARQUETTE RD.)
AVE.
AVE.
ST.

EXPWY.
SOUTH CHICAGO

71ST
CHICAGO
ST.

† St. Columbanus
R. C. Church

75TH
RYAN
ST.

New Covenant
Missionary
Baptist Church †
■ Ingleside-Whitfield
United Methodist
Church

† Carter Temple
■ C. M. E. Church

79TH
DAN
ST.
AVE.
SKYWAY

83RD
KING
JR.
ST.

87TH
STATE
ST.

MARTIN
LUTHER
Vernon Park
Church of God
†
■

COTTAGE GROVE
STONY ISLAND

DR.
95TH
ST.

N

0   ½   1
MILE

CHICAGO

Map 7. Chatham, a comfortable middle-class neighborhood, has been formed by a fifty-year process of racial integration and resegregation. Map by Brian Twardosz, BMT Printing and Cartographic Specialists.

"Ain't Gonna Let Nobody Turn Me 'Round"

The Politics of Race and the New Black Middle-Class Religion

David D. Daniels III

The brilliance of the new black middle-class religion is exemplified in its combination of various elements that have created a new religious moment in the Black Church. Annual concerts of Handel's *Messiah* and the choral performances of Bach anthems and Negro spirituals join an extensive repertoire in contemporary gospel music. The artful compositions of Edwin Hawkins and Richard Smallwood intermingle with the hard-hitting sounds of composers John P. Kee and Mattie Moss Clark. New black middle-class congregations delight in the diversity of music, applauding the talents and virtuosity of the musicians and vocalists. Although a Methodist, Roman Catholic, or Pentecostal liturgy orders the Sunday morning worship, the congregation seizes liturgical space to offer spontaneous refrains such as "Amen" and "Thank you, Jesus." With black depictions of biblical characters gracing the Sunday worship bulletin and with rites-of-passage programs in the youth ministry, these congregations embrace an Afrocentric Christian orientation. They also strive to connect their Sunday morning worship of God to their weekday service to the community. The diversity of cultural styles that these congregations intertwine each week—from European classical anthems to African American gospel music, Protestant and Catholic liturgies to Afrocentric events, and Sunday worship to community service—reflects the distinctive manner of the new black middle-class religion.[1]

A prime example of the new black middle-class religion is Carter Temple Christian Methodist Episcopal (CME) Church, which is in Chicago's black middle-class neighborhood of Chatham. Carter Temple locates African Americans in the lineage of kings and queens of Africa, not of slaves of white plantation owners. It offers the model of the church as an African village, where people share responsibility for rearing children, regardless of whether the child's father is around, and where men take up their rightful obligations—even if the world around them, including most of the churches, is caught up in "Eurocentric individualism." Carter Temple provides a new, positive symbolic context for elements of African American culture (the extended family, intergenerational respect, even the village life of the American South) and of the structure and traditions of the CME Church (the ministry of stewards to members). Rituals (rites of passage, black male role celebrations, African festivals), symbols (kente cloth, black liberation colors), and new Afrocentric scholarship all are woven into a new collective self-image.

Carter Temple's ministry affirms the humanity of African Americans and recognizes their peoplehood. The congregation joins the battle against the denigration of African Americans in the media, literature, and films by promoting positive images of African American people and life. At Carter Temple, African Americans are taught to respect and love themselves as a people through learning about the contributions of Africans and African Americans in history, the arts, and sciences. The cultural heritage emphasis at Carter Temple serves various functions: it counters the claims that Christianity is a "white man's religion," offers a corrective to the biased Eurocentric interpretation and representation of Christianity and world history, and provides African Americans with information that increases knowledge of their heritage.

Afrocentricity redefines the African American cultural heritage and perspective that Carter Temple expresses. As a worldview, Afrocentricity construes reality from the perspective of the peoples of Africa, both in Africa and in the diaspora. Ethicist Robert Franklin contends that Afrocentricity as a cultural approach "seeks to celebrate the halcyon days of the African past and to affirm black identity in the present through cultural displays." Within the framework of Afrocentricity, black social pathologies are sometimes defined as the products of the African American embrace of Eurocentric values and individualistic culture. To cure the social pathologies in the black community, adherents to the Afrocentric worldview maintain that African Americans need to embrace historical black and African communal values. Thus Afrocentricity offers healing and restoration to the black community, and a Christian Afrocentricity offers salvation.[2] At Carter Temple, sermons juxtapose the individualistic character of American materialism against the communal character of African culture, a communalism in line with Christian virtues.

Afrocentricity frames Carter Temple's engagement of racial politics as the struggle for a liberating construction of African American identity within the sociopolitical context defined by white racism. It inverts the hierarchy of cultural values in the production of racial identity from the best of western culture to the best of African and African American culture. According to philosopher Molefi Asante, "The music and dance of the church may be the essence of our Africanity."[3] Now Africa, not Europe, is the measuring rod of civilization, of the cultural best. Carter Temple, for instance, intentionally valorizes Africa and constructively reappropriates African American folk culture embodied in the mores and customs of the black poor and working class. This leads to a positive reevaluation of the black stereotype that is based in the culture of the black poor. Previously, the black middle class had constructed its identity in contradistinction to the poor and its folk culture; now Carter Temple participates in the construction of black identity utilizing the culture of the poor, especially the folk culture of the poor. The new racial identity encourages cultural and moral identification with the poor, in a rejection of the white American cultural norm. The embrace of features of the stereotype of blacks has facilitated the construction of a common identity stemming from a common history of oppression and achievement, common heritage, and common destiny.[4]

Carter Temple challenges Eurocentric individualism through a number of its various ministries. Especially connected to nurturing an Afrocentric communalism are its Save Our Sons, Project Essence, One-Church-One-School, and Boys to Men conferences. The One-Church-One-School ministry, for instance, links Carter Temple to nearby Ruggles Elementary School, which serves many at-risk children and youth. In each of these ministries, one of the goals is to build the self-esteem of the youth so that they can develop into mature, responsible adults and reject destructive behavior such as gang involvement. These ministries play a double role of strengthening the congregational and neighborhood life.

A distinctive element of Carter Temple's Afrocentricity is its identification with and commitment to the African American community as a whole, including explicitly its more disadvantaged members. Carter Temple strives to define community across class lines; they have formed a partnership with the Olive Branch, a South Side homeless shelter, and

Fig. 7-1. The Lord's Supper is part of the Afrocentric art at Carter Temple CME Church, Chatham area, Chicago. Paintings and stained glass depicting white biblical characters have been removed. Photo by Lowell W. Livezey.

hold a "Come as You Are" Saturday worship service, designed to make the homeless feel comfortable. The congregation aggressively promotes a black male emphasis. In their attempt to "reclaim" the black male, they have stressed patriarchical roles for men and supporting roles for black women. They have also reached out to the prison population, which is predominantly male, in order to include these individuals in the reclaiming endeavor.

The symbolic and stylistic innovations, most obvious in worship, co-here with attempts to broaden the constituency of the church and bridge barriers of class, for example, through inclusion of at-risk children and youth in the Carter Temple family and through the new Saturday "Come as You Are" worship service. This cohesion is effected in part by the incorporation of particular styles of preaching (including escalating, rhythmic intonations known as "hooping") and music (gospel, percussion, rhythm) and "expressiveness" into a setting where inspirational preaching, note-perfect singing, and "sweet hour of prayer" quietness might have been expected—and are still preserved as part of the new mix. The church also sponsors extensive programs in Christian education and mutual support that strengthen the communal life of Carter Temple.

Carter Temple's challenge to Eurocentric individualism spurs its project to redefine community, especially black community. The Afrocentric symbolization at Carter Temple represents only part of a deeper shift in the style of worship and collective identity in what has been a thoroughly middle-class congregation in a denomination identified with the black middle class. The Afrocentricity loosens the grip of the older black middle-class culture, especially the religious dimension of that culture, that critics such as E. Franklin Frazier challenged for its social stratification and paternalistic attitude toward the poor. Carter Temple thus moves away from what might be called the "old black middle-class religion" of its past and, with its particular racial politics, contributes to the construction of a new black middle-class religion.

Diversity within Black Middle-Class Religion

This chapter examines Carter Temple and four other congregations located in the central part of Chicago's South Side, an area we shall call Chatham, although it includes the official community areas not only of Chatham but of Greater Grand Crossing and Avalon Park as well. "Chatham" begins about nine miles south of Chicago's central business district and extends from Sixty-seventh to Ninety-fifth Streets and from the Dan Ryan Expressway to Stony Island Avenue. Politically, this area includes most of the Sixth Ward—long a stronghold of the black component of Chicago's "Regular Democratic Organization"—as well as the western half of the Eighth Ward and a corner of the Fifth. During the midtwentieth century, this area switched from a white to an "integrated" to, finally, an African American community. We call this entire area Chatham, because, as a symbol of the black middle class, the image of Chatham dominates the area. The five congregations discussed in this chapter either moved to Chatham during the 1950s or 1960s or, already located there, became majority African American congregations during the 1960s.

In the 1950s the racial politics of the old black middle-class religion inspired many middle-class African Americans to participate in the integration of Chatham. They were pursuing the American dream of home ownership and the African American dream of integration. The dream of integration, however, faded in the wake of white flight. Chatham, which had virtually no blacks in 1950, saw an increase to 64 percent by 1960 and 98 percent by 1970, along with a significant increase in the total population as black people purchased vacant land and built new homes. Thus, by 1960, Chatham had become established as the preferred area among very limited options for Chicago's relatively affluent black people. William Braden, a respected columnist for the *Chicago Sun-Times,* wrote in 1986 that "Chatham is a bastion of Chicago's black middle class . . . represent[ing] perhaps the largest concentration of middle class blacks in America outside of Harlem and Atlanta."[5]

Chatham is part of Chicago's larger black community and a product of African American integrationists' goals, which spurred the African American relocation into white neighborhoods. Blacks moved into the area in large numbers during the 1950s. The earlier black community, from which African Americans relocated, had been mainly a narrow north-south strip from the Loop to Forty-seventh Street. The area eventually extended to Sixty-seventh Street, due in part to the housing shortages that resulted from the "urban renewal" and "slum clearance" of portions of the pre–World War II area. Urban renewal replaced black people's apartment buildings with Michael Reese Hospital, Illinois Institute of Technology, and the upscale housing of Lake Meadows and Prairie Shores. Restrictive covenants, "white only" home-owner agreements, confined African Americans to particular neighborhoods. The residential boundaries, edging south of Sixty-seventh Street during 1949, expanded through a process of competition for space that was motivated in part by white violence as well as white commercial and political interests. In effect, Chatham became a community where African Americans who possessed the financial resources to purchase or rent housing could integrate, however briefly.[6]

Although the flight of white residents and congregations undermined the integration of Chatham and produced the resegregation of African Americans, a number of factors permitted Chatham to become a vital black middle-class community. The new black residents had the financial resources, the leadership skills, the cultural resources, and the social networks to build and maintain a solid community. Moreover, Chicago's industrial sector was still strong and provided a high concentration of well-paying jobs on the South Side—within an easy commute of Chatham.

African American congregations were at the center of the integration and, later, of the new black middle-class community of Chatham.

This chapter contends that the new black middle-class religion, which is represented by three of the five congregations discussed here, signals a shift in the religious culture constructed by African Americans as a response to the reordering of African American society during the 1960s. Sociologist C. Eric Lincoln helps set the stage for our discussion of the new black middle-class religion. In *The Black Church since Frazier*,[7] he contends that during the 1960s a transformation of the Black Church occurred. The pre-1967 Black Church, which has been examined and critiqued in classics such as E. Franklin Frazier's *The Negro Church in America*, collapsed, and a new Black Church emerged. Frazier had been concerned with what I now call the old black middle-class religion. According to Frazier, racial discrimination and segregation defined the social context of the pre-1967 Black Church, which, under segregation, had become a place for African Americans to accommodate to their second-class citizenship. For Frazier, urbanization, social disintegration, social stratification, secularization, and desegregation, especially in the North, marked the twentieth-century Black Church of the pre–Civil Rights era. His project was to distinguish the new social context of the mid-twentieth-century Black Church from the rural location, traditional social organization, predominantly uniform class identification, religious worldview, disfranchisement, and segregation of the post-Reconstruction Negro Church.[8]

Central to Frazier's analysis was the process of achieving status among the black middle class. Two routes to status were occupational and cultural performance. Cultural performance was a vital means to achieving status. The theorists of the old black middle-class religion participated in the designing of a new African American identity. Their cultural production was defined in terms of elite western culture, rejecting African American folk culture and identifying with European and Euro-American elite cultural expressions. The racial politics of old black middle-class church confronted the ideology of African American inferiority through the creative mastery of elite western culture, debunking this debilitating ideology by successfully competing with white Americans on their cultural terrain.[9]

Frazier died before he had the opportunity to witness the change occurring in many black middle-class churches during the 1960s. The theorists of the new black middle-class religion, both reflecting and

promoting these changes, rejected the ideology of African American inferiority outright and refused to privilege elite western culture. They
preached liberation from white cultural, theological, and intellectual
categories and called for the celebration of all things African and
African American. This is not to say that they invented black political
activism, which began in Chicago, for instance, at the advent of the
twentieth century with the pastorates of African Methodist Episcopal
Archibald J. Carey Sr. and Baptist Elijah J. Fisher. But the theorists of the
1960s disagreed with the old black middle-class religion about the role
of black folk culture in their religion. The contest produced a shift in
African American religious culture. Some scholars described the cultural shift as the "birth of a new 'black being.'" Others characterized the
shift as a psychological revolution, the overthrow of "the rule of white
men in our [African American] minds." The old black middle-class religion, then, operated in a social world dominated by western or Eurocentric cultural values that the theorists of new black middle-class religion supplanted with their own creation.[10]

The five congregations presented in this chapter all existed during the
heyday of the old black middle-class religion. They now represent different constituencies within the Black Church. Two congregations are members of historically black denominations, the Christian Methodist Episcopal Church and the National Baptist Convention of America, respectively.
The other three congregations are members of predominantly white denominations: the Roman Catholic Church, the Church of God (Anderson, Indiana), and the United Methodist Church (UMC). Three of the
congregations were founded by African Americans; one congregation is a
merger of a white and an African American congregation; and one congregation began as a white congregation, whose membership became interracial prior to becoming predominantly African American. The congregations vary in membership and attendance at Sunday worship, with
more than a thousand people attending Sunday worship at each of two of
the churches, while six hundred, five hundred, and one hundred persons,
respectively, attend the other three. These congregations bear the marks
of their respective histories.

Carter Temple, a congregation with more than twenty-two hundred
members and a major community institution by virtue of its membership and neighborhood presence, is located in the west-central part of
Chatham on Seventy-ninth Street, a relatively affluent and stable portion
of the neighborhood. Founded in 1921, Carter Temple moved to this lo-

cation and built the present edifice in 1965. Since the Reverend Henry M. Williamson Sr. was appointed pastor in 1986, the church has grown by one thousand members and has added a second Sunday service and a Saturday service. Carter Temple actively supports its denomination, the Christian Methodist Episcopal Church.

Located on Stony Island Avenue at Ninetieth Street on the eastern edge of Chatham, abutting a pleasant residential and commercial area, Vernon Park Church of God was founded in 1955 by its current pastor, the Reverend Claude Wyatt, and his wife, who was later ordained, the Reverend Addie Wyatt. It grew steadily while worshiping in several locations before building its present complex in 1985. At present, it has more than one thousand members and nearly that many in its Sunday morning worship service. It has a wide range of ministries, with an emphasis on pastoral care for both members and nonmembers. Vernon Park is a congregation of the Church of God (Anderson, Indiana) and a member of its National Association, an organization of the denomination's African American clergy.

New Covenant Missionary Baptist Church is located one block west of Cottage Grove Avenue on Seventy-seventh Street (now Reverend Stephen John Thurston Place, in honor of the current pastor). A growing church of fifteen hundred members with a weekly Sunday-worship attendance of more than one thousand, New Covenant was established in 1934 on Forty-fourth Street by the Reverend Elijah Thurston, the grandfather of the current pastor. New Covenant moved to its present location in Greater Grand Crossing during 1956, when only a few of its families lived in its new neighborhood. Its pastor and prominent laypeople are leaders in the National Baptist Convention of America, Inc.

The racial politics of Carter Temple, Vernon Park, and New Covenant represent different trajectories in the new black middle-class religion. For each congregation, racial authenticity became the standard in its liturgy and congregational life. Whether or not an element was authentically black served as a criterion for appropriation. Thus new black middle-class religion adopted gospel music, "hooping," religious dance, expressive and celebrative gestures, and Pentecostal-like spirituality. By the 1980s, the term *Afrocentricity* was employed to provide specificity to racial authenticity. Rites of passage, kente cloth, and African attire were introduced as elements of a specifically African cultural identification. Coupled with the liturgical and cultural elements were emphases on educational ministries related to blacks in the Bible, black religious and social history, and black theology. Instead of attempting to debunk myths of black inferiority through greater adherence to elite western cultural norms, these congregations sought to advance knowledge about Africans as a biblical people and makers of a great ancient civilization as well as a great culture, in order to construct a vibrant religious community buoyed by this knowledge.[11]

Compared with Carter Temple, Vernon Park Church retains more of the characteristics of the "middlebrow," middle-class Black Church, with its note-perfect music, Pastor Claude Wyatt's inspirational preaching, and the pastoral function in all aspects of church life and work. This church exhibits no stereotypical Pentecostal qualities, though its holiness identity is evidenced by the expectation that the gifts of the Holy Spirit should shape the Christian lifestyle more than emotional or expressive forms of praise and worship. Yet, Vernon Park promotes the new Afrocentric perspective that defines the new black middle-class religion. The black liberation flag of red, black, and green hangs in the sanctuary. Kente cloth occasionally adorns the liturgical garments of the clergy. African American art graces the walls of the corridors and the fellowship hall. Black history shapes the educational programs of the church. The ministry supports the PUSH/Rainbow Coalition's goal to create a "just" America, a new America. Afrocentricity at Vernon Park celebrates the achievements and agenda of African Americans. It differs, however, from perspectives that define knowledge by race, are basically separatist in racial orientation, or reinterpret Scripture and the Christian tradition through racial concerns. Vernon Park embraces Afrocentricity along with its progressive political agenda and justice emphasis as a means of empowerment and liberation.

While at Vernon Park there is little systematic differentiation from or critique of "the predominant culture" in terms of race, there is an explicit public concern with the *urban* situation, defined not mainly in terms of race but in terms of conditions and issues that affect everyone. Vernon Park defines itself as engaged in urban ministry rather than in Afrocentric ministry. The church sponsors a food pantry for the poor and a Saturday Academy for youth, an enrichment program funded through the Urban League. At Vernon Park, Pastors Claude and Addie Wyatt model the relevance of political engagement along with other leaders in their congregation, such as the former mayor Eugene Sawyer and the Reverend Willie Barrow of Operation PUSH. Afrocentricity infuses the life of Vernon Park, although it is not central.

New Covenant reflects less of the new black middle-class religion than do Carter Temple and Vernon Park. But it also rejects the old black middle-class religion by appropriating aspects of the black folk church into the new cultural context of the black middle class. New Covenant is also engaged in the redefinition of black religious culture, but the central frame of reference for its innovation is the Black Church in America, not Africa—although the congregation occasionally invokes African symbols. The central lineage of New Covenant members is not the kings and queens of Africa but the Christian slaves who found salvation by trusting in Jesus and—this is crucial—who organized the Black Church. Thus, if African Americans are to find assurance that the Bible is true for blacks today as a minority group in a white, secular culture that dominates them, they must remember that it was also true for the slaves who trusted Jesus.

One might reasonably ask: Where lies the innovation? Nothing being presented about the Black Church is new here, at least not in terms of its history. The innovation is that New Covenant, a historically elite, "upper-class church" (to quote Pastor Stephen Thurston) catering to the very black bourgeoisie studied by Frazier, now seeks to locate itself among the contemporary descendants of slaves who remain oppressed by the dominant culture during the postsegregation era. Rev. Thurston's preaching constantly reminds the congregation that they have arrived not in the promised land but in an alien land. The pastor invites congregants to model an alternative to the dominant culture, not to trust it and certainly not to join it. Those who have not crossed the church's threshold—which is social and cultural as well as physical—may hear its message on its weekly telecast or from a mission group member doing her time of service witnessing on the street or door to door. The congregation welcomes the newcomer into a cultural enclave shaped by the black folk church, one that defines itself over against the dominant culture and embraces all who trust Jesus. Music, preaching, education, and mission combine to define New Covenant as an enclave.

New Covenant's pastor, the Reverend Stephen John Thurston, has expressed his commitment to civil rights through his active involvement in Operation PUSH. To assist the poor, the congregation sponsors a secondhand-clothing store. Although Afrocentricity is not a major focus at New Covenant, in 1993 the church assisted 150 of its youth to visit Africa as a mission-to-Africa trip as well as an activity of religious formation of the youth. Africa represents an important symbol and place in the congregation.

In contrast to the three churches thus far examined, congregations such as Saint Columbanus Roman Catholic Church and Ingleside-Whitfield United Methodist Church have resisted any adoption of the new black middle-class religion in Chatham. Saint Columbanus was built in 1925 on Seventy-first Street in the northwest corner of Chatham, having been created in 1909 for upwardly mobile Irish American residents. The church easily seats one thousand. Since the mid-1960s, Saint Columbanus has been a predominantly African American parish. From the 350 families now registered, perhaps five hundred people attend mass weekly. While the majority of the active members and leadership are age fifty or older, a significant number of younger families with children are active in the parish. Father Phillip Cyscon, a diocesan priest of Polish descent, has been pastor since 1993. With two priests and two deacons, the parish offers daily and three weekend masses. It also operates a highly respected and growing school, whose students come from across the South Side of Chicago.

Saint Columbanus, particularly its older leaders, drew a sharper line between African American culture and Catholic faith than did the African American Catholics who created and promoted the Gospel Mass movement. Saint Columbanus's leadership resisted the developments that endowed African American cultural expressions with religious valence and declined to support campaigns for black cultural liberation within the Chicago Archdiocese, withholding strong attachment to either African religious rituals and holidays or African American religious-based cultural forms. Whereas other black parishes, such as Holy Angels, Saint Sabina, and Saint Benedict the African, celebrated their African and African American heritage liturgically, Saint Columbanus opted to bring the older black middle-class religion into the new religious context.[12]

The parish continues the older black middle-class commitment to racial uplift, defined in terms of social change. It daily opens its gymnasium to the neighborhood youth to provide a "safe place" for recreation. Its parochial school sponsors a before- and after-school program, offering working parents a supervised and structured environment for their youth. To serve the poor, the church stocks a food pantry.

Similar in some respects to Saint Columbanus is Ingleside-Whitfield's adjustment to the new cultural context of the Black Church. A new congregation resulting from the merger of a white and an African American Methodist congregation in 1960, Ingleside-Whitfield is located on Seventh-sixth Street in the central part of Chatham (near New Covenant). Its first African American pastor, the Reverend Edsel Ammons, later a United Methodist bishop, was appointed at the time of the merger. At the time of our study the church had a single worship service, with an average attendance slightly over one hundred. The pastor, the Reverend Danita R. Anderson, was appointed in 1991.

Until the 1990s, Ingleside-Whitfield held to the old black middle-class religion, resisting the appropriation of elements from the black folk church. The introduction of Afrocentric elements and folk worship styles in the last decade of the twentieth century has been divisive. Yet, as with Saint Columbanus, the ties to the old black middle-class religion have included commitment to racial uplift. Ingleside-Whitfield offers a program for younger children sponsored by the Edsel Ammons Nursery School and Kindergarten. A layperson from the church has been the mainstay of the Greater Grand Crossing Organizing Committee, a church-based community organization of modest impact. Saint Columbanus and Ingleside-Whitfield both remain closely aligned to the old black middle-class religion, albeit adapted to the new cultural and social context.

The diversity within black middle-class religion reflects the differing forms of racial politics selected to construct racial identity as well as to advance the full incorporation of African Americans in American society. The post-1967 cultural and social context, while defined by desegregation and later resegregation, reflects the cultural production currently identified with Afrocentricity. Although relative agreement exists on the overall civil rights agenda, widespread disagreement engulfs the cultural agenda of the black middle-class church.[13]

Black Middle-Class Religion in the Age of Segregation and Desegregation

The new black middle-class religion is an heir of the Civil Rights movement, black ecumenism, and black nationalism, and is a product of the black theology movement. It emerged in the 1970s, well after the collapse of the integration of Chatham. Black middle-class congregations supported the integration of communities like Chatham in the 1950s, often relocating their congregations to predominantly white neighborhoods before their memberships did the same (as was the case with New Covenant), thus competing with the "open" white congregations for black middle-class members relocating into these neighborhoods. The racial politics of the old black middle-class religion shaped the aspirations of African Americans moving into Chatham.

By the time African Americans began residing in Chatham, the civil rights activists vigorously promoted integration. They espoused the philosophy of an activist federal government taking "responsibility of making a better life for all its citizens, regardless of race, creed, or color." Encouraged by Franklin Delano Roosevelt's initiatives, they applauded the Supreme Court's efforts to supplant legalized segregation with "an Integrated Equality that included political equality, equality of economic opportunity, and integrated public facilities." They adopted proportionality as a measure of equality and a means to achieve it, advocating open public facilities and even proportional percentages of African Americans and whites in public institutions such as federal housing, public schools, hospitals, and occupations. Since all human beings were the same, they contended that "extensive assimilation and integration of the races was both necessary and desirable."[14]

Housing loomed as a cardinal goal of integration. But housing, like schools, became contested in northern cities such as Chicago. As historian Thomas J. Sugrue demonstrates, in northern cities "the politics of race, home ownership, and neighborhood" spawned the white resistance to integration in the post–World War II era that preceded white flight. Neighborhood civic associations engaged in "defensive localism" and asserted the right to racially homogeneous neighborhoods, a right initially defended even by the HOLC (Home Owners' Loan Corporation) and FHA (Federal Housing Administration) as democratic. During 1946 and 1947, the focal points for this struggle in Chicago were the Airport Homes and the Fernwood Apartments, two temporary veteran housing projects sponsored by the Federal Public Housing Authority and administered by the Chicago Housing Authority.[15]

The people and congregations moving into Chatham in the 1950s were also part of the larger middle-class world of black sororities, fraternities, lodges, and social clubs, with their elaborate rituals and social networks. They had created an alternative world of African American society within the space African Americans cleared in the midst of the racially segregated nation. This achievement demonstrated that African Americans could appropriate and excel at what was considered the best of western bourgeois culture. In the racial politics of the older black middle class, class was defined as culture and status. To traverse the divide between the African American working class and the middle class, African Americans needed to acquire middle-class values and culture. The cultural project of the old black middle-class religion was not mimicry; it involved something new: the creation of African American modern art, dance, music, and literature, by geniuses such as Horace Pippin, Katherine Dunham, William Grant Still, and Zora Neale Hurston.

The old black middle-class church often yoked the social incorporation of African Americans into American society with their cultural productions. The development of an African American middle-class culture served the political purpose of debunking myths about African American racial inferiority through its ability to assimilate culturally. Black pathologies would be exorcised from the black community as a consequence of full assimilation bolstered by a black middle-class culture, proving that these pathologies were the products of social malformation due to racial isolation and racism and were not inherent in black people.[16] Central to the racial project of the old black middle-class church was cultural contact: African Americans had to learn and contextualize the best of white American and European culture.

The hallmark of black cultural production was music. Black middle-class congregations had distinguished themselves in Chicago for their musical productions, ranging from classical concerts to operas, in post–World War I Chicago. Choral study clubs became the primary vehicles for cultural advancement. Historian Michael Wesley Harris notes that these clubs advertised that they were "organized to create a desire for better music among Chicago Negroes and to render musical numbers of the higher type." These clubs excelled in the performances of "Handel's *Messiah,* Gall's *Holy City,* and the choral music of Samuel Coleridge-Taylor." Bethel African Methodist Episcopal Church mounted the first opera sung by African Americans in Chicago with the choir's performance of Friedrich von Flotow's *Martha.* By 1930, the choral study clubs had become the choirs for local congregations. These choirs would sing, in Latin and in English, compositions ranging from Rossini's *Stabat Mater* to Mendelssohn's *Elijah,* from Bach's cantatas to Haydn's *Creation* to Theodore Dubois's *The Seven Last Words.* The complete performance of these works occurred at concerts advertised as "monthly musicales." In addition to European classical music, the choir sang Negro spirituals in choral arrangements by Nathaniel Dett, Hall Johnson, Harry T. Burleigh. The choir members often donned a "black robe with white collar and black cap with tassel."[17]

Yet, in worship, the old black middle-class church did not take the same artistic license. To distance themselves from the stereotype of black religion as sheer emotionalism and ignorance, they de-emphasized rhythmic music, religious dancing, and hooping and stressed note-per-fect singing, quietness, and inspirational and intellectual preaching. Music structured the worship service, with hymns representative of mainline Protestant hymnody and choral selections drawn from anthems and spirituals. Even their singing of spirituals was anglicized. The congre-gational singing reflected little of the urban gospel sound or the rural harmonies associated with long-meter hymns. Black middle-class con-gregations prided themselves on their ability to worship in a manner deemed as dignified as that of white middle-class Protestants.

The preaching style in these congregations was informational and in-spirational, with biblical or theological applications on practical, every-day issues presented in an "intelligent" manner. Vattel Daniel, in his 1940s study of Black Church worship in Chicago, found that black middle-class congregations reflected the social stratification within the black commu-nity, and in contrast to lower-class black congregations, their worship tended to be more "ritualistic and deliberative" than "emotional and demonstrative." Willis Laurence Jones described these deliberative black middle-class churches as Europeanized in decorum.[18]

Carter Temple and New Covenant were proud bearers of older black middle-class religion in the pre-1967 era. By the time New Covenant re-located to Chatham in 1956 the congregation had already replaced its southern black religious ethos with the black middle-class religious style. The congregations' identification with the middle class affected their de-sire to attract middle-class blacks, especially professionals, and to serve as a pillar of the social world of the black middle class; they often restricted leadership positions in the church to the middle-class membership. The Whitfield congregation, prior to the merger with Ingleside during the 1960s, embraced the religious style of the black middle-class church, with its focus on respectability and racial uplift, while Saint Columbanus dur-ing the 1960s embraced the ethos of black middle-class Roman Catholi-cism, with its selective continuation of the traditions, values, and norms of the pre–Vatican II era. These norms related to the status of the parish's parochial school, the activities of the fraternal and social organizations in the parish, and the relationship to the neighborhood, in which Saint Columbanus strove to be a service institution.[19]

The racial politics of the old black middle-class religion found allies in the social and political context in which Americanization or cultural con-formity defined the dominant cultural policy for all racial and ethnic

Fig. 7-2. A 1960s black-tie dinner at New Covenant Missionary Baptist Church, Chatham area, Chicago. Formal events remain important to this and many black churches. Photo courtesy of New Covenant Missionary Baptist Church.

groups and in which racial integration framed liberal social policy, especially in the post–World War II era. The racial advancement of the African Americans in this period seemingly illustrated the effectiveness of the racial politics of the old black middle-class religion.

The ideological, political, and cultural changes in the black community of the 1960s undermined the racial politics of the old black middle-class religion. As noted earlier, the late 1960s was the dividing line between the Black Church under and after segregation. Assimilationism, the liberal cultural policy during segregation, lost its appeal to African Americans through the white American Church's explicit and implicit support of the state-sponsored terrorism waged against the Civil Rights movement. This depletion of the moral and cultural standing of white Christians occurred for a significant segment of African Americans. "The Negro Church is dead," noted Lincoln, "because the norms and presuppositions which structured and conditioned it are not the relevant norms and presuppositions to which contemporary Blacks . . . can give their asserevation and support."[20]

The coalition of the black middle-class church and the black folk church in the Civil Rights movement anticipated this shift by the prominence the movement gave to black folk songs and culture, legitimating the "unanglicized" versions of spirituals and other songs and fashioning individuals into movement people. Black folk Christianity supplied cultural forms, discourse, and music that formed the core of the mass meetings sponsored by civil rights activists, thus further legitimating black folk culture. These meetings, attended by various pastors of Chicago's black middle-class congregations, including Rev. Claude Wyatt and Rev. Addie Wyatt, pastors of Vernon Park Church, employed the spontaneous testimony of the devotional service to narrate the experiences of injustices and activism. They adopted old-fashioned preaching, with its accent on realism, application, and inspiration, and the church-rocking singing of congregational and freedom songs. And they also utilized social analyses, "creating an experience which transformed powerless individuals" into powerful agents of God's new world.[21]

The racial politics of the old black middle class in Chicago was challenged as much by factions within the Black Church as by outside critics. Central to the struggle were the divisions within the old black middle class over the strategies of civil rights campaigns in Chicago. The civil rights struggle over de facto school desegregation and open housing in Chicago led to divisions in Chicago's black middle class in general and in its churches in particular, which were widest in February 1964, after the successful one-day school boycott held on October 22, 1963. The black leadership and congregations were divided over whether to organize a second school boycott. Abstaining from supporting the boycott were the Chicago branches of the NAACP (National Association for the Advancement of Colored People) and the Urban League, Chicago's black Democratic leadership, and many prominent African American congregations, including Olivet Baptist Church, pastored by the Reverend Joseph H. Jackson. Support for the boycott included other representatives of the black middle class and their churches, including Vernon Park Church, Quinn Chapel AME, and First Baptist Congregational Church. Although black leaders and institutions, including churches, were divided over the strategies to promote civil rights in Chicago, part of the black middle and working classes began to support more aggressive measures during 1964. During the second school boycott, a number of black congregations housed the "Freedom Schools." A July 1964 rally drew more than thirty thousand protesters to march. The black middle-class religion found itself divided on the role of social activism to achieve racial advancement.[22]

It was within the emergent Black Church of the late 1960s that the nationalist sentiment encountered its most vigorous reception. African American nationalists had led an active campaign to discredit assimilation and integration as means of racial advancement. This led to the repudiation of the "traditional leadership of the black community, which had typically arisen from the well-educated, hard working, successful women and men of the black middle class," because, according to the nationalists, "the black masses had never wanted integration; that always had been a middle-class dream." Nationalists labeled Christianity a "white man's religion." According to theologian Mark Chapman, a key issue addressed by the National Committee of Negro Churchmen during the late 1960s was "the charge that black clergy were representatives of white Christianity." The clergy who leveled the charge, mostly men, belonged to predominantly white denominations and supported black power as a "precondition for any meaningful reconciliation between blacks and whites." The espousal of black power by black clergy fostered a militance that nurtured the political independence of black clergy from white clergy. The former expressed this independence in organizing black caucuses during 1967–1968 in predominantly white denominations such as the United Methodist Church, the denomination of Ingleside-Whitfield.[23]

Related to the call for the political independence of the Black Church was the question of its cultural integrity. In 1968 theologian Henry H. Mitchell argued that African American Christianity needed cultural integrity as well as political independence to refute the nationalist critique. He defined cultural integrity in terms of the "distinctive quality of black religious culture—its music, preaching, worship style and theology."[24] Mitchell's focus on cultural integrity reflected the cultural shift within black middle-class religion, in which black folk culture supplanted the dominant culture as the ideal.

Ready to embrace the new cultural awareness were the recent arrivals to the black middle class. According to Andrew Billingsley, "The proportion of middle-class families doubled during the decade of the 1960s from 12 percent to 25 percent." These tended to be people who came from the black poor to the middle class during the 1960s. The doubling of the black middle class overwhelmed the old black middle class as a group and undermined their cultural hegemony, challenging middle-class leadership and discrediting their organizations. The contest cleared space for the new black middle class to define itself.[25]

The social and political context in which the racial politics of the old black middle-class religion had thrived was changing. The new context inverted the hierarchy of social and cultural values and created an ethos in which the new black middle-class religion would invent itself within the emerging Black Church identified by C. Eric Lincoln. The racial politics that the new black middle class would craft allied itself to the new racial identity and black cultural awareness advanced during the Black Power era.

Conclusion

The black middle-class religion redefines itself in the age of resegregation. The racial politics of these five Chatham congregations play not only a crucial economic, social, and political role in their resegregated community but also a cultural role. The structural changes affecting the neighborhood since the white flight from and the resegregation of Chatham have created a different community by the 1990s than the community some of these black congregations integrated in the 1950s and 1960s. Chatham has been significantly underinstitutionalized due to local and global economics. It is a throwback to the bedroom communities of the 1950s, without many social amenities. There are relatively few community-based organizations and social service agencies. It lacks strong public schools and is without a trauma center or major hospital. The area no longer includes a major shopping center, nor are there nearby employers capable of replacing the steel mills and stockyards.

The role of the new black middle-class churches in this economic context is complicated with regard to their mission, resources, and organizing skills, as well as the larger restructuring occurring in the U.S. economy and society. On one level, these churches provide a major countertrend to the underinstitutionalization of this neighborhood: that is, there are churches here (including those we have studied) that attract people from outside of the neighborhood. While few people come into this neighborhood to work, shop, or go to public school, many come to worship at neighborhood churches and attend parochial schools. These churches are anchor institutions of the community.

Regarding the role of the new black middle-class religion in the racial construction of neighborhoods, there has been a shift away from the devaluing of racial separation and the valuing of integration. While resegregation of neighborhoods by whites is abhorred, the relocations of African Americans to black neighborhoods are interpreted as a positive expression of self-determination and black solidarity. Although whites are welcomed to the neighborhood, they are not needed to give the neighborhood value. Ideals of interracial cooperation and harmony are avowed, but a quest for interracial residential communities is not a focus. The focus is the quest for racial justice and a racially just city and society.

Race is an issue that all five churches confront. None of them takes the racial subordination and abasement of African American people as a given. They all seek, in different ways, to engage in the racial advancement of African Americans. They affirm African Americans and valorize the African American community, and they do so by invoking specific dimensions of their religious life. In some of the congregations, this valorization of African American culture is part of the redefinition and evolution of black religious culture. Its importance extends not only to the vitality of the Black Church (one of the strongest sectors in American Christianity) but also to its prospects for sustaining community when other neighborhood institutions are under siege or fail to undergird it.

Innovations in Christian worship and ministry also contribute to the construction of racial identity and the redefinition of black religious culture. These innovations undermine differentiation in worship styles associated with social stratification and class. The poor and working class can join the middle class in worship and in social-justice endeavors without adopting middle-class religious culture as a prerequisite. The new black middle-class religion actively appropriates elements of black folk religion to fashion its racial and religious identity. This process strengthens black solidarity across class lines. While it also widens the divide between African Americans and whites, it defines the cultural difference in terms of black versus white culture rather than in terms of education and intelligence. By intentionally adopting elements of black folk culture, the new black middle-class church dispels the branding of this culture as inferior and therefore as a sign of African American social inferiority. Thus previously untapped religious and cultural resources are now available for utilization by the new black middle-class religion.

The racial politics of the new black middle-class religion involves more than the differences in cultural strategies between itself and old black middle-class religion. It emerges from the competition between various moral discourses informed by Christianity and by assimilationism, black nationalism, and Afrocentricity. Each moral discourse describes a different role for race to play in the realization of racial justice, as well as a different conception of humanity and culture. The racial politics of the new black middle-class religion coincides with the wider struggle of the identity politics movement that engulfs American society. Although the battle over multiculturalism fails to exhaust the challenge of identity politics in movements for bilingual education, racial and ethnic designations in the federal census, and culturally diverse textbooks for public schools, it nevertheless functions as a focal point for the culture wars raging across the country. The racial politics of the new black middle-class religion stands in the vanguard of the identity politics movement to reshape American society in the late twentieth century.

The new black middle-class religion intersects with myriad social currents such as identity politics, urban revitalization, and social activism. Through its racial politics it participates in reconceiving the dynamic interplay of race, class, and culture within the Black Church. The creation of a new religious and cultural moment in the African American community and American society stands as a result.

NOTES

1. On new black middle-class congregations, see Mamiya, "Social History"; Lawrence, *Reviving the Spirit.* On the new black middle class, see Landry, *New Black Middle Class.*

2. Franklin, *Another Day's Journey,* 42, 59–62.

3. Asante, *Afrocentricity,* 74.

4. Dyson, *Reflecting Black,* 78–87; Asante, *Afrocentricity,* 74; McClain, "What Is Authentic Black Worship?"

5. Chicago Fact Book Consortium, *Local Community Fact Book 1990,* 121, 174, 177; Braden, "Chatham." The 1990 U.S. Census indicates that of Chatham's 36,779 residents, 97 percent are African Americans, with the rest made up of 363 Euro-Americans, 312 Hispanic Americans, 29 Asian Americans, and 23 Native Americans; Greater Grand Crossing population totals 38,644, of whom 99.2 percent are African Americans.

6. Braden, "Chatham," 341; Chicago Fact Book Consortium, *Local Community Fact Book 1990,* 119–121 and 175–177.

7. Lincoln, *Black Church since Frazier.*

8. Frazier, *Negro Church in America,* 89; also, e.g., Mays and Nicholson, *Negro's Church.*

9. Banner-Haley, *Fruits of Integration,* 3–26.

10. Ibid., 37.

11. For example, Carter Temple displayed and sold publications by healing evangelist Kenneth Hagen; Lawrence Mamiya on Bethel AME, Baltimore; Walter McCary's *Black Presence in the Bible;* Charles Copher's *Black Biblical Studies,* among others.

12. See Rivers, *Soulful Worship;* Hovda, ed., *This Far by Faith.*

13. The black neoconservative platform is the major challenge to the civil rights agenda. See West, *Race Matters.*

14. Condit and Lucaites, *Crafting Equality,* 167, 171, 169, 192, 170.

15. Sugrue, *Origins of the Urban Crisis,* 557.

16. Frazier, *Negro Family in Chicago* and *Negro Family in the United States;* Scott, *Contempt and Pity.*

17. Harris, *Rise of Gospel Blues,* 106–108; Ferguson, *History,* 66.

18. Frazier, *Black Bourgeoisie,* 65–71; Lincoln, *Black Church since Frazier,* 73; Daniel, "Ritual Stratification."

19. Lincoln, "Black Methodists"; Irvin, *Unsung Heart,* 32–49; Davis, *History of Black Catholics.*

20. Lincoln, *Black Church since Frazier,* 106–107.

21. The black folk church and the black middle-class church are two segments within the Black Church. The black folk church is recognized for its use of long-meter hymns and congregational songs, as well as for its jubilant preaching. Often associated with the black working class, the black folk church differs from its black middle-class counterpart more by its religious culture than by mere economic and educational factors. See Washington, *Black Sects and Cults;* Boyer, *How Sweet the Sound.*

22. Anderson and Pickering, *Confronting the Color Line,* 125, 118, 133; Travis, *Autobiography of Black Politics,* vol. 1, 319, 327–336, 338, 335; Jackson, *Story of Christian Activism;* and "Joseph H. Jackson," in Paris, *Black Religious Leaders,* 65–98.

23. Condit and Lucaites, *Crafting Equality,* 195; Chapman, *Christianity on Trial,* 38, 77, 82. Black caucuses were formed in the Presbyterian Church (U.S.A.), Presbyterian Church U.S., United Methodist Church, United Church of Christ, Disciples of Christ, Protestant Episcopal Church, American Baptist Churches in the U.S.A., American Lutheran Church, Lutheran Church–Missouri Synod, Reformed Church of America. Also see Lincoln and Mamiya, "The New Black Revolution: The Black Consciousness Movement and the Black Church," in *Black Church,* Chap. 7, 164–95.

24. Mitchell, "Black Power and the Christian Church," 105.

25. Billingsley, *Climbing Jacob's Ladder,* 51.

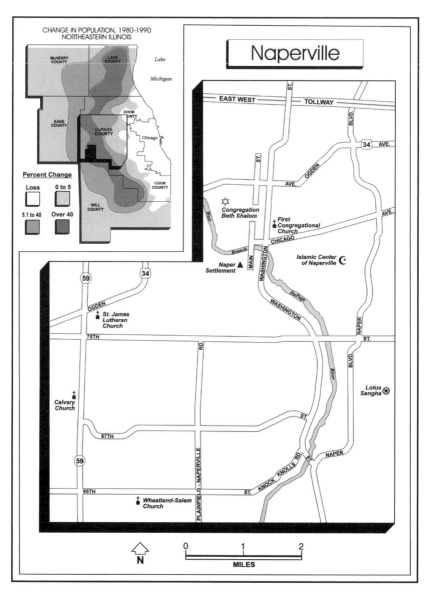

Map 8. Naperville, Illinois, is one of metropolitan Chicago's fastest-growing edge cities. Map by Brian Twardosz, BMT Printing and Cartographic Specialists.

Change, Stress, and Congregations in an Edge-City Technoburb

Paul D. Numrich

Naperville has become a popular place. During its first summer of operation in 1996, the city's Internet web page received more than twenty-two thousand hits. Three hundred people move into Naperville every month, making it the tenth-fastest-growing municipality in the country. "Naperville has a good reputation," a real estate agent remarks in one of countless local newspaper stories about Naperville's recent growth. "People just want to live here."[1]

Naperville has even established a place for itself in the literature on contemporary American society, with feature articles in the *Atlantic Monthly* and *Inland Architect* and a book-length study of women forging life on the postindustrial frontier. The portrait of Naperville drawn in these pieces, however, tends to be more ambivalent than real estate agents would wish. Nicholas Lemann titled his 1989 *Atlantic* article "Stressed Out in Suburbia," while Sally Helgesen's recent book *Everyday Revolutionaries,* acknowledging its analytical debt to Lemann, describes the overextended lives of Naperville's women, who nevertheless remain optimistic and energized about the opportunities afforded by life here. Michael Ebner's article in *Inland Architect* points out the structural stress on Naperville during its transformation from small town to "technoburb" over the past forty-five years.[2]

This chapter also examines life in contemporary Naperville, but unlike previous studies, it grants institutional religion a central position.[3] Naperville's congregations have participated in the change and stress of the city's recent transformation and, like some edge-city observers, often harbor ambivalent feelings about life in such a popular place.

Their spiritual perspectives on edge-city life certainly help members to alleviate the strains; but do they strike to the underlying causes?

Naperville, Yesterday and Today

The city's namesake, Great Lakes steamship captain Joseph Naper, founded Naperville in 1831.[4] Befriended by local Potawatomis—and protected by Fort Payne on the highest point in the area—Naper's settlement survived the Black Hawk Indian War the following year. Naperville received rail service when the Chicago Burlington and Quincy (today's Burlington Northern) came through in 1864, establishing an economic lifeline for the town. A public library was dedicated in 1898, and in 1913 the Naperville Lounge Company changed its name to Kroehler Manufacturing Company, which would later become the nation's largest furniture manufacturer.

It took three decades for Naperville's turn-of-the-century population of twenty-six hundred to double. The city's centennial fell early in the Great Depression, during which a county guidebook described Naperville as reminiscent of a New England village.[5] But area development accelerated immediately after World War II. Historian Michael Ebner identifies Argonne National Laboratory, built in 1947, as the "high-technology seed" from which sprouted Naperville's present status as the hub of Chicago's technoburb (Robert Fishman's term). "Technoburb" and Joel Garreau's notion of "edge city" insightfully describe places like Naperville—self-contained socioeconomic territories on the urban periphery, dense with high-technology industries, corporate headquarters, retail space, and residents. As Garreau notes, such a place "has it all" today, yet it is nothing like it was only a few years earlier.[6]

According to Ebner, Argonne's arrival in 1947 corresponded with Naperville's new commitment to providing quality public education comparable to prestige school systems around the country. Commuter ridership on the Burlington line increased in the 1950s; parking near the downtown depot became a problem; and the East-West Tollway brought interstate access to Chicago in 1958. From this point it took only about one decade for Naperville's population to double.

Packer Engineering (1962) and Northern Illinois Gas (1963, now Nicor Gas) initiated an influx of technology-based companies. In 1966, AT&T opened a major research facility, Bell Labs (now Lucent Technologies), that would supplant Kroehler Manufacturing as the area's largest employer, employing in the 1990s more than ten thousand people on six campuses in Naperville and adjoining Lisle. Fermi National Accelerator Laboratory, Amoco Research Center, and Nalco Research followed. By the mid-1980s, when Governor James Thompson designated a stretch along the East-West Tollway as the Illinois Research and Development Corridor, Naperville had become what Ebner describes as "the geographic center of Chicago's version of California's Silicon Valley."[7]

Naperville's municipal territory expanded from twelve square miles in 1970 to fifty square miles by the early 1990s, while its population exploded during the same period from just under twenty-three thousand to more than one hundred thousand. Projections call for 135,000 Napervillians by the year 2005 and 160,000 by 2020, an anticipated percentage increase more than three times that of the metropolitan region as a whole. The city's senior planner predicted that up to 75 percent of all future population growth would occur in South Naperville's so-called Sector G.

Indian Prairie School District 204, bridging Aurora and Naperville (including Sector G), is the fastest-growing school district in Illinois and trails only Chicago's public school system in student diversity in the state. Its English as a Second Language program accommodates students from nearly one hundred countries. Enrollment is not expected to peak until the year 2008. With a price tag in excess of $60 million, Neuqua Valley High School, named after one of the friendly Potawatomis who ensured Naperville's early survival, opened in 1997 as the most expensive public school in Illinois history, funded by the state's largest referendum.

Naperville remains a predominantly White community, although Blacks (2 percent) and Asians (over 5 percent) comprise a significant new presence. Naperville's Blacks rank sixth in per-capita income among Blacks in all local communities, while only two suburbs have more Asian residents than Naperville. Asians make up more than 10 percent of Lucent Technologies' work force.

Median family income for Naperville in 1995 was nearly $67,000, $12,000 higher than the DuPage County median, which itself ranks twenty-fourth among all U.S. counties. Less than 2 percent of Naperville residents lived below the poverty line, and the average home value stood at $191,000. A marketing analysis conducted by Virginia-based Claritas Inc. categorized Naperville as an "elite suburb" with predominant "lifestyle clusters" of kids and cul-de-sacs on the one hand and executive suites on the other. Respectively, according to Claritas, people with such lifestyles "buy trivia games, own a piano, read parenting magazines" and "play racquetball, own a video camera, listen to jazz radio."[8] The traditional American nuclear family of two parents with children still characterizes DuPage County demographics more than the national profile. Contrary to a thirty-year trend of decreasing mobility among the American public overall, during the period 1985–1990 over one-fourth of Naperville's new residents relocated from outside of the Chicago metropolitan region.

By most measures, Naperville offers its residents a high—and highly touted—quality of life. Commenting on plans to revive a Black community on Chicago's South Side, Chicago's mayor Richard M. Daley promised that children will feel "like they are in Naperville." Indeed, Zero Population Growth, a Washington, D.C., organization that examines the relation between population growth and quality of life, named Naperville the nation's most child-friendly city. Dining, entertainment, and the arts, once the exclusive purview of downtown Chicago, now lie close at hand for Napervillians.

Thus the Naperville area epitomizes Joel Garreau's edge city, a recent growth area on the urban periphery that offers all the essentials of modern life—job, home, market, education, culture.[9] Naperville strikes many observers as a postindustrial metropolitan success story, having made the transition from quaint small town to thriving technoburb. The old Kroehler factory near the heart of town speaks volumes in this regard: once it cranked out couches for Sears; today it houses upscale restaurants, shops, and condominiums.

But the other side of Naperville's success is visible as well. Vocational anxieties, social problems, congestion from rapid development—to some these signify growing pains soon to be overcome, to others red flags that qualify claims about the satisfaction offered by such edge-city technoburbs.

As Lemann wrote in 1989, "In Naperville the word 'stress' came up constantly in conversations. . . . They complain that between working long hours, traveling on business, and trying to stay in shape they have no free time."[10] A decade later Sally Helgesen filed the same report, noting that life for Naperville's women had become characterized by "the disappearance of time."[11] Lurking behind all of this stands the specter of corporate downsizing, threatening to end Naperville's technoburban heyday. When AT&T announced a nationwide layoff of forty thousand employees in the mid-1990s, the *Chicago Tribune* commented that some workers in

Naperville saw it as "yet another thunderclap in a place often shaken by such storms." Moreover, some of Naperville's high-tech luster certainly dimmed with the recent discovery of twenty cases of brain tumors among former and current Amoco Research Center employees.

In the four-year period 1993–1996, when Naperville's population grew by 12 percent, reported incidents of domestic abuse in Naperville increased over three times that rate. Likewise, although a comprehensive health assessment found the county to be "very healthy," with "good medical and support services," nevertheless negative behavioral choices (e.g., alcohol consumption and cigarette smoking) and pockets of poverty among the overall affluence of the county remained areas of concerns. A 1996 survey of Naperville teens revealed dramatic increases in substance abuse, with marijuana usage significantly higher than the national average. One estimate suggested as many as 150 homeless people in Naperville. With high monthly rental rates and a housing market geared to white-collar residents, one report concluded, affordable housing and home ownership are problematic for a significant portion of Naperville's population.

Contention over Naperville's rapid change and new diversity surfaces periodically, for example, in home-owner resistance to an apartment complex that could tarnish the city's image, in protests of School District 203's minority hiring practices, and in Asian Indian voters' claims of discrimination over a nominating petition for a city council candidate. DuPage County's board chairperson identified growing diversity as the county's "biggest problem."

As in edge cities across the country, the phenomenal development that created today's Naperville carries inherent threats to the overall quality of life of its residents. One county study identified traffic congestion and an imbalanced jobs/housing ratio as key concerns, characterizing Naperville's jobs/housing ratio as "extremely out of balance." Each day nearly 180,000 DuPage residents leave the county for work, while even more— another 220,000—enter the county to work. Add to this the more than 245,000 DuPage residents who commute to work within the county, and the burden on the area's transportation infrastructure becomes obvious, as does the stress on commuting workers.

As a solution, the county planning commission suggested slowing the growth of jobs in the area. The ambivalence of other area planners, however, surfaced in Naperville's decision to allow construction of a four hundred–unit "upscale" apartment complex that would provide affordable housing for interim corporate workers along the Research and Development Corridor. The Naperville City Council approved the complex over the objections of its own planning commission, which saw the parcel of land as a prime location for even more office, research, and industrial development.

Religion in Naperville

Noted church consultant Lyle Schaller, a local resident, identifies some trends about religion in Naperville. At the end of World War I, Naperville had only nine churches, all northern European Christian in heritage. Today Naperville has about sixty congregations, many still northern European Christian but many more of the homegrown American variety, such as Mormons, Jehovah's Witnesses, and Pentecostal groups. Today's congregations place less emphasis on denominational identity and hierarchical polity than the churches of previous generations, and laypeople play a much greater role now, exercising their prerogative of joining the congregation of their choice. Today, Naperville's congregations tend to be bigger and much more competitive than their predecessors in attracting members—like the stores in nearby shopping centers.[12]

Korean and Chinese Christians, along with Jews, Muslims, Baha'is, and Buddhists, have increased Naperville's religious diversity in recent years. New religious facilities sprout up as fast as new subdivisions, and solicitation of new members through mass marketing techniques is commonplace. Pollsters have reported either steady or declining worship attendance nationwide in recent years, but that is the exception rather than the rule among Naperville congregations of all religious identities.

The following congregational profiles illuminate key dynamics of edge-city life in Naperville. How have these congregations participated in the change and stress that characterize life in such places today?

First Congregational Church

On the highest point in town, not far from the site of old Fort Payne, sits Piety Hill, local lingo for the cluster of Naperville's oldest churches. One bears the name First Congregational Church (United Church of Christ), tracing its origins to a weekend gathering of mostly New England Puritans in July 1833. In the early years worship services rotated, with worshipers meeting in a variety of venues—homes, barns, schools, the

Fig. 8-1. First Congregational Church on "Piety Hill" is one of the oldest churches in Naperville, Illinois. Photo by Paul D. Numrich.

courthouse, a Baptist church. Disagreement over a permanent location led to the congregation's first split. A faction withdrew to build their own church south of town, whereas in 1846 First Congregational erected a wooden-frame structure on donated land at its current Piety Hill location, the donor stipulating that the church must always have a cupola and bell. A limestone structure replaced the original church in 1906.

First Congressional's membership declined in the 1960s, but by the early 1970s it began a sustained upturn that would last two decades—precisely the period of Naperville's coming-of-age as an edge-city technoburb. The church's latest schism is directly related to this growth and change.

In 1993 the congregation's Long Range Planning Board (LRPB) concluded that maintaining the church's status quo at the Piety Hill location should not be a long-term option. The next year the LRPB broached the idea of a split-site operation, and in January 1995 it brought a formal recommendation asking that the congregation "aggressively and prayerfully pursue a step-by-step plan to relocate the entire membership to a new facility and establish the [downtown] facility as a Church-led Community Center." The LRPB targeted the high-growth area of South Naperville as the site for the new facility, and the denomination appeared ready to lend financial support to the venture. By a simple majority vote, the congregation approved further study of the LRPB's recommendation.

But ensuing congregational debate about the future of the church proved emotional and, ultimately, schismatic. Other options were discussed, including razing the historic facility and erecting a new one on the site, a notion many could not abide. Rejecting the recommendation of a split-site operation, a previous chair of the LRPB wrote in an open letter to the congregation, "We must support the preservation of our heritage through the delivery of our entire ministry in the downtown location." "We must value organic growth over numerical growth," the letter continued, countering a key rationale for relocation to South Naperville—attraction of young families in the residential boom areas. "Bigger is not necessarily better," wrote one church member, while still another argued that "the church should remain at its present site . . . [since] God doesn't need another big church in a cornfield; He has enough of them already." This last member even raised possible legal ramifications of relocation, given the implicit wish of the nineteenth-century donor of the downtown property that there always be a church, with cupola and bell, on that site. Members who cherished First Congregational's social mission orientation feared that aspect of the church's liberal heritage would be lost through relocation away from downtown Naperville.

After months of debate, it became clear that the faction favoring relocation could not garner the required two-thirds majority congregational vote for the necessary allocation of funds. Forty families subsequently left First Congregational to found Hope Church, which in September 1998 dedicated its new multi-acre site in South Naperville's booming Sector G. Both churches thrive today, having succeeded in attracting different segments of the edge-city baby-boomer population. First Congregational focuses on rechurching the disaffected, many of whom, according to the current pastor, appreciate the historic sanctuary on Piety Hill. It feels like "home," they say, reminding them of the churches of their childhood.

Wheatland Salem Church

"That's it over there," the construction supervisor told me in the summer of 1996, pointing to a slight knoll amid the stakes outlining phase two of Mission Oaks subdivision in Sector G. The knoll betrayed no indication that it had once been a church cemetery, nor even that it had once been surrounded by farmland. The supervisor mentioned that during phase one of development a few Mission Oaks home owners had asked permission to take some of the headstones, presumably for use as yard ornaments. With advice from the local genealogical society, church leaders eventually decided to cover over the graves and remaining markers and to erect a single monument honoring the pioneers of their congregation.

Like its old cemetery, Wheatland Salem Church (United Methodist) nearly passed into oblivion around 1980. The church's remarkable rescue from the brink of institutional demise can be traced to the fortuitous appointment of the right pastor at exactly the right time of residential growth in South Naperville.

Wheatland Salem's roots lay in two congregations of Pennsylvania German farmers affiliated with the Evangelical Association in North America. Copenhagen Church (also known as Salem Church), established in 1852 at the crossroads of Copenhagen Road and today's Illinois Route 59, and Emmanuel Church, established in 1860 several miles to the southwest in Wheatland Township, merged in 1907 to build a new church halfway between the two, at Ninety-fifth Street and Route 59. One old-timer reminisces about going to the church as a child by horse and buggy down Route 59, then a gravel road.

The congregation declined after World War II, and by 1979 membership had dropped to eighty-seven. In 1980 the United Methodist bishop appointed the Reverend Scott Field to preside over Wheatland Salem's imminent closure.

Pastor Scott, as he is often called, did not listen to the bishop. And no one—certainly not the farmers who founded the church—could have predicted what was about to happen in Naperville's Sector G, where the church was located. In 1987, when the area was still considered Naperville's "boondocks," the prestigious White Eagle subdivision opened just to the north, with its signature Arnold Palmer golf course. Less than a decade later, more than thirteen thousand residents lived in the sector. Route 59, the one-time gravel road, expanded to six lanes of fast-moving traffic.

Wheatland Salem's resuscitation paralleled the growth around it. In 1986 the church expanded its facility by three times the original size. The next year the administrative council committed the congregation to a development strategy that shifted the laity into ministry roles and the pastor into the role of manager of ministry. By 1989 the church broke the two hundred mark in worship attendance, and in the 1990s church programming began bursting the seams of the expanded facility. During a

personal prayer retreat in 1993, Pastor Scott concluded that further improvement of the current site was much too timid a plan for the future.
Besides, he says today, the old farm church would have been a "retrograde
fit" in the new development slated around it. When Pastor Scott challenged the congregation to think big and relocate, he was pleasantly surprised at the overwhelmingly positive response.

In the fall of 1997 those big thoughts culminated in the opening of a
$6 million "church for the twenty-first century," located on fourteen
acres of former farmland east of the old site, in the middle of what Pastor Scott, playing on downtown's Piety Hill, calls Naperville's new Piety
Row. The church battled two municipalities and a major land developer
over annexation and utilities problems at the new location, and congregational leaders make no bones about using the large mortgage as a
"poison pill" tactic against the loss of Pastor Scott through appointment
elsewhere.

The new Wheatland Salem Church fits comfortably into its edge-city
milieu. Pastor Scott is savvy to the ways of his members' information-age
world and adept at strategizing for a twenty-first-century church. "We are
using this time of societal and technological change to build a place to
serve Christ's Gospel now and in the future," states a professional-quality
prospectus on the new church facility. The only "retrograde" features are
the stained-glass windows brought over from the old church and the new
address, 1852 Ninety-fifth Street, commemorating the year the church
was founded.

Pastor Scott is also adept at applying evangelical theology to a congregation often clinging to the edge of their technoburban lives. During the
children's sermon one Sunday, he held up a McDonald's cup that bore the
likeness of flamboyant Chicago Bulls basketball player Dennis Rodman,
noting that some members of the congregation had contributed to the
cup's marketing. (Rodman's hair changed color with the temperature of
the beverage in the cup.)

"Do you ever worry?" Pastor Scott asked the children.

"Yes," a few answered, sheepishly.

"Do your parents ever worry?" "Yes!" the children all shouted, un-
coaxed. Pastor Scott then broached his evangelical topic for the day: "Give
all your worries over to Jesus." The sermon for the adults bore the title,
"When Maalox Moments Become a Way of Life," and Pastor Scott declared the communion table a "worry-free zone," where the dreaded concept of "Monday" could be left at Jesus' feet.

Pastor Scott holds no naive sentiments about some universal edge-city thirst for intimate relationships that can be quenched by church programming. As he writes:

> Our discovery has been that while friendliness is important to everyone, many newer members are not particularly concerned about "the closeness of the church" in the first place. The primary organizing principle which holds them to this congregation is not the constellation of close relationships built up over years spent together but an attraction to particular programs for themselves or their children, engaging worship experiences, and/or the opportunity to participate in meaningful Christian volunteer opportunities. These members certainly expect to be treated warmly and cordially in their relationships with other church folks, but they also seem to value a degree of distance and privacy.[13]

Such are the needs of many edge-city congregations.

Calvary Church

The person from First Congregational who spoke of big churches in cornfields certainly had this one in mind. Calvary Church (Assemblies of God)[14] is big by any standard, with a massive facility that dominates 116 acres of former farmland and accommodates nearly three thousand worshipers each Sunday.

The church's history parallels Naperville's edge-city growth. Sandwiched between the openings of Bell Labs and Amoco Research, Calvary began its corporate life in 1967 by purchasing a wooden-frame church near the center of town (which now houses Calvary's ministry to the poor); then, in the late 1970s, it erected an eighty thousand–square-foot facility in an early boom area of South Naperville (which now houses Calvary Christian School). The church's current $20 million complex is a stone's throw from the prestigious White Eagle subdivision in Naperville's Sector G.

Calvary Church qualifies as a "megachurch" in its large attendance figures; its full-service programming for a consumer-oriented clientele, including numerous fellowship groups that mete out the big-church experience in manageably small doses; its architectural overtones, reminiscent of a shopping mall or convention hotel. Yet Calvary's unapologetic Pentecostalism cuts against the grain of the most influential megachurch model: Willow Creek Community Church, with its "seeker-targeted" or

Fig. 8-2. Calvary Church and campus in Naperville, Illinois. Calvary is a growing Pentecostal "megachurch," which participates in Naperville's rapid expansion. Photo courtesy of Calvary Church.

"seeker-oriented" sensitivity to today's unchurched, skeptical, disaffected, yet spiritually searching baby boomers. Calvary retains many "cringe factors" that might drive seekers away. A free-standing, forty-foot-high cross outside the main entrance stakes Calvary's Pentecostal claim in full view of busy Route 59. Sunday services feature long sermons replete with extensive biblical expositions. Members prefer songs with unambiguous Christian lyrics, ranging in genre from traditional hymns such as "Blessed Assurance" and "Trust and Obey" to catchy contemporary Christian music. Offering plates are passed with unflinching admonitions to Christian commitment. People speak in tongues occasionally, and many raise their hands in typical Pentecostal fashion during the prayers. Services climax with an old-fashioned altar call for the unsaved to come forward and give their lives to the Lord.

When I asked the assistant pastor if all this might frighten off unsuspecting visitors, he admitted that Calvary's Pentecostalism is "seeker hostile," and that the message of the cross runs counter to the secular humanism and self-centered values of the typical baby boomer. But he also pointed out that even non-Pentecostal Christians have initial misgivings about attending a Pentecostal service. The key is whether a person's pain is great enough to risk anything to find healing, even walking into a Pentecostal church.

Naperville is a "scary" place for many people, the founder of Calvary's counseling ministry told me—an assessment at odds with the usual portrayal of the town. Calvary's youth ministry, which draws hundreds to midweek services that feature rock music with Pentecostal lyrics, exhorts teenagers to take a stand for righteous behavior in their schools, to reject drug-and-sex lifestyles fueled by the ethics of tolerance that dominates modern society, and to encourage nominal Christians in their schools to join them in righteous living. Calvary also offers a ministry to single adults, some of whom are parents struggling to raise the youth just mentioned. Many singles throw themselves into their work, the singles pastor told me, seeking life's entire meaning there. Others add friends and regular workouts at the health club to their work, but this still leaves a spiritual void that Calvary seeks to fill.

I attended one of the church's fellowship group meetings. Seven couples ranging in age from their twenties to their fifties gathered on a Friday night at a home in one of South Naperville's new subdivisions. The group sat in a large circle in the living room, first sharing a time of "praise reports and prayer requests," the latter being the more numerous. One couple had just learned they were expecting a baby, a cause for praise. But another woman shared her dismay at how greatly her extended family was enmeshed in sexual sin without even realizing it (specific details were supplied). Two men spoke of work-related stresses. In one case, high level managers were being terminated without explanation. The man prayed for peace of mind for the most recent casualty. Several people asked prayers for good health and impending surgeries. After this impromptu individual sharing, the group entered into a time of more formal prayer, punctuated by frequent exclamations of "Yes, Lord," "Thank you, Jesus," "Praise God," and the like. The group then sang several contemporary Christian songs and shared more individual prayer requests.

A Bible study would have ensued had there not been a Chicago Bulls playoff game that evening. The group ate popcorn and pizza and analyzed the game like any number of Naperville fans gathered that evening. The difference had been in this group's Pentecostal pregame warm-ups.

Saint James Lutheran Church

Saint James serves as a counterpoint to the visible and exponentially growing congregations of Naperville, such as Calvary and Wheatland

Salem. The church struggles with problems of location and membership loss, in addition to addressing the stresses of edge-city life.

Saint James (Evangelical Lutheran Church in America) began in 1979 as a denominational mission enterprise in the home of its founding pastor. The congregation met in a public elementary school at the intersection of Routes 59 and 34 (Ogden Avenue) before moving to its present site, about one block east, in September 1989. At that time the church and an adjacent landscaper had the only structures in the area, but eventually they were joined on the west and north by commercial developments piggybacking on nearby Fox Valley Center mall. Moreover, Routes 59 and 34 have become major traffic arteries, and a residential subdivision will likely be developed soon on open land immediately to the south.

This site has become a source of concern for the congregation. Although the location would appear choice for attracting new members, the church building itself, a small, A-shaped sanctuary with an attached multipurpose wing, is engulfed by surrounding development to the point of near obscurity. Particularly galling for some is the view approaching from the west on Route 34, which is dominated by a flooring store that the current pastor, the Reverend Roger Timm, calls "a two-story monstrosity."

The congregation has mounted efforts to overcome this visibility problem, for instance, through flyer distributions in nearby subdivisions. An Advent caroling party in 1995 doubled as a time to decorate the front of the church in order to catch the eyes of passersby. Newly dedicated stained-glass windows led the pastor to reflect in 1996, "It really has added to [our] morale. We have always feared that our church looks like part of a strip mall, but these windows are a sign that we are a church."

Much of the recent low congregational morale derives from the forced resignation of the founding pastor in February 1992, which caused a great upheaval in the church and a precipitous decline in membership. Early in his tenure at Saint James, the present pastor held cottage discussions and other activities in order to determine the mood of the congregation. The church's current motto—"A welcoming place for sharing the love of God"—developed out of those discussions, and the pastor feels that the congregation has now appropriated this view of itself. By 1996, membership loss appeared to have bottomed out.

Most of the congregation are middle-class professionals who suffer from vocational stress, overextension, and anxiety about corporate downsizing. Saint James has responded by trying to create a comfortable,

Fig. 8-3. Saint James Lutheran Church, eclipsed by commercial developments in Naperville, Illinois, attempts to be a respite from the stress of edge-city life. Photo by Paul D. Numrich.

face-to-face community where harried, unappreciated, and anxious people can take heart that God loves them and calls them to a life of love in an often unloving society. People know each other here and share a friendly Christian fellowship together. The pastor's sermons emphasize God's loving care and its transformative power in people's daily lives. Posing the question in one sermon "Would it make any difference if Saint James didn't exist?" the pastor answered that the result would be one less place "to gather to worship and to listen to the message of God's love for us and God's will for our lives, . . . one less place in our fast-paced, impersonal world where we can experience personal caring."

The pastor's approach to job loss and transition within the congregation illustrates this emphasis. He addresses such issues about once a month in his sermons. He feels the church's role is to maintain people's sense of self-esteem by showing them that they are loved throughout their ordeals. People can get help with their résumés elsewhere—the church is where they feel worthwhile in spite of a situation where they are made to feel otherwise. Christian commiseration is key. What does one do, the pastor asked in a sermon, if one's position requires letting other people go at their place of employment? The answer:

No easy answer. Quitting in protest wouldn't do much good except to add one more person to the unemployment rolls. Can you lay someone off lovingly? Words of sympathy and appreciation may seem hollow, and your authority to act may be limited. But concern for justice, fairness, and compassion can shape how you act and what support is offered to the people affected.

One lay leader spoke about the role Saint James plays in many members' lives. This person sees the local church as providing an alternative to the corporate and residential contexts in which people work and live. The church allows people to express their faith and to enrich their lives in ways not found on the job or in the neighborhood. One simply does not discuss certain things with one's neighbors, who typically are more passing acquaintances than close friends. Also, since many members have no extended family in the area, the one continuity in their transient lives becomes church membership. In this lay leader's own case, the family had lived in five different states, but in each new area they found a church to join.

Congregations Reflecting Naperville's New Diversity

The *Naperville Sun*'s sesquicentennial edition in 1981 captured some of the town's growing religious diversity, featuring Unitarian (established 1955), Jehovah's Witness (1956), and Mormon (1966) congregations in addition to many of the earlier and mainline churches. Much more diversity would come to town in the 1980s and 1990s. For instance, DuPage Korean United Methodist Church, the largest of eight Korean Christian congregations in the area, has shared space in one of Naperville's original Piety Hill churches since 1986. The congregation's membership of nearly one hundred is predominantly professional and well educated, including several engineers from Argonne National Laboratory. In 1996 a Chinese Lutheran congregation bought Naperville's historic Nichols Library. As one member put it, "I really do feel this is the place God wanted us to be in."

Three relatively new congregations—Jewish, Muslim, and Buddhist—have particularly poignant tales to tell about their place in edge-city Naperville.

Congregation Beth Shalom, affiliated with the Jewish Reconstructionist Federation and one of two DuPage County synagogues, began in 1972 through the efforts of local Jewish residents, virtually all of whom have since moved away. In 1985, Beth Shalom purchased a former Evangelical Free Church facility north of downtown Naperville, which it eventually outgrew. The congregation constructed a new building in 1998, DuPage County's first synagogue to be built from the ground up, on a donated site not far from Naperville's Piety Hill.

Rabbi Michael Remson characterizes his congregation as mostly young, relatively economically secure, corporate employees. Several work at Amoco, Argonne, and Lucent. Were it not for the mobility of the membership, the rabbi says, Congregation Beth Shalom would not exist. The membership is a conglomeration of religious backgrounds—Reform and Conservative Jews, even many Christians through marriage—for whom the synagogue's Reconstructionist affiliation may be the most workable institutional compromise. Beth Shalom does not represent the "home synagogue" for most members, a fact evident when many return to their childhood synagogues to celebrate Jewish holy days.

One constant for most members is their choice to live in Naperville. "We west-suburban Jews are a self-selected community," the rabbi pointed out at a forum held in Chicago's heavily Jewish North Side. "We like it in Naperville," he explained. Jews remain a small minority, and they must endure occasional ignorance about Judaism as well as the "seasonal pain" of Christmastime, but Jewish life in Naperville is unpretentious and less intense than in other settings, and other minority religious groups are around to deflect attention. As one member of Beth Shalom explained, the town is rather homogeneous on most levels: "Jew or not Jew, look who's living in Naperville. We're not all that different from the rest of the folks who live in Naperville."

Still, to be a Jewish community in Naperville has a unique social geography. I noticed the unconscious language used by virtually every person interviewed at Congregation Beth Shalom: they talked about being Jews "out here" in the western exurbs, implying a qualitative difference from Jewish life "in there," that is, in the thickly settled Jewish northern suburbs and the North Side of Chicago. After moving to Naperville from Wilmette in the early 1980s, Beth Shalom's lay president would quip to friends and family that he had joined the Diaspora.

Since Congregation Beth Shalom is "the only show in town," to quote one member, it devolves upon the synagogue to bring Judaism to bear on Naperville's edge-city lifestyle. Some in the congregation fear that the influence runs too much in the opposite direction. A synagogue board member with nearly thirty years of teaching experience at an area public school lamented the priorities of many members' lives, in this order: house, car, vacations, work, and Judaism. When I asked about potential conflicts between school athletic events and Sabbath services on Friday nights, he replied that there is no conflict, since the kids are at the game.

"Throughout this year, I have had quite a hectic schedule," wrote one tenth grader in her culminating essay for confirmation class. "High pressure and academic demands have been my life!" We might speculate about what her adult life will be like, given her hectic life already as a sixteen-year-old, yet she contends: "I know how [difficult] it is to hold a busy schedule and [still] attend Sunday School, but it is possible."

For several years Beth Shalom has run a Havurah (fellowship) program of adult small groups. According to the program's founder, these groups fill a void in many members' lives. Naperville is more like California than the Jewish North Side of Chicago, he explained. Life here is so spread out, and there is no strong sense of "community," but it can be created within congregations like Beth Shalom. Another member gave unexpected confirmation of this opinion during an interview. A committed Jewish feminist who remembers Beth Shalom's beginnings, she bemoaned the small number of like-minded feminist members today. Yet, when asked why she stays, she pointed to the symbolic significance of the synagogue and also to a certain "richness" in the relationships she has developed here.

Workplace anxiety—and not a little anger—struck several of Beth Shalom's members when both Amoco and AT&T downsized. The congregation's adult members also suffer the added anxiety of being the "sandwich generation," that is, concerned about the quality of life of both aging parents and maturing children. In his 1995 newsletter message to the congregation during Sukkoth, the Jewish festival in which temporary shelters (*sukkah*s) were traditionally constructed, the rabbi advised: "The sukkah reminds us that life is not secure; that worrying is part of the human condition. . . . So, at least we aren't crazy for being afraid. Come; eat in the sukkah. If life is insecure at least it can be fun."

On the other side of town from Congregation Beth Shalom, the Islamic Center of Naperville occupies the former Jehovah's Witnesses Kingdom Hall. Like other American mosques, the Islamic Center of Naperville features a communal prayer room oriented toward the holy city of Mecca. Because of the Chicago area's historical pattern of building on a north-south-east-west grid, such an orientation means that the focal point (*mihrab*) of the prayer room is the northeast corner, the direction to Mecca following the curvature of the globe. Thus, symbolically, American Muslims in prayer place themselves slightly askew of the dominant culture. To be a Muslim congregation in a place like Naperville thus carries a unique sense of spiritual distinction.[15]

The Islamic Center of Naperville emerged from discussions among mostly Indo-Pakistani professionals in the late 1970s. Around 1980, leaders from several western suburbs formed an organization for the purpose of building a mosque, but a proposed site in Woodridge never materialized. Instead the community established a short-lived Islamic school while continuing to raise funds for a mosque. When Muslims in nearby Villa Park opened their mosque and school in 1983, Naperville Muslims joined that venture.

The distance to the Villa Park mosque proved inconvenient to many, however. A small group began meeting in Naperville homes for evening prayer, and employees of Bell Labs reserved a conference room for Friday's midday communal prayer, signing in non-employees as visitors. The present mosque facility was purchased in 1992 and offers all five daily prayers, as well as an Islamic school in the afternoons. The congregation now comprises Arabs and other ethnic groups in addition to the Indo-Pakistani majority.

Perhaps, a founding member told me, the Islamic Center of Naperville would not have experienced problems with its neighbors had the congregation not sought to renovate their facility. But the subsequent contention between the center and its non-Muslim neighborhood has brought the marginal status of immigrant Muslims into focus. "Every Friday in a quiet Naperville neighborhood," opens one of many newspaper accounts, "a weekly clash of communities begins just before 1 p.m." The issue has to do with traffic congestion at prayer time, which the neighbors fear will be exacerbated by the proposed renovations. Still, when a neighbor purportedly exclaimed to members, "Why don't you go back where you came from?" the intent likely was not to send them back to their own suburban neighborhoods.

The notion of "neighborliness" has been invoked many times. The center's president, an Arab engineer, has consistently maintained that his members try to be "good neighbors" to the area. Parking attendants protect access to residential driveways and curbside mailboxes, for instance, banning mosque attenders who disobey their rules of parking etiquette three times. Still, the center may not be long in this neighborhood, since it hopes eventually to build a new facility in another location.

Come what may, we can expect the mosque's president to be consistent with his *khutbah* (sermon) theme during a recent Eid Ul-Adha holy day service. There is no better prayer than to pray to be a good Muslim, he said—better than to pray for a new house, a new car, or even children. Being better Muslims will make us better people, he stressed, and the community around us will be a better community.

Lotus Sangha (established 1995) gathers regularly in a private residence in one of Naperville's newer subdivisions.[16] Followers of well-known Vietnamese monk Venerable Thich Nhat Hanh, the immigrant Vietnamese members of Lotus Sangha are simply too busy to establish a full-fledged Buddhist temple, according to the group's coordinator. Lotus Sangha arranges periodic visits by out-of-town Buddhist monastics who apply Hanh's Zen Buddhist insights to members' lives and concerns during extended meditation/teaching sessions. People attend from throughout the metropolitan area, attracted by Lotus Sangha's particular combination of ethnic identity and Buddhist practice.

I observed three sessions that typify Lotus Sangha's approach. The first, a day-long mindfulness retreat, featured different forms of meditation in the morning and afternoon. In the evening, sixteen adults attended a two-hour *dharma* (teaching) talk by a Buddhist monk from San Diego, though the style was much more dialogical than a traditional Buddhist *dharma* talk. The session began with everyone introducing themselves and identifying where they live. After a brief ritual honoring the Buddha, the group heard the monk's message about clearing their minds and meditatively cultivating a peacefulness that is "empty" of either excessive happiness or depression. The key here, the monk explained, is to do everything with complete concentration.

A man who identified himself as an architect pressed the monk on how to accomplish this. It is easy to talk about concentration, he proposed, but difficult to put into practice. The man found it particularly difficult in his occupation, where he faces tense situations and even anger, where fellow workers argue with him and challenge his work. He feels he must not back down, otherwise he will be labeled a "loser," anathema in today's work world. The monk suggested ways to discuss issues without becoming angry, since anger will consume a person and create negative results in family and other relationships. Others in the room eagerly joined the discussion, though not in English. A time of singing followed. One woman offered a solo in French; another woman sang several emotional solos "about our homeland and how we miss it," as she announced in English. The title of the final group song translated as "Get Together" or "Come Closer," an expression of Lotus Sangha's cohesiveness around the compassion and mutual understanding they find in the Buddha's *dharma.*

At the second session, the same monk from San Diego gave an hourlong *dharma* talk to the children. True understanding and true happiness come from being a Buddha, he said. The lotus flower grows in ponds in Vietnam, the country of your parents, and it is like your mind: the true mind or Buddha mind rises above the mud of the ordinary world and is pure. Practice mindfulness meditation in everyday life—if you are mindful, you will discover something beautiful already within your body and mind. We should get in touch with the energy of a clear mind in order to become intelligent, happy, and loving people. Be good children so your parents will be happy, and you will be happy too. The essence of Buddhism is to live with true understanding, to live mindfully, to help others, to refrain from doing bad things or making people angry.

The third session marked Ullambana or Vulan, the Vietnamese Mother's Day. Two Vietnamese nuns from Michigan led the dialogue about how to maintain a peaceful mind in everyday life. The question arose as to how to have a peaceful family, especially if you are the only one in your family who meditates. One fiftyish man, an accounting manager, described his daily practice in detail. His stressful week involves long commutes and very demanding work. He listens to peaceful music (from Thich Nhat Hanh), pauses for focused breathing exercises before getting out of the car to go into work, meditates during his breaks, and stops at a park on the way home for fifteen to thirty minutes of practice. He and his wife both practice, and because of this they have no marital problems, he testified.

The nuns gave advice throughout the evening. It is not easy to practice daily, but we should use our time wisely. Don't eat or fight in the car, rather use that time to practice. When you feel a physical pressure in your chest, it indicates some kind of worry in your life. But the mind controls everything in this world—a good mind makes everything around you good, but a "devil mind" (my translator's term) makes everything around you bad.

Conclusion: Ambivalence over Edge-City Life

Like other corporate entities, congregations participate in the social and structural dynamics that create edge-city technoburbs like Naperville. Some congregations contribute directly to the physical reconfiguration of such places, riding the crests of residential growth patterns and building new religious facilities consistent with the new landscape. Wheatland Salem Church (which owes its continued existence to the building boom in Sector G), Calvary Church (whose history parallels Naperville's coming-of-age as an edge city), and Congregation Beth Shalom (with a membership turnover of virtually 100 percent since its establishment) stand out in this regard. All three recently opened new facilities architecturally appropriate to their edge-city niches—even Calvary's "big church in a cornfield" would not strike typical edge-city commuters as out of place as they whiz past it on Route 59. Other edge-city congregations try to buck the reconfiguration trends swirling around them, but they evolve vis-à-vis those trends nonetheless. First Congregational Church (which split over the issue of relocation from its historic downtown site) and Saint James Lutheran Church (which has suffered from poor visibility and a downward trend in membership) provide cases of relative ill ease or ill fit with edge-city transformations.

Edge-city congregations also contribute to the increasing social and cultural diversity of these "places apart" within the restructuring metropolis of contemporary America. Most residents of outer-ring or exurban enclaves may still be Christian, but some of their Christian neighbors now hail originally from Asia instead of Europe. And other neighbors now profess non-Christian faiths such as Islam and Buddhism, in addition to the more familiar Judaism. The cultural landscapes of places like Naperville now include synagogues, mosques, and temples alongside churches. To a great extent, the congregations served by these religious institutions were formed by the dynamics of edge-city technoburban development and are affected by those same dynamics, no matter whether they call themselves Christians, Muslims, Buddhists, or Jews.

Edge-city congregations confront the stresses of edge-city life, offering religion's transcendent perspective and spiritual comfort to people in need in the midst of general material abundance. Naperville is a popular place, yet its congregations are not always happy about what Naperville has become. The hectic pace of life, anxieties in the workplace, social problems, congestion from rapid development—these represent the downsides of prosperity, the costs of successful transition to technoburban status. But religion has always measured "success" by more than one yardstick. At heart, the search is the same no matter the denominational label—the search for spiritual meaning in "the most materialistic community in America," in the words of one local Baptist pastor. The ambivalence of edge-city religion is that it nearly bites the hand that feeds it, so to speak; for in the midst of obvious material success, edge-city congregations ask: Is this worth the costs? Is this all there is to life?

Intriguingly, religion's ambivalence over edge-city life is shared by many edge-city analysts, despite their relative lack of interest in edge-city religious life. From a mall owner's perspective, religious facilities may represent simple "noncompeting low-density [land] use," but Joel Garreau suggests that religion is an important purveyor of "community" and "connectedness" amid the centrifugal forces of edge-city life, and thus religion helps make an edge city a livable place. Provocatively, Garreau points to religion's rather uncomfortable fit in the edge-city environment—after all, what need is there for religion's vision of a life more abundant in the midst of such material abundance?[17]

As Garreau sees it, these exurban enclaves are the wave of the future, though it remains to be seen what kind of future this wave will bring in its wake. "Are we satisfying our deepest yearnings for the good life with Edge City?" Garreau asks. "Or are we poisoning everything across which we sprawl?"[18] Whereas Garreau's concern for the good life may be motivated largely by civic and aesthetic considerations, edge-city congregations pose the same questions for spiritual reasons, seeking satisfying answers in sermons, fellowship, and programs of various types. The case studies presented in this chapter suggest that congregations in edge-city technoburban milieus may tend to offer spiritual palliatives for individuals rather than structural alternatives for edge-city technoburban life. Fellowship, prayer, and meditation mitigate the stresses of this lifestyle. They do not advocate substituting a less stressful, alternative lifestyle.

NOTES

My thanks to Nancy L. Eiesland for her helpful comments on an earlier version of this chapter. Research for this chapter began in October 1995.

1. In the interests of space and readability, newspaper reports, primary documents, and personal interviews are cited sparingly. These sources include numer-

ous articles published between 1995 and 1998 in the *Beacon News* (Aurora, Illinois), the *Naperville Sun,* the *Daily Herald,* the *Chicago Sun-Times,* and the *Chicago Tribune.* Primary documents were provided by the city of Naperville, the Fox Valley Genealogical Society, the DuPage County Regional Planning Commission, the DuPage County Development Department, and Indian Prairie School District 204.

2. Ebner, "Technoburb"; Helgesen, *Everyday Revolutionaries;* Lemann, "Stressed Out in Suburbia."

3. Ebner does not consider religion, while Lemann devotes one paragraph to Naperville's congregations. Helgesen considers religion throughout her book, but her analysis takes a predominantly individualistic perspective.

4. Historical information from Towsley, "View of Historic Naperville"; Keating and Lebeau, *North Central College and Naperville.*

5. Ebner, "Technoburb," 56.

6. Fishman, *Bourgeois Utopias;* Garreau, *Edge City,* 7. Eiesland, *Particular Place,* surveys the literature on such places.

7. Ebner, "Technoburb," 59.

8. Claritas divided the United States into sixty-two lifestyle clusters based on census data, opinion polls, and product purchases, assigning each cluster a clever nickname. Reardon, "New Geography," reports the view of the National Opinion Research Center director that these nicknames both are "too cute" and tend to imply that the difference between these types are greater than they are. Even so, the labels do capture aspects of Naperville's lifestyle.

9. See Garreau, *Edge City,* 428.

10. Lemann, "Stressed Out in Suburbia," 42.

11. Helgesen, *Everyday Revolutionaries,* 51–53.

12. Lyle E. Schaller, phone interview with Paul D. Numrich, February 7, 1996.

13. Field, "'Let My People Go,'" 84–85.

14. For a fuller treatment of this congregation, see Numrich, "Pentecostal Megachurch on the Edge."

15. See Numrich, "Facing Northeast."

16. Though not in Sector G as Helgesen, *Everyday Revolutionaries,* 226, reports.

17. Garreau, *Edge City,* 63–65, 288, 291–94, 454.

18. Ibid., 11–12.

Religion and the New Metropolitan Context

Map 9. Old Saint Patrick's Roman Catholic Church draws members from through-out—and beyond—the Archdiocese of Chicago, while also serving as a local parish. Map by Brian Twardosz, BMT Printing and Cartographic Specialists.

Catholic Spirituality in a
New Urban Church

Elfriede Wedam

"They welcomed a stranger . . . that's how Abraham and Sarah got started. . . . I think the church ought to model for the world that virtue of hospitality." So responds Father Jack Wall, the pastor of Old Saint Patrick's Church, to the question of how to meet the challenges of pairing old understandings with new times. Hospitality is only the first step, but it suggests an older virtue that may affect the uneasy balance between the changes many urban Americans have made and those to which they have been subject. The religious practices of American Catholics have always stood at the junction of faith and world, and this chapter assesses what has happened in one urban Catholic church in an attempt to learn where current change might lead.

In the mid-1960s, the west side of Chicago's business district was home to skid row. There were no residences, and the area had retained few of the commercial activities that were generated by overland rail and Great Lakes ship traffic during industrial growth of the city. But Old Saint Patrick's Catholic Church, the oldest public building in Chicago, founded in 1846 by Irish railroad workers, remained. The church's yellow bricks, joined in a Romanesque revival style, contain museum-quality stained-glass windows that use motifs from the *Book of Kells*.[1] Each of its mismatched towers, representing eastern and western Christendom, is topped by a Celtic cross.

Succeeding waves of Italians, Mexicans, and other immigrants were served by Old Saint Patrick's Church as they passed through this tenement district, which was also the home of Jane Addams. In 1931, the local archdiocesan newspaper wrote that Old Saint Pat's served "the Loop workers and transients because of its convenience to the hotels in the central part of the city."[2] The printers from the South Loop Printers Row came for the 3:30 A.M. Sunday mass, created for them after their shift. Today the church has made a place for a new transient population—middle-class urbanites, both returnees from the suburbs who now prefer to live in the city again and young adults who work in the Loop.

The current story began in the mid-1980s, when Old Saint Patrick's was redefined as a regional or magnet church. Because the church had been designated a historic landmark in 1964 it had remained open, although used more as meeting space than as a functioning parish, since only one residential building was located inside the parish boundaries. But Old Saint Patrick's captured the interest of Fr. John J. Wall, a diocesan priest whose own Irish bloodlines were connected to both the Catholic and the political history of the city. A church at a major expressway interchange that was also within walking distance of the Loop suggested to him centrality and access—a way to create a second-generation, postimmigrant urban church.

Since few people live within the parish territorial boundaries, fluid membership categories were deliberately created. One could simultaneously belong to Old Saint Patrick's and to one's neighborhood parish, or just belong to Old Saint Pat's, or simply participate in one of the church's many opportunities for volunteering or socializing. By the mid-1990s the church had fifteen hundred registered members, the majority from various city neighborhoods and about 25 percent from the suburbs. The 1998 rolls reveal twenty-eight hundred members and a mailing list of over twelve thousand. New building construction and conversions of lofts and warehouses added residences where there were none before. The members are predominantly white, with a handful of African Americans and an occasional Asian or Hispanic, and are overwhelmingly white-collar professional and business people, and young adult and middle-aged. Church programs on work and faith, spirituality, and young adult issues, as well as social events and community outreach, attract from hundreds to thousands of participants. Successful fund-raising, anchored by the popular but increasingly secular "World's Largest Block Party" each July, has produced an annual budget over $1 million. The church has turned more to stewardship as the staff strives to reduce the financial dependence on vagaries such as the weather and the popularity of the rock bands at the block party. Old Saint Pat's recently undertook a multimillion-dollar restoration of the architectural and artistic features of the

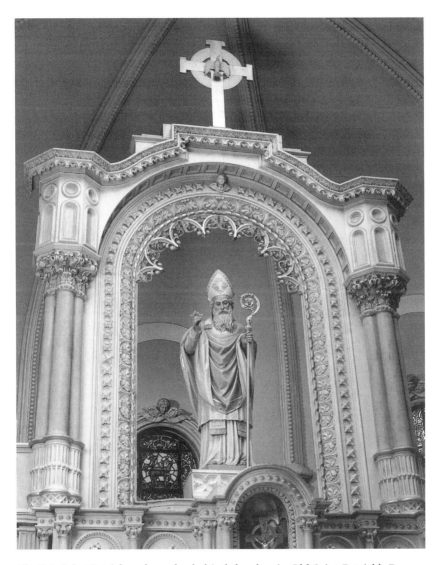

Fig. 9-1. Saint Patrick and reredos behind the altar in Old Saint Patrick's Roman Catholic Church, Chicago. The Celtic cross symbolizes the church's understanding of the relationship to the city: the circle represents the city boundary and the cross, the meeting point of the people. Photo by Erin Jaeb. Used by permission.

church, entirely financed through the parish's own efforts. Their elementary school, the first to open under Catholic auspices in twenty-five years in Chicago, has a substantial waiting list. While not the only post–Vatican II model of "being church," the successful revival of Old Saint Patrick's has been much noticed in an archdiocese that has struggled mightily to keep open the doors of its urban parishes.

A New Organizational Form

A Catholic parish is a manifestation of universal Catholicism at the most local level, and Old Saint Patrick's has been innovating and experimenting with alternative forms of that manifestation. When the social and cultural structures that support a particular model of parish relationships change, members of parishes begin to seek new models. Scholars have noted that the story of this local expression—the "origins, size, activities, inner dynamics and how they responded to the religious needs of their members—has not yet been told."[3] This chapter is about a parish that is responding to the changed urban realities by evolving a new ecclesiology that will continue to support communal relationships not tied to the territorial parish.

The innovation inevitably raises important questions: What is essential to the idea of a parish? Which elements of a parish can be changed before it is no longer a parish? The question was put positively by theologian Langdon Gilkey:

> How can this center, that is, the parish remain vital in a "revised" ecclesia that recognizes historical change and hence change in all the church's structures and expressions, including its forms of ultimate authority, its liturgy and liturgical sacramental rites, its exclusive rules of participation, and its surrounding ecclesiastical dogmas?[4]

When vitality of parish life becomes the goal, as at Old Saint Pat's, there is much room for creating and changing structures to support it.

One of the changes in ecclesiastical dogma that has given Old Saint Pat's the opportunity for innovation and growth is the status of parish territorial boundaries. The 1983 Revised Code of Canon Law states that "as a general rule a parish is to be territorial . . . whenever it is judged useful, however, personal parishes are to be established."[5] Yet this increased flexibility in practice suggests a change in religious identity. If a baptized

Catholic chooses what parish to belong to, does that mean she is in some sense choosing Catholicism and therefore creating a Catholic identity, rather than accepting historical circumstances as a given? Furthermore, can she reject that identity just as easily? While the answer may seem obvious to Protestant and modern secular observers, it is a question about a Catholic self-concept—this ascriptive or inherited status—that has been tied to the assumption of membership in the geographic parish. So now, with parish boundaries less decisive for where and how Catholics belong to their church, the theological and ecclesiological question arises of whether the meaning of being Catholic has changed as a result.

Another question is whether and how culturally constructed (as opposed to geographic) boundaries that demarcate the rules of participation can foster the communal relationships historically associated with the Catholic parish. When a parish like Old Saint Pat's shifts the emphasis from geographic to cultural and social boundaries, what happens to the cohesion of the group? When identity becomes less ascribed and increasingly a matter of choice about whom members associate with, what kinds of relationships will result?

Our ethnographic observation of Old Saint Patrick's Catholic Church mainly provides evidence on the sociological questions about communal relationships, although there are interesting clues for the ecclesiological and theological questions as well. This is in part because Old Saint Patrick's connects the meaning of the cultural and social boundaries to personal identity as a Catholic.

The "loss" of community and the excesses of American individualism are historical themes that crystallized in the imaginations of the present generation through the 1985 publication of Robert Bellah and colleagues' *Habits of the Heart.* Applying these themes to the Catholic Church in *Religion and Personal Autonomy,* Phillip Hammond argues that when choice of parish is available, Catholics lose the primary-group ties that anticipate the obligations parishioners have for one another. The group ties give way to a drive for personal expression, to preoccupation with the question "What am I getting out of this?"[6]

In this study of Old Saint Patrick's Church, I argue not only that this fundamental shift accords with Vatican II but, more important, that it need not result in the loss of the communal character of Catholic parish life. The kind of participation Old Saint Pat's asks of its members respects the broad pluralism of everyday urban life; at the same time, it refuses to build a church simply around their needs. Nevertheless, this new integration is a work in progress, with gaps in concept and execution. This new form reveals losses as well as gains in modifying tradition—serious considerations as the American Catholic Church undergoes the "most significant changes in parish life since the U.S. church mobilized to meet the needs of immigrants."[7]

Old Saint Patrick's is in some respects what R. Stephen Warner calls a "*de facto* congregation," an informal polity of a "gathered assembly," members who are drawn together rather than required to be there—a practice Warner says is becoming increasingly common in America, even among Catholics and others whose religion has historically been ascribed and whose institutions express strong central authority.[8] Yet, Old Saint Patrick's demonstrates that a *de facto* congregation may be quite collective in its actions and communal in its social networks, depending on the propensities of the members and which traditions they draw on. Old Saint Patrick's respects the voluntary commitment that makes a congregation but at the same time consciously seeks to rebuild a corporate foundation to support all aspects of parish life. This rebuilding attempts to respond to urban realities with a new model of parish that will work in a metropolitan—not just a neighborhood—context.

Church Practice in an Urban Setting: Theology and Social Theory

Styles of parish life are determined in part by the theological mission of a particular diocese, the quality of lay and clerical leadership, and the desires of the Catholics in the pews. Intersecting with these factors is the process of "inculturation," which requires innovation to achieve "the proper relationship between faith and culture" in each local setting.[9] Thus the local context helps determine the particular shape and voice of the local churches, so there are different legitimate cultural modes of expressing the "ancient faith" in the contemporary understanding of faith and cultures. Since the Revised Code of Canon Law cited above, several types of nonterritorial parish models have been developed (or redeveloped) around ethnic identification and language, young adult ministries, and urban outreach. One type is like Old Saint Patrick's, located in the downtowns of aging industrial cities without large residential populations. These nonterritorial parishes have open boundaries but still focus on the theological mission of the communion of the church.[10]

The social character of Catholic identity is expressed in many ways that do not depend on territory. For example, gathering around the table, the communion feast, is a collective expression.[11] Yet Catholic churches vary in their communal expression. Phillip Hammond describes a three-stage move of church affiliation from that of a primary-group model to a secondary- and voluntary-group model. Old Saint Pat's is, in many respects, an example of "individual-expressive" relationships, in which secondary- and voluntary-group ties form the basis of its associational life. This contrasts with the "collective-expressive" model, which represents inherited relationships with several overlapping primary-group ties.[12] The collective-expressive model of human agency emphasizes the obligations of the human condition—being a member of something, such as the parish, that is greater than the individual ego and makes claims upon it.

However, Hammond argues, when people *choose* their religious affiliation, including whether to affiliate at all, the nature of religious expression and hence its role and impact on individuals changes. This is the basis of his critique of the increasingly voluntary nature of American religion. While Protestants have long celebrated the "voluntary principle"[13] in American religious affiliation, it is mainly since the 1960s that choosing whether and where to affiliate has increased as a form of personal autonomy for Catholics. Hammond argues empirically that personal autonomy correlates with an erosion of local, primary ties and an acceptance of a new morality based heavily on individual conscience and choice. Personal autonomy among Catholics is revealed in how they choose personal parishes over territorial ones and evidence lower rates of parish involvement. The decline of involvement in parish life is accompanied by a change in the meaning of that involvement; that is, increasingly, parish involvement is a vehicle for self-expression only.[14]

Although Hammond notes how personal autonomy resulted from structural and cultural changes, his formulation is nevertheless nonreflexive. His collective-expressive model assumes that people are Catholic because they have always been Catholic and go to church out of habit. He argues that this mode permits the church to mediate for its members against the autonomy of the state and the market. The church's authority rests on its claim that its members constitute a perduring group and do not just come together to pursue temporary interests. In contrast, observers like José Casanova note that although the Catholic Church has not, for example, been able to shape public policy on abortion, it has been extremely effective in stimulating, informing, and focusing a public debate.[15] Universal education enhanced the ability of ordinary Catholics to decide whether or not their parish fosters the development of their inner spiritual life. Their reform efforts echo the Council of Trent, which determined that parish territorial reform was needed "for the spiritual good of souls."[16]

Phillip Hammond's collective-expressive view of the church is consistent with a theological interpretation of parish that "the church is not an object that they, as individuals, may freely accept or reject."[17] Some Catholic writers have argued that the church is not "merely a private reality, solely at the service of its members. It is the divinely constituted Body of Christ in history, an essentially public entity."[18] In this view, assent is more a matter of fulfilling a destiny of faith than of engaging a positive preference.[19] But choosing to attend a particular Catholic church is different from choosing to live as a practicing Catholic. Does being a practicing Catholic imply attendance at one's territorial parish? Not necessarily. Unlike Protestants, who may change denominations in the process of choosing a congregation, for Catholics, institutional identity does not change with a change in parish affiliation.

Catholics are retaining a fundamentally institutional identity, regardless of what parish they choose to join or attend. For example, national (that is, ethnically defined) parishes are not territorial either, despite the convenient clustering of European immigrants in ethnic enclaves, often encouraged by pastors to foster commitment to "their" parish (but not necessarily for theological reasons).[20] The primary-group ties created by shared language, national culture, and immigrant status are dependent on a particular historical circumstance. In the typically large ethnic parishes of two thousand or more families, the intimacy implied in primary group ties would have been difficult to find. I hesitate, therefore, to link members' "choosing" of Old Saint Patrick's with "wanting" rather than "having" to go to church. These Catholics *have* to go to church, but they find Old Saint Patrick's contemporary style is intellectually, aesthetically, and spiritually more satisfying than that in their neighborhood parishes. The same can be said of ethnic immigrants' desires to worship in national parishes where a common language and cultural style were and continue to be valued. This is also an expression of choice, but I question that such voluntariness reduces the ability to fulfill one's destiny as a baptized Catholic.

Nevertheless, Hammond's analysis points to important concerns. What is the consequence for community when removed from territory?

What is the further consequence, then, for identity? While American Protestant congregational life is strong and extensive, its social character is different from that of Catholicism. One reflection of this is the difference in commitment to locale, especially to the neighborhood and one's neighbors. I agree with John McGreevy that Catholics' theological and social commitments to neighborhoods had negative consequences for race relations in the United States, but he and other scholars still point to certain positive consequences for security, safety, and the building of civic infrastructure.[21] Sharon Zukin is right that "men and women still want to live in specific places,"[22] that is, a geography they can point to and identify with. Place continues to have meaning, and the construction of meaning cannot rest solely on issues and relationships about which people can freely choose. Personal identity is partially derived from where one lives and the kinds of ties one makes there.

Old Saint Patrick's can be usefully compared to the medieval cathedral churches which were built in the major towns and served the entire region, particularly on liturgical holidays. Similarly, Old Saint Patrick's members are revising—regionalizing—the geographic basis of (social) ascription. They may reject their inherited relationships (with neighbors they, in fact, do not know), but Old Saint Patrick's is nevertheless a necessary expression of their theological inheritance: they *must* go to church, and they must go to a Catholic church with other Catholics.

Old Saint Patrick's: A Model for the World

At Old Saint Pat's, the whole city of Chicago is construed as a metaphor for the territorial parish, and the church is the "meeting at the crossroads" symbolized by the bars on the Celtic cross. The cross is surrounded by a circle, a symbol used on ancient city maps to represent the walls protecting the city residents. Old Saint Pat's has reinterpreted and used this symbolism to connect the church with the city as a whole, reaching beyond traditional parish boundaries. The church draws on Vatican II, which redefined a universal conception of the church so as to make porous the boundaries of the parish center, making the parish "open to the world."[23] Consequently, the focus of the parish is continually outward-looking rather than parochial.

The church is organized around the mobility of young adults for whom "the whole country is their backyard," as associate pastor Father

John Cusick put it. By creating programs around their transitory circumstances rather than lamenting their unpredictability, the church has
opened new patterns of attendance and involvement. Outreach efforts
then call for the development of new—or rediscovered—virtues, beginning with hospitality.

Hospitality is not only highlighted in the church's mission statement
but articulated in every liturgy, particularly by the clergy when they welcome the congregants. The liturgy begins with a greeting to "neighbors"
surrounding the worshiper in the pew. This "encounter" with the stranger
is vested with spiritual meaning. "Everything is meeting a stranger, is
opening yourself up to that gift of the stranger," continued the pastor.

Hospitality has more valence in the church than does the discussion of
building a community—the relationship among intimates commonly at-
tributed to the traditional parish. At the same time, the tension between
welcoming the seeker, the traveler, or simply the curious and addressing
the continuing assembly, who have put down their roots, enrolled their
children, and volunteered on a steady basis, is self-consciously balanced.
For example, support for family programs has been increased by the addition of staff and a family mass. At the same time, a renewed emphasis
on young adults in their twenties has resulted in new programming because of a leveling off of membership.

In part, this tension exists because of the continual movement and im-
permanence, or at least very conditional stability, of urban life. Old Saint
Pat's shares this sense of movement rather than the more fixed sense of
neighborhood or traditional "community." The Near West Side surroundings lack an identity, including a "turf." In exchange, the church has
centrality and accessibility, which make its programs available for a metropolitan constituency.

Because this is a downtown church with a mission to reach the Loop
workers, the church has organized its programs and activities around the
schedules and rhythms of the business world. This includes the timing of
activities but also the mode of addressing members, who may be transferred to another city or country next month. Many programs are organized with built-in end points—"so people know how to get out of something before they commit to it," Fr. Cusick explained.

Old Saint Pat's has diverse programs for many kinds of Catholics.
Through the many community volunteering programs and social programs, its members have reinterpreted their roles as lay Catholics for
their own generation. Volunteering is a direct expression of the outward-

looking mission of the church, explicitly designed to get away from a clublike model of "meeting members' needs." One volunteer described the involvement of himself and his wife as a calling to "share their gifts."

The entirely lay-run Community Outreach Group is the church's cornerstone mission project, with more than five hundred members. It has reduced bureaucratic demands on participants—there are no bylaws or regular meetings—so they can focus on relationship building with those they serve, and on efficiently achieving their goals. One can volunteer for any level of commitment, and exiting is built into the system. The group offers a variety of venues to work in—elementary school tutoring in a black Catholic parish, adult literacy and employment training at both Catholic and non-Catholic locations, pediatric visits at a non-Catholic hospital, working at two Franciscan homeless shelters, an athletic program for Hispanic youth in a Latino parish, holiday sustenance drives, and even a wine auction to raise funds for a home for the mentally handicapped.

A built-in transience is also evident in the content of parish programs, which have none of the traditional membership requirements such as running for office and having monthly meetings; nor is a continuous commitment expected. Instead, this programming resembles an active conference center wherein a variety of lectures, forums, and discussion groups are held—often over an affordable breakfast, lunch, or dinner—and speakers address issues interesting to professional workers. These programs focus on spiritual, ethical, and civic concerns and, together with the archdiocesan young adult ministry led by Fr. Cusick, programs for young adults addressing relationship issues.

The rich mix of activities at Old Saint Pat's means that the parish is a vital social center, continuing the intensive and extensive group life that American Catholics have created as a legacy of the "immigrant church."[24] To be sure, contemporary practices are less devotional and more social than those of the nineteenth century.[25] Nevertheless, they continue to be expressions of faith and are certainly no less collective in character. Indeed, those nineteenth-century devotional activities were also a pursuit of personal spiritual growth, albeit less critical of church ecclesiology or doctrine.

The metaphor of the parish as a community is used sparingly at Old Saint Pat's. The ideal moral construction of community as a relationship among intimates may not adapt well to the kinds of relationships these urban people actually have. Joseph Fichter suggested this in the mid-1950s: "I say an urban parish cannot be a community—it can't be; it's too

Fig. 9-2. Old Saint Patrick's Roman Catholic Church and "the World's Largest Block Party," which raises over half a million dollars each year for parish activities. Photo by Gail Pollard, courtesy of Old Saint Patrick's Roman Catholic Church.

big. The typical urban parish is a secondary association within which there are maybe a dozen to twenty or twenty-five primary groupings; and this is all to the good."[26]

Old Saint Patrick's Church contains different combinations of primary and segmental relationships of the sort Fichter and others since have observed.[27] Its activities foster overlapping friendship groups. The welcoming atmosphere at meetings, for example, is deliberately organized but appears to emanate spontaneously from the attendees. Rather than a solemn atmosphere before the beginning of each mass, the pews buzz with friendly conversation, and a priest can often be spotted socializing in the aisles. The peace greeting during the liturgy is an occasion for warm and enthusiastic exchanges among the priest celebrant and members spilling into the aisles.

The mass celebrations exhibit immediacy, a sense of participation, and informality. One Sunday the celebrant suggested that because two choir members got married the day before, the choir was a little hung over. Congregants talk about the church as an attraction—something they look forward to, something "you didn't want to miss." But their vibrancy may derive less from intimacy than from the rich variety of intellectually stimulating opportunities that the church offers, including preaching that responds to events in congregants' lives in an intellectually engaging way.

In only a matter of weeks I easily identified familiar faces in a half dozen different church venues, suggesting that many of the members know one another in multiple contexts, partially offsetting the segmental character of urban social life. Such multifaceted arrangements have always characterized urban life; whereas urban relationships are less spatially proximal than in rural areas, Claude Fischer argues that they are not less solid or intimate. The urban environment is one of higher density and more massive scale and separates our relationships into specialized roles. Our neighborhood friends and our work friends, for example, are not likely to know each other. But the relationships around occupation or ethnicity or religious membership are often intimate, face to face, and deep.[28] Old Saint Pat's provides a site for these relationships to form and thrive.

Pluralism, Experimentation, and the Laity

Old Saint Pat's members are thoroughly invested in an incarnational theology that values spirituality over dogma, experience-centeredness rather than rule-centeredness, and presence in this world more than preparation for the next. The theology is inclusive and pluralistic, best seen in the establishment of the Jewish-Catholic Dialogue Group, a dual worshiping group of mixed-marriage couples. Clergy from Old Saint Pat's and a Reform rabbi from a downtown synagogue share ministry to this group. Innovative activities include dual-faith liturgies, such as a naming ceremony and baptism. The family that originated the ceremony described it as "the most meaningful thing we have ever done. It was a real turning point in our religious lives." The dual-faith religious education program for primary-grade children, entirely written and taught by the members, received an award from the Archdiocese of Chicago for its innovative content and quality of lay leadership. Some families in the group emphasize one faith over the other, but others respect both equally, and the content of the religious education school and curriculum reflects the latter approach.

Typically, couples seek out the dialogue group when looking for help in holding a dual-liturgy marriage ceremony. One point of pride is the number of nonpracticing Jews and Catholics who returned to observance after joining. But the deeper response has been the unalloyed relief among couples who have discovered they do not have to yield to marriage the faith of their birth or abandon faith altogether in the desire for familial harmony. They have found a "third way." They can connect their concrete, personal, and pluralistic life situation with what their bylaws call "a meaningful way to find God."

Through their leadership with the dialogue group, Old Saint Patrick's clergy express a theological—not just an ecumenical—pluralism. The group works effectively because clergy help them explicate the role of Christ as a Jew in Jewish history and seek out the symbolic, universal meaning of Christ. For the annual talk on the relationship between Passover and the Lenten-Easter season, the group invited a priest-theologian, who challenged the wall of hostility between the faiths erected over the historical events. He said Jesus "was born a Jew, lived and died as a believing Jew" and then explained how integrating such an idea into the ritual practices of both Christians and Jews directly reflects the content of Jesus' personal ministry.

When asked how this approach stands the test of evangelization, Old Saint Patrick's clergy say they prefer that people be brought into spiritual awareness and practice rather than into doctrinal adherence or conversion. They also point out that a small number of Jews and Protestants have become regular members.

The search for new models of an urban church depends heavily on lay initiative, enabled by Vatican II's reversal of the four hundred years of lay passivity the Tridentine reforms had effected.[29] Many of Old Saint Pat's programs are developed because a layperson suggests a need such as discussion groups focusing on inner spirituality, which are the sodalities of the twentieth century. In Progress (young adult issues), Sunday Suppers (speakers for the "seasoned" adult), the Men's Spirituality Group, and Pray Allways (prayer group) are examples of this. Others, especially the volunteering groups, are more outward-looking. The mission statement orients the effort of Old Saint Patrick's to "serve the life and work of the laity in the world." Staff provide opportunities based on members' experience rather than a prescriptive model of what people "should" do. Yet, while the communal experience is enriched by the bazaar of activities available, a certain busyness may obstruct the ability to achieve deeper self-insight.

A lay-initiated group heralding from a previous era but being redefined by the current membership is the Council on Working Life, which was once an activist organization concerned with the problems of blue-collar workers. Currently, the members have shifted their focus from public issues to individual members' struggle to understand the current economic environment. Reported one member: "What the Council is willing to talk about is ways to humanize the workplace, advise and encourage people to shape the small space which they occupy in their work into something they can live with and keep their sanity." Although some on the Catholic Left will criticize this shift, Monsignor Daniel Cantwell, the chaplain to the group, whose credentials include the labor movement and civil rights, redefined activism in other terms. He declared that being "psychologically and spiritually involved" in everyday life is preferable to testing the correctness of people's positions.

Much of the discourse in the church's programs, as in the wider culture, centers on the notion of interests rather than commitments, and this comes at a cost. The pursuit of self-interest weakens a communal model, because interests are based on individual needs that will change as they become fulfilled, forcing churches (and other institutions) continually to adapt.[30] Therefore, the pursuit of individual interests may fracture communal well-being. For example, interests draw like-minded and like-status people together; hence, while pluralism in Old Saint Patrick's is an expressed ideal, homogeneity of race and class still predominates. The rhetoric of inclusion is part of the self-presentation of Old Saint Pat's, but that presentation appears not to connect with the non-English-speaking or the poor or the nonwhite. For example, exchanges of choirs on Martin Luther King Jr.'s Birthday do not bring African Americans into the congregation. Old Saint Pat's high quality liturgical choir with professional-level soloists and orchestral accompaniment, appeals to middle- and upper-middle-class whites but has not attracted middle- and upper-middle-class African Americans and Hispanics.

Despite the 30 percent nonwhite component in the elementary school, the nonwhite parents are not visible in the congregation. Despite the extensive volunteering in the poor areas of the city, it is hard to spot anyone without a middle-class appearance. While the metropolitan locality constitutes the de facto parish boundaries for inclusion in this church, other symbolic boundaries—middle-classness, professional job status, like-mindedness in taste and style—form the exclusive boundaries.

These choices are probably not intentionally exclusive. Singing music that reflects one's ethnic heritage or taste is a meaningful experience. But the consequences for groups or individuals not privileged to be included can be overlooked or ignored. The metropolitan reach created by Old Saint Pat's overcomes the limitations of access that parishes of the "club mentality" tend to foster. But it promotes an ideology of access without creating the necessary structures to implement it. Such criticism is familiar to the leadership at Old Saint Patrick's. "I want concrete strategies, not condemnations," complained Fr. Cusick to me. "Tell me how to do it!"

In spite of these potential and existing areas of exclusivity, some Old Saint Pat's members who grew up in ethnic or national parishes recounted how Old Saint Patrick's provides an inclusivity they had not previously experienced. One member cited how cliquishness and vested interests in her home parish created "us versus them" styles of relationships. Yet the shift from the boundaries of ethnicity to the boundaries of class, while a freeing experience for many, replaces rather than eliminates definitions of "otherness." At the annual, well-attended Seder Supper, Fr. Wall asked members to make their offering for the needy in order "to expand our community." He reflects an awareness of the limits of the congregation's self-identity but does not directly challenge it. Nevertheless, Fr. Wall acknowledges that Catholics in general are "missing out on the multicultural experience."

Old Saint Patrick's has developed an urban church that is universalistic, theologically pluralistic, fluid, and outward-looking. There are some costs—a certain kind of familiarity, shared identity based on ethnicity, language, historic memory, or even long-term membership, does not exist. Transitory and segmented relationships and a consumer orientation to participation mitigate against an integrated continuity of relationships. Through appropriation of Celtic aesthetics, the church celebrates an Irish heritage that has more to do with the Saint Patrick's Day parade and political connections in the city than with the Irish religious heritage. Pluralism in race and class has not been achieved. The fluidity of membership offers choices, but choices also limit the construction of broader visions that might require a more demanding discipline. "Commitment to relationships is one of the most daunting challenges of our culture," writes Philip Murnion. "Parishes need to keep calling people into commitment to family and friendship, to parish and public life."[31]

What is gained, though, is an inventiveness in the creation of programs inspired by the outward-looking orientation of both the leaders and the members. Music, theater, and artistic expressions in the liturgy are well developed and sensually pleasing. The emphasis on the practical, nondogmatic, nonmoralistic, and holistic understanding of spirituality challenges middle-class, well-educated Catholics with an approach that is worldly and pluralistic. This "non-ideological" theology, as Fr. Cusick calls it, also permits the word from the homilist to be more publicly critical of contemporary society and politics, as when he criticized the warmongering of both the United States and Iraq during the 1991 Persian Gulf War, and to be more cognizant of the ironic than if he were preaching a dogmatic theology. In offering their non-ideological theology, the pastors invoke the Vatican II document *Pastoral Constitution on the Church in the Modern World* in support of a critical understanding of the world by Catholic believers, who are expected to become more open to the world, not to retreat from it.[32]

A non-ideological theology can also limit the range of discussion. At Saint Patrick's, for example, tension points within Catholic dogma—a married clergy, ordination of women, and the abortion issue—are rarely discussed. The effort to avoid moralism and rigidity results in avoiding conversations in which the issues contain stark and oppositional views. The so-called culture wars debate shows the limits of our language to interpret and communicate experiences that contain morally different resolutions, so it may not be surprising that at Old Saint Pat's such conversations are avoided. Leaders at Old Saint Pat's have observed that the young people who come to the church are interested in their relationships and in work; by contrast, "the ordination of women is not high on young people's list of importance." But recent ethnographic studies have also shown how groups actively seek to overcome polarization.[33]

Church programs that focus on workplace issues are under the leadership of the Crossroads Center for Faith and Work, the brainchild of former staffer John Fontana, a self-styled "religious entrepreneur."[34] The center provides forums for professionals to discuss topics ranging from the costs of downsizing to the economic necessity of redeveloping Chicago's poorest neighborhoods. These discussions are infused with the language of transformation: "The church is a reflective community engaging in public dialogue to transform the world." "How can we transform religious convictions into public issues?" "The purpose of the church is not to do ministry but to be captured by mission." In practice, however, the appeal is usually to individual rather than social tranformation. As Fontana concludes, "Discussion often comes back to small transformations in each layperson in accordance with roles, responsibilities, and the use of power and authority in their worlds of work, family, community life, and citizenship."

Charles Shaw, the developer of Lake Point Tower and other upscale Chicago high-rises, has spearheaded a development in North Lawndale, a poor African American neighborhood on the West Side. He speaks compellingly on the necessity of a commitment to the urban core. At Civic Forum, a regular series sponsored by the Crossroads Center, Shaw reminded his audience that in great part the infrastructure of the outlying areas was built at the expense of the city. He stated his belief in both the free market and social responsibility and suggested that we "must know how to blend them together." His vision, however, is focused on the "fundamental power of individuals." Similarly, the moral issues surrounding the responsibility of CEO members of the church who order massive labor cuts is avoided. Questions about responsibility for social justice are answered with "These are educated people. We cannot tell them what to do. Instead we show them the Gospel and encourage their understanding of the power to live out the Gospel." The language of transformation usually refers to the influence one has over the small area around oneself, yet members of the elite, whose sphere of influence is considerably larger, are not challenged to extend their responsibility likewise. The church's principal response is a retreat to spiritual personalism.

The program presentations I was able to observe were mute on the suggestion that Catholicism or Christianity or Christ should permeate or direct decisions in members' work lives. The In Progress series is devoted to discussions on issues that "touch the lives of young adults in the

1990s." There was little discussion about how religion could be a resource to solve problems in the work life. To some extent, these members saw the church as a haven from the unethical or amoral work environment.

Other programs on faith and work focused on the psychological costs of work-life problems—identity crises, consumer numbness, lifestyle hollowness, which result from work chosen for the income it may provide, regardless of intrinsic worth or the collective costs. One speaker repeated the now-familiar warning that "a lifestyle is not a life." When audience members probed for alternatives, he suggested only that individuals elevate satisfying work choices—"do what you really like to do"—above financial considerations and "hope for the best." He did not, for example, suggest that a refashioned union movement could be a fruitful approach, even though his answers to other questions reminded his listeners of the taken-for-granted benefits of past labor struggles.

In a similar way, the problems of corporate downsizing were addressed with a reactive and adaptive perspective, focusing entirely on survival strategies and advising members to "adapt to changes in the business environment." Such shunning of prescriptive approaches makes religious values difficult to articulate. Labor perspectives received a couple of slots during other Civic Forum seasons, but only one speaker suggested any serious role for religion. He was a labor lawyer who included churches with unions as types of organizations that can mediate between the individual and the changes occurring in the global economy. An Old Saint Pat's member likened the non-ideological approach of the church to that which "comes up to the doorway, but does not cross the threshold."

The church's relationship to change is complex, eagerly looking forward yet somewhat stymied by the cultural compromises it finds itself making and the limitations of a focus on personal spirituality. The explicit consensus is that Old Saint Pat's is not involved in structural change. One member commented that the priests of Old Saint Pat's want to ameliorate abuses but not change structures. If members want a challenge, they can find it, but it's not a requirement for participation. Invited speakers have addressed the death penalty, consumerism, unionism, and poverty. Homilies have addressed war and racism. But as one member voiced, "We can talk about issues here, but there is no collective experience that can lead to change."

New ways of connecting individual with collective forms must be constructed. Most Americans speak comfortably the language of individualism as their "first language," asserted the authors of *Habits of the*

Heart.[35] The language of collective expression, however, is more difficult to find and is mostly located where most Americans are not, that is, in "communities of memory." Such groups share a tradition and a past that are continually retold to its members through ritual and story but also through interdependent sharing and decision making. Critics of *Habits of the Heart* have pointed out that while in many ways the language of the collective has been held hostage by the limitations of our current therapeutic, individualistic culture, it can be found in the process of telling the story, more so than in the structures of the group per se. These critics argue that transcending individualism can occur, for example, in the narratives that families pass down and in communities of choice in which the rituals and activities of the members help them interpret their lives and pass the stories on to others.[36] Different forms of communities, those that do not depend on history and tradition, can develop a moral discourse about their shared life with deliberate and self-conscious strategies.

Volunteering is a type of practice that offers the possibility of transcending the self. First, volunteering with others is a way to experience, however fleetingly, a different life. This exposure creates possibilities for volunteers to deal with issues in their own personal situations in a totally different way. Second, it is a way to express altruism, even if it is minimal. At an adult literacy and employment training program in a poor area near the church, a small but tenacious and resourceful staff direct the professionals from Old Saint Patrick's who volunteer each evening. Sister Virginia Phillips, the Catholic nun who runs this program, is impressed with the church for a membership that "has gathered for others." She thinks the Catholic yuppies and their parents who come to Old Saint Patrick's are hungry to serve others, and that is why the church is growing and successful. Sister Virginia views the social-service approach vis-à-vis the more activist social-justice model positively. When volunteers witness small victories in the lives of individual poor people, these suggest larger hopes. The interaction between the Old Saint Pat's members and the members of the center leads to communication and sometimes friendship. Sister Virginia pointed with delight to the warmth and sociality among the Christmas party guests at the large annual event, which brings social mingling between the volunteers and the people they serve. One church staff member reminded me that "outreach is a human thing. It's vested in a human person, not just a program." Through their own reflection, Old Saint Pat's volunteers bring what they have learned to their

work settings, where there may be a long-term, though likely not an immediate, potential for wider social change.

Old Saint Patrick's is also attempting to transcend the limits of therapeutic culture by suggesting that members reflect on the experience of
others as they reflect on their own experience. The creative potential of
this approach was demonstrated in a courageous presentation by Father
Larry Craig, director of Maximilian Kolbe House, the ministry to prison-
ers at Cook County Jail. He offered a Catholic view of capital punishment
on the eve of the sentencing of John Wayne Gacy, the most notorious ser-
ial killer from Chicago since Richard Speck. He asked the group of two
hundred Old Saint Patrick's professionals how many favored capital punishment; more than half raised their hands. Through a narrative describing issues faced by the prison inmates to whom he ministers, Fr. Craig
raised questions—without taking an explicit position—about the uses of
death in the American criminal justice system. The result was to make his
listeners uncomfortable as they reflected on their own positions.

Labor and civil rights activist Msgr. Cantwell was in residence at Old
Saint Patrick's when he died of cancer in early 1996. He was known to
have spoken out for women's ordination during his homilies. Staff members felt privileged by his presence but also noted his singular courage.
Nevertheless, Msgr. Cantwell was not disappointed in the absence of a
countercultural stance among Old Saint Pat's members. "A certain kind
of activism turns me off," he explained, "especially the kind that comes in
from the outside telling [people] what to do." The role of leadership, he
felt, was to "encourage people to do what they want and help them see
how it fits into the larger whole" of what they want to accomplish. He
noted that the strong involvement of young adults in Old Saint Pat's was
distinctive—"we're making other parishes wonder what happened to
their young adults"—as well as hopeful for the church in general. "There
is life here," he told me.

Conclusion: "What the Church Is For"

Old St. Patrick's changed its name from "parish" to "church" to reflect its
mission to serve all Catholics who choose to come here. While Old Saint
Pat's members voluntarily identify with the church, they continue to
carry out a corporate identity of obligations. Voluntarily joining the
church has not made attending church less obligatory. Moreover, while

choice does not automatically translate into commitment, the latter can be developed in parishes like Old Saint Patrick's, in part because of what Nancy Ammerman calls the "consonance" of individual choice with individual identity and purposiveness.[37] Even religious inheritance, which translates into religious identity, does not automatically result in commitment. Andrew Greeley estimates that about 15 percent of cradle Catholics leave the church.[38]

Catholic identity is not just inherited; it is also constructed by a combination of achievement and ascription. How one grew up was mediated by the interpretative abilities of the earlier generation to connect theology with the social context of their time. It is the same for the next generation. Furthermore, one's identity as a Catholic is the result not just of continually reinterpreted history and tradition but also of religiously legitimated parish and archdiocesan planning (see chapters 5 and 11). The inculturation process connects in an ongoing dialogue the institutional with the personal through the action of the local church.

There is no singular unfolding of history in the development of Catholic parishes. As noted above, the earliest church models were urban but not territorial. Lay initiative was responsible for much of the development of the early American church.[39] Yet current ecclesiological structures emerged from systems of relationships that are now either antiquated—the feudal agrarian model of European parishes—or rare—the small-town American congregations.[40]

Many Catholics, not just those from Old Saint Patrick's, have rejected ideologies of the left and the right on public issues in favor of a focus on and commitment to their private work and family lives. Perhaps they are avoiding larger society-wide moral obligations; alternatively, they may truly be looking for new ways—"for new insights," suggests Fr. Cusick. Creating common understandings about societal obligations in a pluralistic society will require changing our understanding of community and its connection to territory. To accomplish this, the individual-expressive and collective-expressive modes of relationship may need a new fusion. While analytically distinct and clarifying for many purposes, both modes have always been present in some combination and to different degrees, the emphasis shifting with different historical and cultural epochs. When the collective mode had primary agency, individuals tended to become passive, as the recent history of American Catholicism demonstrates. To compensate, individuals exercised choice by being only tangentially related to parishes, as in "Christmas and Easter Catholics." Many pastors have noted that the active core of parishioners consists in only about 10 percent of the members.

Old Saint Pat's acknowledges that it sits in the tension between recourse to individual conscience and the teaching power of the church in moral matters. There, too, it draws on a theological tradition revised and reemphasized in the Second Vatican Council's *Declaration on Religious Freedom*. Thus Old Saint Patrick's signifies one type of the individual-expressive mode of being church. As a case study, it gives evidence of a level of activity and commitment considerably above what is found in the "typical" parish. This evidence is contrary to Hammond's finding that high parish activity and commitment correlate with local ties and implicit acceptance of collective authority in matters of moral issues. Also contrary to Hammond, Old Saint Patrick's demonstrates that the individual-expressive model can be a center of social life and community service, and not just a deliverer of services to members. Old Saint Patrick's may well represent the fusion I argued for above, although the form is still emerging.

Yet there are worries among some members that the church may fall victim to its own successes. Despite the positive atmosphere and high rates of participation, some have noticed a two-class system coming to hand. As one member remarked, a "furs and hats" crowd has developed, some of whom receive celebratory treatment because of their financial giving. Some of the social events carry a big price tag and further stratify the congregation. Moreover, the church is "too packed to be pleasant," especially on holy days, she said. And she worried that people who come for the prestige element are not "volunteering and participating in the regular life of the church." This member fears "the loss of intimacy" as the social cost for Old Saint Patrick's institutional success. Another member ruefully admitted regarding the World's Largest Block Party, while "it's great to have so much money that will sponsor such great programs, the block party is not a Catholic event any more." These are important concerns because, as John McGreevy recently pointed out, the danger of a religious consumerism based on individual autonomy is that it offers "little resistance to 'absorption by business culture.'"[41]

The challenge for the members of Old Saint Patrick's, as for every Catholic church, is to answer the question of mission posed by Fr. Wall, "how to stay focused on what the church is for, and not to somehow respond in the narrow way to one's own needs." This requires "searching for new elements of the transcendent . . . by listening with a 'third ear' to the

symbolic and moral content of existing religious traditions which res-
onate with the contemporary scene."[42] Although the case is hopeful, it is
yet unclear whether the emerging identity of Old Saint Patrick's provides
a model of an urban church based on a dialectical relationship between
the current social context and the theological teachings of the church or
is primarily an adaptation to the prevailing ideas of materially prosperous members.

The members of Old Saint Patrick's Church are middle-class, city-cen-
tered people who participate in several forms of community—segmental
yet multidimensional, through primary *and* secondary relationships. As a
parish, the compliance with parish territorial boundaries is subordinate to
more practical, critical questions of effective church mission and effective
connections with individual spiritually hungry Catholics. So, although Old
Saint Patrick's Church may be a *de facto* congregation, it retains and reen-
acts some of the essential qualities and functions of a parish. In short, I believe it is responding to the restructured urban setting by using the inherited Catholic tradition, the innovations of Vatican II, and the resources of
the city itself to construct multivalent connections among its members in
order to develop new metropolitan forms of belonging.

NOTES

For comments on earlier versions of this chapter, I thank my Religion in Urban
America Program colleagues and, Penny Becker, Kevin Corn, Art Farnsley, John
Hickey, Robert Lammers, Rhys Williams and Patricia Wittberg.

1. Barton, "Celtic Revived."

2. Quoted in Koenig, *History of the Parishes,* 757.

3. Coriden, *Parish in Catholic Tradition,* 18.

4. Gilkey, "Christian Congregation," 113.

5. Coriden, Green, and Heintschel, eds., *Code of Canon Law,* canon 518,
418–419. See also Warner, "Place of the Congregation," 79.

6. Bellah et al., *Habits of the Heart;* Hammond, *Religion and Personal Autonomy.*

7. Murnion, review of *The Parish in Catholic Tradition.*

8. Warner, "Work in Progress"; and Warner, "Place of the Congregation," 63,
68, 73.

9. Schreiter, "Faith and Cultures."

10. For additional examples in Chicago, see Marciniak and Droel, "Future of
Catholic Churches."

11. Michael Novak cites Aquinas on the social nature of Catholic thought in *Catholic Ethic*, 301.

12. Hammond, *Religion and Personal Autonomy*, 3–11.

13. Handy, "Voluntary Principle in Religion," 129–140.

14. Hammond, *Religion and Personal Autonomy*, 171.

15. Casanova, *Public Religions.*

16. Coriden, *Parish in Catholic Tradition*, 31.

17. Hammond, *Religion and Personal Autonomy*, 3.

18. Linnan, "Re-thinking the Urban Parish," 5.

19. Gilkey, "Christian Congregation," 105–106.

20. For an elaboration of this complex subject, see McGreevy, *Parish Boundaries*, 19; Conzen, "Forum," 112.

21. McGreevy, *Parish Boundaries;* also McGreevy, "Faith and Morals," 247.

22. Zukin, *Landscapes of Power*, 275.

23. Linnan, "Re-thinking the Urban Parish," 25.

24. Avella, *This Confident Church.*

25. Orsi, *Madonna of 115th Street.*

26. Quoted in Linnan, "Re-thinking the Urban Parish," 7.

27. Fischer, "Subcultural Theory of Urbanism" and *To Dwell among Friends;* Gannon, "Religious Tradition and Urban Community."

28. Fischer, *To Dwell among Friends.* Also see Ammerman *Congregation and Community*, 354.

29. Coriden, *Parish in Catholic Tradition*, 32.

30. Bellah et al., *Habits of the Heart;* also Hammond, *Religion and Personal Autonomy.*

31. Murnion, "Parish," 7.

32. See Linnan, "Re-thinking the Urban Parish," 25; and Coriden, Green, and Heintschel, eds., *Code of Canon Law.*

33. See examples in Becker and Eiesland, *Contemporary American Religion.*

34. Fontana, "Religious Entrepreneur," 1420.

35. Bellah et al., *Habits of the Heart.*

36. Hall and Neitz, *Culture*, 38–43. See also Reynolds and Norman, eds., *Community in America.*

37. Ammerman, *Congregation and Community*, 354.

38. Greeley, *Catholic Myth*, 111.

39. Dolan, *American Catholic Experience.*

40. Green, ed., *Churches, Cities and Human Community.*

41. McGreevy, "Faith and Morals," 248.

42. Gannon, "Religious Tradition and Urban Community," 299.

Map 10. Indo-Pakistani immigrants and religious centers are widely disbursed in metropolitan Chicago, with concentrations based more on class than on language or country of origin. Map by Brian Twardosz, BMT Printing and Cartographic Specialists.

Recent Immigrant Religions and the Restructuring of Metropolitan Chicago

Paul D. Numrich

America's most recent immigrant religions face many of the same dynamics of Americanization encountered by their classical counterparts. Confronted by the cultural travail that necessarily accompanies migration to another country, immigrant groups transplant familiar Old World religious practices and institutions to their New World communities. Of course, exact duplication of the Old World cannot be accomplished; although traditional roots may be put down, transplantation inevitably becomes transformation as growth and change occur in a new sociocultural environment.[1]

Classical and recent (post–World War II) immigrant religious groups differ, however, with regard to the respective urban contexts that they entered and helped shape, and which in turn shaped them. Since World War II, urban restructuring has created a new American metropolis characterized by deindustrialization, regional reconfiguration, socioeconomic polarization, and demographic diversification. This chapter thus has a dual purpose: first, to identify classically "immigrant" aspects of the recent immigrant religious experience; second, to examine the interrelation of recent immigrant religions and the post–World War II restructuring of metropolitan Chicago.[2] We highlight Indo-Pakistanis here, due to their relatively large numbers and current scholarly interest in their experiences.[3]

We begin with case studies of three Indo-Pakistani immigrant congregations in the Chicago region. The first two, a Hindu temple and a Muslim mosque, have self-consciously sought to bridge ethnoreligious differences within the immigrant community; the third, a Sikh *gurdwārā*, maintains its distinctive ethnoreligious identity. The Hindu and Sikh congregations have built commuter religious centers in relatively well-off exurban locations; the Muslim center is located in an area of transition within the city of Chicago and serves both a neighborhood and a commuter clientele. Institutionally, all three congregations are well integrated into the larger American society. These case studies illustrate the classical functions fulfilled by recent immigrant religious centers, wherein Old World traditions and identities are both transplanted and transformed in a New World context. These case studies also provide local texture to the dynamics of post–World War II urban restructuring.

The Hindu Temple of Greater Chicago
(Southwest Cook County)

More intentionally than perhaps any other Indian congregation in the Chicago area, The Hindu Temple of Greater Chicago (HTGC) pursues what has been called an "ecumenical adaptive strategy."[4] HTGC accommodates the various sectarian and regional/linguistic groups within the Indian immigrant community by facilitating multiple expressions of Hinduism. The inclusive name chosen for the temple bespeaks this, as other local temples specify their particularist emphases—for example, Sri Venkateswara (Balaji) Temple of Greater Chicago (a South Indian temple) and Chinmaya Mission of Chicago (a sectarian temple).

HTGC's membership draws on immigrants from all regions of India, and the temple offers various region-specific programs as well as classes in several Indian vernacular languages. Two other Hindu congregations meet in HTGC's facility. When asked about the distinct groups associated with HTGC, leaders stressed the larger, shared identity as Hindu Indians. As one said, "It depends on how you look at it. I have come, and we have come, [from] far away, so we can see India from above, from the point of view of the whole." HTGC also cultivates broader interreligious dialogue—it served as a cosponsor of the 1993 Parliament of the World's Religions and has representation in the DuPage (County) Interfaith Resource Network.

HTGC's priests provide daily *pūjās* (worship services) and *āratīs* (light ceremonies) for individuals, families, and groups visiting the temple, usually several hundred people per week. Special *pūjās* are held on a regular basis throughout the year, and the temple offers various *samskāras*, or religious ceremonies marking life-cycle passages such as birth and marriage. Hinduism's major religious celebrations, such as Shivaratri (a vigil to the god Shiva) and Diwali (a festival of lights), all of which follow a traditional lunar calendar, can draw as many as four thousand people.

HTGC's Cultural Committee, often working with other area organizations, coordinates many events featuring Indian arts and customs. Well-known Indian artists perform at the temple periodically. Also, a popular summerfest called Greeshma Mela, offering regional Indian cuisines, clothing and jewelry sales, entertainment, and free health screenings, has been organized since 1991. The Humanitarian Committee tends to the social and personal needs of the temple's elderly, most of whom have joined children and grandchildren through family reunification provisions of the immigration laws and who often feel lonely and unproductive in their new surroundings. It also coordinates relief efforts for the economically needy in both India and the United States.

"As the children in these new families grew older," HTGC's own written history observes, "it became important to preserve traditional religious and cultural values." One observer elaborates on the broader phenomenon of local temple-building: "So the temples of Chicago have become the focal point of culture propagation among second-generation Indians, something that the first generation sees as a very critical issue, if not *the* single most important issue, at this stage in their development as an ethnic group."[5]

Through its Education Committee and some twenty-five volunteers, HTGC offers Sunday school classes twice monthly. The Sunday school began in 1984 with only four children but today serves well over one hundred. The children learn various subjects, such as scriptures, *bhājan* (a sacred devotional song), and vernacular Indian languages. Two Sunday school teachers we interviewed stressed the importance of language instruction. It is much easier, they insisted, to teach traditional Indian values through the native languages of Indian culture than through English. Language instruction allows the children to discover their cultural roots, they continued, and in knowing their roots, children can begin to take pride in their identity. Such pride is imperative for those children who experience anti-Asian or anti-Indian prejudice in the public schools.

In 1991 high school and college-age youth formed a group called In the Wings, which by 1995 had some three hundred members. As a flyer puts it, "'Waiting In the Wings' means waiting to take over; these youths are the future of our temple." In the Wings organizes twenty to twenty-five programs annually, including social events, sports activities, and a summer camp. The group also schedules a discussion series called Youth Speaks to address topics such as prejudice, drugs and alcohol, and AIDS.

Marriage appears to be a very touchy subject between the youth and their parents. Ironically, during our interviews at the temple we heard an adult leader predict that marriages with non-Indian Americans would soon become common, whereas a youth leader stated that most of the temple's young people would prefer to marry a fellow Indian.

Every committee has youth representation, though some youth complain that their elders often do not take their opinions seriously. An adult liaison brokers disputes with the board of trustees. One youth leader reported to us that "most of the time [the liaison] successfully resolves the conflict and almost always there is a compromise." As the children become more Americanized through the influences of peers and popular culture, the temple serves as the venue for both challenge and compromise vis-à-vis their Indian heritage. Confrontation most often occurs when individualistic values of the youth clash with Indian values regarding family and respect for elders. Adults may show dismay over the situation, but at the same time they have taken steps to address it positively. For instance, one temple committee has organized open forums to help parents answer their children's questions about Hinduism's relevance in modern America. Moreover, adults have shown a willingness to concede to changes in traditional practices. In commenting on why doughnuts are served during Sunday school as part of *prasāda* (the food consumed at the conclusion of a *pūjā*), one person generalized that such accommodations to the tastes of the younger generation must be made if the temple is to retain these children as its future leaders. "It is impossible," this person pointed out, "to impose strict, conservative, Indian values on American-born kids."

Another group of note in HTGC is Akshaya ("Perennial"), made up of adults in their twenties and thirties "who are seeking to explore, learn, and expand upon their knowledge of the Hindu religion," as the group's flyer puts it. "We are affiliated with The Hindu Temple of Greater Chicago (HTGC)," the flyer continues, "and our goals are to begin the transition to future leadership of the temple and increase public awareness of the HTGC and its goals."

The Hindu Temple of Greater Chicago traces its origin to discussions among South Indian community leaders beginning in 1977. Two important decisions were made in the organization's early years. First, Sri Rama was chosen as the principal deity for the temple. One of the popular *avatāra*s (literally, "descents," savior figures) of the god Vishnu and the title character of the *Ramayana* epic, Rama was seen by temple leaders as a pan-Indian deity that all Hindu immigrants could recognize and honor.

The second important decision concerned a suitable location for the proposed temple. The organization considered more than thirty sites around the metropolitan region and eventually purchased an eighteen-acre parcel of undeveloped bluff property near southwest suburban Lemont. Three considerations sealed the choice, according to the temple's written history: "[a] its proximity to I-55 and other major highways, [b] its quiet spot secluded from thickly populated residential and commercial areas, as well as [c] budgetary constraints." Considerations [a] and [b] clearly presupposed a commuter clientele.

For several years the organization gathered building funds from a variety of sources, including local fund-raising activities and loans from both an Indian-owned Chicago bank and the Tirumala Tirupati Devasthanam, a popular and wealthy Sri Venkateswara temple in South India.[6] In 1982–1983 temporary facilities for ritual practices and community gatherings were set up in west and southwest suburban locations, first in a Lombard residence, then in rented halls in Downers Grove and Romeoville.

By 1983–1984, however, the strain of the project began to show. Several years had passed, the temple's history reports, "and yet there was nothing concrete on the Lemont site, [thus] the patience of the devotees was getting exhausted." A group headed by Telugu professionals pulled out of the Lemont project to build a South Indian temple in west suburban Aurora, with Venkateswara (Balaji) as its principal deity. Groundbreaking for that temple took place in May 1985 and dedication the following June.[7] This split off of the Aurora temple poignantly testifies to the challenges inherent in HTGC's ecumenical agenda. As Padma Rangaswamy summarizes in rather dramatic terms, "The history of temple building in Chicago is also the story of bitter infighting among rival groups."[8] And as Raymond B. Williams notes specifically with regard to HTGC, "The difficulties encountered in developing the plans and in raising the funds for the temple indicate how hard it is to unite people from the various regions and sects in support of one project."[9]

The Lemont group carried through with its plans nonetheless. June 1984 saw the chief minister of the Indian state of Andhra Pradesh lay the foundation stone for the Rama temple. The *kumbhābhishēkam* (dedication ceremony) was held on the Fourth of July 1986.

The temple compound today rises impressively above Lemont Road, two miles south of Interstate 55. The white exterior of the Rama temple exhibits key architectural features of traditional South Indian temples—a

Fig. 10-1. Gopuram of Rama Temple, The Hindu Temple of Greater Chicago in Lemont, Illinois. Photo by Paul D. Numrich.

large, pyramid-shaped entryway (*gopuram*) as well as smaller towers sur-mounting the cubicles of three of the temple's deities. The main hall on the upper level features shrines to several deities, including Ganesha and Hanuman. A room to one side contains images of Krishna and Radha; an opposite room contains Venkateswara and two goddess consorts. The focal point of the hall itself is the sanctum, with its images of Rama and his brother Lakshmana and wife Sita. The ceiling in this part of the hall drops dramatically so that the worshiper approaching the sanctum will experience a sense of entering the *garbhagriha* (womb chamber), the sa-cred center of the spiritual mountain symbolized by a Hindu temple.[10]

The Hindu Temple of Greater Chicago recently completed a project transforming the original building on the site into a temple honoring the deities Ganesha, Shiva, and Durga. The *kumbhābhishēkam* for this temple was performed in the summer of 1994. The tower surmounting the Shiva sanctum here follows the North Indian architectural style, so the two tem-ples together express HTGC's pan-Indian ecumenism. HTGC plans next to build the Kalyana Mandapam and Community Center, a large, three-level facility housing an auditorium, dining hall, and multipurpose classrooms.

With its traditional Old World architectural symbolism and its inclu-sive ecumenical approach, The Hindu Temple of Greater Chicago functions like a regional "cathedral" for the widespread immigrant Hindu community of metropolitan Chicago. Its impressive physical plant bespeaks a significant resource base within that community, particularly among exurban Indian professionals. At the same time, many less-well-off Hindus living around Devon Avenue on the North Side of the city of Chicago cannot easily travel to the southwest suburban Lemont temple to perform their ritual practices. For these Hindus, the ISKCON (International Society for Krishna Consciousness) temple in the Rogers Parks area of Chicago has taken on increasing importance in recent years. The ISKCON temple conducts all the prescribed daily Hindu services, including the 4:30 A.M. service that the Lemont temple does not provide. The ISKCON temple also adds special weekend services for the convenience of those who work during the week. Gujarati Indians predominate at this temple, most of them small-business owners and working-class people.

Fig. 10-2. International Society for Krishna Consciousness (Hare Krishna Temple), formerly a Masonic lodge, is clustered with Catholic and Protestant churches in Rogers Park, Chicago. Photo by Paul D. Numrich.

Muslim Community Center (Albany Park, Chicago)

Muslim Community Center (MCC) is the oldest of the Chicago region's Indo-Pakistani mosques. From its inception, MCC has articulated its mission in light of both recent immigration trends and the Islamic theological ideal of *ummah,* that is, the greater Muslim community that transcends differences of nationality or ethnicity. Looking back on MCC's history, the program booklet for its twenty-fifth anniversary celebration explained: "Its birth was part of the global vision in which Muslims from diverse cultural backgrounds welded into one with one common goal: the establishment of a dynamic and vibrant Islamic Community in North America." A banner hangs today at the front of MCC's prayer hall proclaiming, in both Arabic and English, the Qur'anic injunction "Thus We [Allah] have made you a model community that you may be witnesses to the nations." Commenting on the typically negative perception of Islam held by the American public, MCC's president challenged the Muslim audience at the anniversary celebration to present a balanced picture of Muslims in America. If other Americans saw Muslims as people who do more than just sit around all day reading the Qur'an, he suggested, then knee-jerk negative reactions such as those in the aftermath of the Oklahoma City bombing would be less likely to occur.[11] MCC served as a cosponsor of the 1993 Parliament of the World's Religions and is a member of the Council of Islamic Organizations of Greater Chicago.

MCC has a substantially mixed ethnic congregation. At Friday *jum'ah* prayers, which draw two thousand people during the sacred month of Ramadan, MCC's worshiping body is approximately 70 percent Indo-Pakistanis, 25 percent Arabs, and 5 percent Blacks, Whites, and others. Attendance at daily prayers runs half-and-half Indo-Pakistanis and Arabs. MCC's highest leadership has always been predominantly Indo-Pakistani, but a special committee organizes all programs for Arab members. The center has no appointed *imām* ("exemplar," the Muslim equivalent of clergy), an unusual situation partly explained by a concern that an *imām* might favor one Islamic school of thought (*fiqh*) over others. Each week a different person gives the Friday sermon (*khutbah*) at the center in both Arabic and English, the latter the common language among worshipers. In 1994, MCC elected its first non-immigrant president, a Harvard-educated Black convert, thus expressing the center's awareness of the racial diversity of America's largely urban Muslim community.

MCC facilitates the living of a full Islamic lifestyle by its members. All five daily prayers are observed at the mosque. During Ramadan, many Muslims gather in the evening for the special prayers (*tarāwīh*) and to break the daily fast. The center's Rehab and Welfare Committee organizes the collection and redistribution of the obligatory Islamic alms (*zakāh*). In 1993 these funds totaled about $83,000, more than 90 percent of which came from Indo-Pakistani donors; more than three hundred individuals and families (65 percent of them Black, 20 percent Arab) received the funds. The Darul Qadah Committee offers counseling and handles disputes among the Islamic membership, including divorce cases. The Women's Committee holds health fairs, study groups, and clothing and food sales. Weddings, social events, and funerals take place regularly at the center; members who cannot afford funeral expenses may receive financial assistance.

MCC pays special attention to programming for children and youth. In its guidelines for classroom behavior, MCC's School of Islamic Studies reminds each student, "As a Muslim you are expected to behave in a dignified, respectful manner at all times." Students and parents both sign the guidelines with this vow: "I have read the rules of classroom behavior and will Inshallah [God willing] abide by them to help me learn more about Islam and be a good Muslim." MCC's Arabic Saturday school draws nearly three hundred students, virtually all Arabs, and a Sunday school conducted in Urdu and English serves an equal number of Indo-Pakistani students. The weekend school's curriculum is extensive, as this sampling from a tenth-grade theology class reveals: Qur'an (scripture), Hadith (traditions from the Prophet Muhammad), Fiqh (schools of thought), Sharia (Islamic law), Haram and Halal (prohibited and acceptable actions), and Contemporary Social Problems (e.g., homelessness, drugs, sex, and abortion).

In 1989, MCC opened its full-time day school, the Muslim Education Center (MEC), in a former public elementary school in near north suburban Morton Grove. The school offers both a preschool and an elementary school program through the fifth grade and has an enrollment of 150 students from city and suburbs, the majority Indo-Pakistani. (MEC also runs a weekend school for 250 students.) Much of the impetus for establishing MEC came from parents concerned about "losing" their children to the surrounding non-Islamic culture, as this wording from MEC's statement of philosophy reveals: "The school's foremost objective is to provide an Islamic environment for the education of young Muslims . . . [that] affirms in our children their identity and pride in the Islamic legacy. . . . As is widely accepted, the education of our children in an

Islamic environment is the only genuine alternative to public school education to avoid their exposure to un-Islamic mannerism[s] and practices
such as sexual permissiveness and undue emphasis on materialism."

The precise parameters of an "Islamic environment" are often negotiated at MEC, given its various constituencies and their variant interpretations of and degrees of adherence to Islamic requirements. For instance,
on the matter of separation of the genders in the school, three views may
be found among MEC parents: no separation at all, total separation, or
separation only after the fourth grade. At the time of our field study,
MEC did not separate the students at all. An issue facing Muslim girls in
American society is whether or not to wear the traditional head covering
(*hijāb*). Confronted with peer ridicule in the public schools, some girls
leave home covered but uncover themselves at school. Such daily dilemmas compel some Muslim parents to enroll their daughters in MEC.

Muslim Community Center runs an annual summer youth camp in
rural Illinois for as many as one hundred youth, ages twelve and older. As its
flyer explains, "Muslim Youth Camp is one week during the entire year
where a young person can live with other young Muslims in an Islamic atmosphere of learning and fun." MCC's organizational structure includes a
Youth Council, and its board of directors is required to include two youth
representatives. In his keynote address at the twenty-fifth anniversary celebration, MCC's president outlined his aspirations for expanding youth programming. For instance, a $1 million athletic facility is being planned that
will provide Muslim youth a controlled Islamic environment for recreation.
Also, the president challenged MCC to develop Islamic high schools to
combat negative social influences on Muslim youth, as well as to consider
establishing an Islamic university. Instead of sending our Muslim children
to a Catholic school like Notre Dame, he asked, why not send them to a
Muhammad University or something of the kind?

Muslim Community Center was established in 1969 primarily by
Indo-Pakistani immigrants and students, who initially gathered wherever
they found space, such as at the University of Chicago and the Illinois Institute of Technology. In the early years MCC developed a close relationship with other Muslim centers already in the Chicago region, but according to an MCC source, these groups eventually parted company over
the issue of multiethnic membership.

MCC purchased its first facility in 1972, a former Danish community
center on Kedzie Avenue in the Humboldt Park area on Chicago's West Side.
The site was available and affordable, and the area had some Muslim pres-

ence, but MCC experienced vandalism and harassment there. By 1975, MCC had appointed a planning committee to study the possibility of relocation. In January 1977 the committee recommended constructing an Islamic complex in a "Proposed Muslim Neighborhood" within specific boundaries on Chicago's North Side, in order "to answer the challenge faced by the Muslim community in its efforts to lead a truly Islamic life in a non-Muslim environment." The neighborhood in question—roughly within the areas of West Rogers Park, North Park, and Forest Glen (the upper part of the break-out portion of Map 10)—fulfilled several of the committee's criteria, including attractive urban conditions, availability of housing, proximity of jobs, and adequate transportation. MCC's eventual choice in 1982, a former movie theater in Albany Park, about a mile south of the designated area, fulfilled two other criteria in particular: (1) a relatively dense and potentially expanding Muslim population and (2) a suitable facility. In 1993, MCC purchased fifteen hundred burial lots for Muslims in Rosehill Cemetery, which may be seen as part of its intention to establish a Muslim neighborhood on Chicago's North Side. Previously, North Side Muslims buried their dead inconveniently in the western and southern suburbs.

Clearly, serving a neighborhood community was an important factor in the decision to relocate to Albany Park, and today the majority of MCC's primary ethnic constituencies (Indo-Pakistanis and Arabs) live near the mosque. Nevertheless, during the annual Eid religious holidays these two groups part company, as Arabs travel to Mosque Foundation in southwest suburban Cook County to celebrate with fellow Arabs, while Indo-Pakistanis gather at McCormick Place, Chicago's largest convention center. Independent Arab mosques have operated on the North Side of the city twice in recent years, apparent indication that North Side Arabs wish to have a nearby mosque "of their own."

Most of MCC's leaders have been immigrant professionals—its past presidents include several engineers and two college professors—and suburbanites. The center thus serves an affluent and influential suburban commuter clientele in addition to its majority of typically less affluent city dwellers. A controversy stemming at least partly from this dichotomy arose over the location of the Muslim Education Center. Eventually, those favoring a suburban site over a city site prevailed, as MCC purchased the Morton Grove facility despite significant opposition in that municipality. Also regarding the issue of suburban influence in MCC, we note that MCC claims to have established several "daughter" mosques to serve residential concentrations of Indo-Pakistanis in the northern and western suburbs.

Fig. 10-3. Muslim Community Center in the Albany Park neighborhood is one of the largest of Chicago's mosques. Once a dinner club and theater, it accommodates 1,500 for weekly prayers and 600 children for weekend school. Photo by Paul D. Numrich.

Muslim Community Center and its suburban daughter institutions have mustered the resources necessary to renovate existing facilities for use in worship, education, and other programming. The purchase of the Morton Grove school marked a clear step in the direction of moving MCC itself away from the city, yet speeches at MCC's twenty-fifth anniversary celebration betrayed continuing ambivalence over the issue of city/suburb siting. The current president spoke of hopes to open a retreat center someday in Wisconsin, away from the "cesspool" of the city's un-Islamic influences. Yet a former MCC president pressed for the erection of a "grand *masjid*" (namely, a mosque with Old World Islamic architecture) in MCC's North Side vicinity as a "permanent landmark of the community." If such a mosque materializes, it will become the first Old World–style "cathedral" erected within the city limits of Chicago by any Indo-Pakistani congregation.

Sikh Religious Society of Chicago (Northwest Cook County)

The United States has lately become the preferred destination for emigrants from the worldwide Sikh diaspora.[12] Even so, "the Sikhs remain a largely unknown ethnic group to most Americans."[13] Unfortunately, when Sikhism emerges into American public consciousness, misconceptions and prejudices often ensue. Ethnic Sikhs in America have sometimes suffered from stereotyping as "terrorists," especially around the time of the Golden Temple incident and its aftermath in 1984.[14] Oddly, Chicago Sikhs experienced difficulties a few years earlier, during the Iranian Revolution in 1979—mistaken for Iranians, some Sikhs were accosted with shouts of "Ayatollah go home," and vandals broke many of the plate-glass windows in the Sikhs' newly constructed suburban religious center. In December 1994 the local Sikh community was thrust into headline news after the tragic murder of a Sikh child at that center by a mentally disturbed Sikh visitor to the area. Sikhs once again faced the task of clarifying the nature of Sikhism to a generally uninformed American public—a Chicago TV news anchor initially identified the site of the slaying as a Hindu temple—despite years of cultivating local civic and interreligious connections, including through the Asian American Coalition, the Parliament of the World's Religions, and municipal events. In fact, the civic activism of one area Sikh youth had resulted in national legislation exempting turbaned Sikhs from military uniform requirements.

As one member summarized, the Sikh Religious Society offers a "psychological niche" of solidarity and solace for the immigrant generation within the community, as well as a "strong cultural anchor" of Punjabi-Sikh identity for the American-born and -raised generations. The society's goals include a stress on worship, education of the second generation, and "unity among our community." The matter of communal unity among ethnic Sikhs in America has taken on added significance since the Golden Temple incident, and the Sikh Religious Society of Chicago prides itself on having one of the more harmonious *gurdwārā*s in the country.[15]

"The *gurdwārā* ['gateway or doorway of the guru'] has always been a crucial institution for knitting together the Sikh community, . . . it has been a multipurpose institution: a place of worship, a political center, an educational institution, and a center for hospitality and service."[16] On average, approximately 250 congregants gather in the *darbar sahib* (worship hall) of the Sikh Religious Society's *gurdwārā* for each of two Sunday morning religious services. For the most part, men sit on one side of the hall, women and children on the other. The women typically dress in traditional Indian fashion. Perhaps one-third of the men are *sahajdhārīs*, their clean-shaven faces and trimmed hair marking them as either uninitiated into the Khalsa or (more likely) assimilated into Western society through abandonment of the five Ks.[17] Religious services usually include *kīrtan,* devotional singing of praise and love to God under the leadership of trained musicians and singers (*rāgis*); *gurbāni,* reading of passages from the Guru Granth Sahib (the Sikh scripture), followed by a homily interpreting and applying the meaning of the passages; and *ardās,* congregational prayers. A *granthī* ("Granth-keeper," the Sikh equivalent of clergy) presides over the service, though lay Sikhs are allowed to read from and expound upon the Granth. Toward the conclusion of the service, all participants receive *parshād,* a small piece of warm, sweet dough. After the service, the congregation gathers downstairs for the *langar,* a communal meal open to all.

Four key events from Sikh history call forth major celebrations at the *gurdwārā,* each drawing as many as fifteen hundred people. The birth of founder Guru Nanak (b. 1469) is honored around the full moon of October/November. In December/January the tenth Guru's birth is honored. Baisakhi, in April, both commemorates the establishment of the Khalsa and marks the beginning of the Indian lunar New Year. This celebration demands several months of preparation each year and involves some two hundred performers. Last, the martyrdom of the fifth Guru is commemorated in June. Life-cycle religious ceremonies such as marriages and funerals also take place regularly at the *gurdwārā.*

Sikhism considers service to others, or *sevā,* a religious obligation. *Sevā* takes many forms at the *gurdwārā,* from checking coats and shoes at the entrance to preparing and serving the Sunday *langar* meals, the latter a formidable task considering the numbers attending on a typical weekend. In an effort to reclaim the original meaning of the *langar* as a *sevā* to all persons, regardless of caste or other distinctions, and also as an expression of concern for the poor, *gurdwārā* volunteers organize a monthly food distribution through the Salvation Army in the Uptown area of Chicago. The Sikh Religious Society also conducts an annual on-site blood drive, contributes to local and national disaster relief efforts, and supports various charitable organizations.

A sign announcing rehearsal for the singers who lead congregational worship every third Sunday of the month reads: "Bring a friend, make friends, meet old friends, and JAM with Kirtan!!!!" Their elders may feel that the sign's tone lacks a proper respectfulness for the religious tradition, but in this and other ways the second generation at the *gurdwārā* hopes to make that tradition both attractive and meaningful to young Sikhs. For an hour each Sunday morning, some sixty children receive Sunday school instruction in scripture, Sikh history, and the Punjabi language. A week-long summer Gurbani Camp—analogous to a Christian "Bible Camp"—has been organized locally for over a decade. Also, the *gurdwārā* facilitates discussions among older Sikh youth concerning issues of peer relationships.

During our interviews, adult members openly shared their concerns about the next generations of Sikhs, as well as their hopes that the *gurdwārā* will expand its programming for them. It appears that high school and college youth tend to drift away from the *gurdwārā*. For some, Punjabi culture has lost its appeal. Others complain that the immigrant generation is unwilling to relinquish control of the institution. Among the younger children, however, there seems to be a revival of interest in Sikh traditions and values. In years past, one interviewee noted, summer camp participants tended to be skeptical of Sikhism's relevance to an American context. Now they show a keen desire to be "good Sikhs," which has at times evoked prejudice in their schools, especially toward Sikh boys wearing turbans. Moreover, Sikh youth sometimes express dissatisfaction with their parents' emphasis on occupational success and material values and long for something more spiritual.

Most of the first Sikhs to settle in the Chicago region were students in the 1950s who met together socially in each other's homes and apartments, often with non-Sikh Indians in attendance. One University of Chicago couple set aside a room for the Guru Granth Sahib, the only such facility in the area at the time. According to one local source, the Sikh Study Circle was formed in 1956 and evolved into the Sikh Religious Society of Chicago in 1972.

Professionals, particularly physicians and engineers, dominated the first local wave of post-1965 Sikh immigrants, many of whom eventually settled in the western and northwestern suburbs. As the community grew in numbers in the early 1970s, social/religious gatherings moved from homes to rented facilities such as the Park District center in west suburban Lombard. Once the decision was made to secure a permanent location, debate emerged over whether to renovate an existing structure in Chicago or to locate in one of the suburbs in anticipation of further suburban Sikh settlement. The latter opinion won out, and in 1972 the community purchased an affordable parcel of land in the northwestern suburb of Palatine and

Fig. 10-4. The *gurdwārā* of the Sikh Religious Society of Chicago, Palatine, Illinois, is home to metropolitan Chicago's largest Sikh congregation. Photo by Paul D. Numrich.

began planning construction of a *gurdwārā*. According to one source, ten Sikh individuals (nine medical doctors and a taxi driver) put up $30,000 each to guarantee the mortgage. Groundbreaking took place in 1976; the first services were held in 1979.

The Palatine *gurdwārā*, tucked away unobtrusively in a modest residential area, does not have obviously "religious" architectural features. Reportedly, its Sikh architect sought to express the openness and simplicity of Sikhism through an uncomplicated design.[18] The upstairs *darbar sahib* feels spacious and airy, with glass on all sides. One's attention is drawn toward the front of the room to the *manji sahib,* the canopied place of honor for the Guru Granth Sahib. Around the perimeter of the lower-level *langar* hall one notices striking expressions of Sikh identity and concerns: a display of key events in Sikh history, including graphic photos of the Golden Temple incident and its aftermath; a sign proclaiming Khalistan as the "Sikh Homeland" (Khalistan is a name given to the Punjab region by those seeking an independent Sikh territory); and a list of "Our Gurus," from Guru Nanak to the Guru Granth Sahib.

Recently the Sikh Religious Society began a major fund-raising campaign to expand the Palatine *gurdwārā*. Phase one will see construction of larger facilities to accommodate the *langar* meal. Plans for later phases focus on a new center for the educational program and the library, both currently housed next door to the *gurdwārā* in the chief *granthī*'s residence.

The local Sikh community typifies many of the dynamics of the metropolitan region's Indian immigrant community. A second wave of Sikh immigrants came beginning in the mid- to late 1970s. Today, according to one community source, only spouses, students, asylum seekers, and illegals continue to enter the United States. Clustering especially near Devon Avenue on Chicago's North Side, most of these newest Sikh arrivals differ from the earlier immigrants in socioeconomic status. Thus a bimodal Sikh community has developed, with the more established and better-off professionals living mostly in the western and northwestern suburbs and the less well-off newcomers living mostly in the city. It would not be unusual to hear members of the former group disparage the status of the latter, and members of the latter group begrudge the fortunate circumstances of the former. Due to the dispersed Sikh settlement around the greater metropolitan Chicago region, many in both groups find it either difficult or inconvenient to travel to the Palatine *gurdwārā*. This partially explains the opening of several new *gurdwārā*s in the late 1990s: in the West Rogers Park area of Chicago,

Fig. 10-5. Gurdwara Sahib of Chicago is a Sikh religious center in the space above this carpet store in West Rogers Park, Chicago. Photo by Paul D. Numrich.

serving less affluent North Side Sikhs living around Devon Avenue; in Oak Brook, serving more affluent western suburban Sikhs, for whom the drive to Palatine may take an hour; and in Milwaukee, Wisconsin, and Merrillville, Indiana. In addition, a Sikh *dera* (spiritual mission center) has been established in Island Lake, Lake County, Illinois.

Recent Immigration and Unprecedented Urban Diversity

The three case studies just presented illustrate certain patterns in recent U.S. immigration history and the resulting unprecedented ethnic and religious diversity now found in our largest cities. Prior to World War II, America's immigration "door" stood nearly shut for Asian groups.[19] Relatively small numbers of Asians entered the United States as measures such as the Chinese Exclusion Act (1882), the Gentlemen's Agreement with Japan (1908), the Asiatic Barred Zone (1917), and the Oriental Exclusion Act (1924), as well as Supreme Court decisions denying U.S. citizenship to Asians in the 1920s, effectively served notice that this country did not welcome such groups. The reversal of Chinese exclusion (1943), passage of the War Brides (1945) and McCarran-Walter Acts (1952), and growing civil rights sentiments in the post–World War II period brought a steady, though still relatively small, influx of Asians into the United States. The 1965 Immigration Act (implemented in 1968) opened wide America's immigration door to previously excluded or restricted groups. The number of Indo-Pakistani immigrants, for instance, increased approximately 4,000 percent between 1965 and 1984.[20] The 1990 census counted just over 815,000 Indians and eighty-one thousand Pakistanis in America. Thus, since World War II, and particularly since the 1960s, immigration patterns have been sculpting a "new face" for the American people, significantly less European in its contours than in the classical period of American immigration.

A remarkable socioeconomic diversity characterizes post-1965 immigrant groups. Professionals, technicians, and skilled workers predominated in the early years, as the 1965 act gave preference to such occupations and thus precipitated a "brain drain" of valuable human capital from certain Third World countries. Since the mid-1970s a more occupationally and educationally varied mixture has characterized the immigration flow, especially through "chain migration" of relatives of the earlier immigrants and the influx of large numbers of Southeast Asian refugees after the end of the Vietnam conflict in 1975. The post-1965 wave of

American newcomers, Alejandro Portes and Ruben Rumbaut observe, is far more diverse in origins, motivations for migration, and adaptation strategies than any wave of immigrants in U.S. history.[21] Whereas most immigrants during the classical period entered American society at the lower socioeconomic strata,[22] recent immigrants "cluster bimodally in both blue- and white-collar occupations": "Today's immigrants include first generation millionaires and topflight engineers and scientists; at the other extreme, they also include destitute refugees and undocumented workers."[23] Relatively speaking, Indo-Pakistanis have been a successful group, with many professionals and small-business owners among them, though the latest immigrants include less elite subgroups.

Post-1965 immigrants have tended to settle in America's largest metropolitan regions.[24] Chicago, which typified America's classical immigration, now ranks fourth behind New York City, Los Angeles, and Miami in the total number of recent immigrants received.[25] According to the 1990 census, the top nine Asian groups in the six-county Chicago metropolitan region are Filipinos, Indians, Chinese, Koreans, Japanese, Pakistanis, Vietnamese, Thais, and Cambodians. Chicago ranks second to New York as the preferred urban destination for Indians;[26] it also has a slightly higher ratio of Pakistanis to Indians (about 1:6) than the national ratio (about 1:10).

This new diversity of immigrant groups has created an unprecedented diversity of religions in America's urban areas. Estimates of the numbers of adherents of selected recent immigrant religions are controversial and vary widely depending on the source. Though arguable, the following figures capture the new diversity of religions in metropolitan Chicago:[27] more than three hundred thousand Muslims (making Islam the second-largest religion, slightly ahead of Judaism though still far behind Christianity); 131,000 Buddhists (over half the number of Orthodox Christians in the area); eighty thousand Hindus (more than the number of Anglicans in the Episcopal Diocese of Chicago); five thousand Jains; five thousand Sikhs; and five hundred Zoroastrians. Non-European Christian groups add to the variety. For instance, the majority of the thirty-six thousand Koreans in metropolitan Chicago are Protestants, and the patriarch of the Assyrian Church of the East has established that church's headquarters in Chicago, where a reputed sixty-five thousand adherents now live.[28]

As the foregoing paragraphs imply, the diversity of the recent immigrants creates a complex, interrelated web of social identity according to ethnicity, race, and religion. Taking the Indo-Pakistani case, we note that Pakistani immigrants are predominantly Muslim, though they represent Sunni, Shi`i, and heterodox (e.g., Ahmadiyya) traditions within Islam, while some Pakistanis are Christian. "Hinduism" is the religious tradition of the majority of Indians, though that term only loosely ties together a variety of practices and emphases sharing a religious family resemblance; additionally, India is home to millions of Muslims, Sikhs, Jains, Zoroastrians, and Christians. Indian immigrants in America distinguish themselves according to homeland regional/linguistic provenance and religious tradition. A regional/linguistic group can include several religious traditions (e.g., Gujaratis can be Hindu, Muslim, Jain, or Christian); by the same token, a religious tradition can include several regional/linguistic groups (e.g., Gujarati, Tamil, and Telugu Hindus). Sometimes several regional/linguistic Hindu groups are subsumed under the broader designations "North Indian" and "South Indian" because of shared cultural characteristics.

"Ethnicity" has to do with a "sense of peoplehood [that] rests mainly on such things as language, custom, and the perception of shared ancestry."[29] It is socially constructed and therefore changes as groups migrate from one society to another. The terms *South Asian* and *Indo-Pakistani*, for instance, take on new meaning for immigrants to the United States. Certainly, for Indo-Pakistanis to be subsumed under the label "Asians" and thus lumped together with Southeast and East Asians stems from their newfound American context.

Whether by ethnicity, race, or religion, most recent immigrant groups occupy a minority position in America and thus face the prejudice and discrimination, both actual and potential, that continue to characterize U.S. society. The largest and most visible of the non-Christian religions practiced by the recent immigrants—Buddhism, Hinduism, Islam, Sikhism—suffer from generally poor public images.[30] A recent national survey, for instance, ranked Buddhism and Islam just after atheism and Scientology as the most negative influences on American society.[31] Despite their collective socioeconomic success as a recent immigrant group, South Asians still face personal harassment and vocational "glass ceilings,"[32] which may stem largely from public ambiguity over the racial identity of South Asians. A U.S. Supreme Court decision in the 1920s ruled that although Indians may technically be Caucasians, they were not "White" under U.S. law and thus not eligible for either citizenship or land ownership. A 1978 national survey showed that 11 percent of respondents saw Indians as White, 15 percent as Black, 23 percent as Brown, 38 percent as Other, and 13 percent did not know what race Indians were.[33] In 1993 the Illinois Chapter of the Association of Indians in America established a Council on Education and Legal Defense to deal with incidents of prejudice and discrimination.

Minority status and other dynamics of post–World War II urban restructuring help explain the prolific differentiation of recent immigrant religious centers according to ethnic, subethnic, and sectarian religious identities. A notable fact about metropolitan Chicago's recent immigrant religious centers is that most serve single-ethnic constituencies, that is, one ethnic group comprises more than 80 percent of the congregation. Yen Le Espiritu and Ivan Light summarize the situation on a general level:

> Partially as a result of urban restructuring, . . . America's immigrants confront a more complex political, economic, and social landscape than did earlier generations of immigrants. These complex and often threatening conditions encourage them to band together around common linguistic and cultural identities in order to influence their life chances and living conditions.[34]

Even more than during the classical period of predominantly European immigration, immigrant institutions today perform vital functions vis-à-vis the larger society. They serve as safe havens from antagonisms of minority daily life and often stand "over against" the majority society, offering social criticism of American values and behaviors—Hindus criticize the individualism, Muslims the moral breakdown of American society, for instance. But at the same time these institutions help broker an advantageous relationship between their constituents and the larger society. As Williams explains:

> The formation of religious groups by immigrants, even those with the most narrowly conceived ethnic or hierarchical boundaries, do [*sic*] not function primarily to separate persons from the rest of the population, but rather to provide the necessary basis on which the individual and group can negotiate effective relations with the majority population as variously defined.[35]

Coalitions for a variety of purposes have arisen among the recent immigrant groups, though success has been uneven. For instance, several religious groups have sponsored the local Asian American Coalition and the Parliament of the World's Religions (the latter held in Chicago in 1993). Intrafaith coalitions include the Buddhist Council of the Midwest and the Council of Islamic Organizations of Greater Chicago. Many population groups remain isolated, however, either unwilling or unable to forge relationships with other groups. As we attempted to compile comprehensive lists of religious centers, it appeared that even within a single ethnic population, one religious segment was unaware of (or unwilling to identify) other religious segments.

Siting of Recent Immigrant Religious Centers

Map 10 plots the sites of religious centers serving eighty-nine predominantly Indian and Indo-Pakistani congregations in the six-county Chicago metropolitan region, broken out by religious identity (Muslim, Christian, Hindu, etc.).[36] The map reveals much about the dynamics involved in the siting of recent immigrant religious centers.

One-third (thirty of eighty-nine) of the religious centers are located within the city limits of Chicago (break-out portion of Map 10). Distribution across the city is highly circumscribed, with centers found in only twelve of Chicago's seventy-seven "community areas" and significant clustering of centers found only on the city's North Side. Their placement typically shadows Asian settlement patterns—ten of the twelve community areas contain more than fifteen hundred Asian residents each—and typically avoids the predominantly Black areas on Chicago's South and West Sides, continuing immigration trends from the 1960s and 1970s.[37] Nevertheless, five of the twelve community areas now have a Black population of 20 percent or more, mostly as a result of simultaneous Black in-migration to immigrant port-of-entry areas. Moreover, nine of the twelve areas have a combined Black and Hispanic population of 20 percent or more. A striking example is Rogers Park, discussed in chapter 6. These facts point to an important shift in settlement patterns among recent immigrant groups, namely, their growing inability to avoid the traditional American minority areas of the city. Also, markedly larger percentages of the Muslim (about half) and Christian (more than one-third) centers are found within the city limits of Chicago than is the case with other Indian (Hindu, Sikh, etc.) religious centers (about 10 percent).

Turning to the suburban centers (Map 10), comprising two-thirds of the metropolitan total, we find that the great majority cluster in two of the region's six counties (Cook and DuPage). Siting generally shadows recent immigrant settlement preferences for predominantly White north-

TABLE 1

Congregations per Religious Group Meeting in Areas
above/below Regional Median Family-Income Level
*Community Areas of Chicago and Suburbs**

Group	City: #Above	City: #Below	Suburbs: #Above	Suburbs: #Below
Indian Christian	0	10	16	3
Indian Hindu, Sikh, etc.	1	2	19	3
Indo-Pakistani Muslim	2	15	12	6
Other Muslim	2	5	1	2
Buddhist	5	12	9	3
Totals	10	44	57	17

* Income figures reported in Chicago Fact Book Consortium, *Local Community Fact Book,*
1990; the regional median family-income level for 1990 was $42,292.

ern and western suburban areas over predominantly Black suburbs, again continuing trends from the 1960s and 1970s.[38] Nevertheless, as with the situation in the city of Chicago, we also see an increasing inability of recent immigrant groups to avoid settling in traditionally American minority areas, indicated by the fact that four suburbs with a Black population of 20 percent or more and eleven suburbs with a combined Black and Hispanic population of 20 percent or more have Indo-Pakistani religious centers. At the same time, unlike the situation in the city of Chicago, where the religious centers largely perpetuate the classical model of "neighborhood" or "parish" institutions that normally serve surrounding residential communities, the diffuse settlement and increased mobility of suburban immigrant populations have given rise to several "commuter" religious centers that draw much (sometimes virtually all) of their congregations from outside the municipalities in which they are located. Less than half (thirteen of thirty-one) of the suburban municipalities with large Asian populations (more than 1,500) have Indo-Pakistani religious centers; conversely, fifteen suburban municipalities with very small Asian populations (less than 250) do have Indo-Pakistani centers—obviously, such centers draw "commuter" congregations. We note again here that Indo-Pakistani Christians and Muslims lag behind fellow ethnics (Hindus, Sikhs, etc.) in establishing religious centers in the suburbs.

Indications of the socioeconomic status of the various religious groups may be seen in Tables 1 and 2. Two additional religious groups—"other" immigrant Muslims (namely, non-Indo-Pakistanis) and immigrant Buddhists—have been added to the analysis for comparative purposes.

Table 1 shows the number of congregations in each religious group that meet in locations either above or below the regional median family-income

TABLE 2

Suburban Congregations per Religious Group
*Meeting in Desirable Municipalities**

Group	Total Congregations	#Desirable	%Desirable
Indian Christian	19	9	47%
Indian Hindu, Sikh, etc.	22	12	55%
Indo-Pakistani Muslim	18	7	39%
Other Muslim	3	1	33%
Buddhist	12	7	58%
Totals	74	36	49%

* A "desirable" municipality has both an income above the regional median level (see Table 1) and a crime rate lower than the median rate for all regional municipalities. Crime-rate data from *Chicago Regional Report*, which does not disaggregate the rates for Chicago's seventy-seven community areas.

level, broken out by community areas of the city of Chicago and suburban municipalities. For virtually all groups, regardless of religious identity, the tendency for suburban centers to be located in higher-income areas and city centers to be located in lower-income areas is dramatically evident. Religious identity appears to be salient in the Muslim case, where the percentage of centers in higher-income areas, particularly in the suburbs, lags markedly behind other groups, including fellow ethnics in the case of Indo-Pakistani Muslims vis-à-vis Indians of other religions.

Table 2 focuses exclusively on the suburbs and provides a caveat against a simplistic dichotomization of city versus suburban conditions. Overall, less than half of the suburban groups meet in municipalities that qualify as "desirable" in terms of both income and safety from crime. Religious identity appears to have salience here again: Muslims lag significantly behind the other groups, Indo-Pakistani Muslims behind their fellow ethnics.

The foregoing discussion illuminates the interrelation of recent immigrant religions and the post–World War II restructuring of the Chicago metropolitan region. Ethnic residential enclavism, characteristic of the classical period of American immigration,[39] has given way to a socioeconomically determined, bimodal geography, as poorer, less assimilated, and less successful immigrants cluster in depressed and transitional metropolitan areas, while better-off, more assimilated, and more successful immigrants gravitate to attractive city locations or disperse throughout exurbia.[40] This typifies "the widening 'social divide' [that] is a striking feature of the post-industrial metropolis."[41] Significantly, this "social divide" includes ethnoreligious features. Bluntly stated, in the Indo-Pakistani case, one's chances of worshiping in a desirable area of the city or suburbs increase in roughly the following sequence: from Muslim to Christian to Hindu, Sikh, and so forth.

Some observations about facilities elaborate this analysis. Most recent immigrant congregations rent or rehabilitate existing facilities to serve as religious centers, a practice also followed by some classical immigrant groups.[42] The variety of converted places—for example, homes, apartments, businesses, schools, churches—reveals both the dynamics of urban restructuring and the practical constraints on these religious groups when securing suitable facilities. Recent Christian immigrants offer an interesting variation on the theme of facility adaptation. Like their non-Christian counterparts, these groups typically cannot yet afford to erect new buildings. As Christians, however, they share the religious identity of the majority in American society, which provides an option typically unavailable to non-Christian congregations: renting a facility from an Anglo-Christian congregation. Fox Valley Muslim Community Center in far west suburban Kane County provides an exception; it rented space from a Christian church. After several years it constructed its own mosque.

In post–World War II metropolitan regions like Chicago, where land is at a premium and construction costs are considerable, erecting a new religious facility, particularly in an Old World architectural style, has become the prerogative of the successful and thus a less realistic dream for many groups than it was during the classical period of American immigration. Very few "cathedrals," new structures whose architectures carry Old World religio-symbolic power, serve the recent immigrants of metropolitan Chicago or attract regional pilgrims. For instance, local immigrant Buddhists have erected only one such structure and immigrant Muslims, four (two of them Indo-Pakistani), whereas non-Christian Indian religious groups (Hindus, Sikhs, etc.) have been proportionally more productive, with as many as six already completed and two more under construction. Of all these "cathedrals," only one is located within the city limits of Chicago, a Japanese Buddhist temple built in 1971 in fashionable, affluent Lincoln Park. Assuming that the urban "social divide" continues to widen, many recent immigrant religious centers will remain in impoverished metropolitan areas. Upward social mobility and geographic relocation to attractive neighborhoods, whether city or exurban, are not inevitable for all recent immigrant groups or subgroups.

Conclusion

As this chapter demonstrates, Chicago's recent immigrant religions follow many patterns from the classical period of American immigration. Through cultural celebrations, religious activities, and educational and other programming, the newest religious centers preside over the transplantation and transformation of Old World traditions. In so doing, these centers perpetuate ethnically, racially, or religiously distinct identities even more prolifically than did their classical European counterparts. Today's Indo-Pakistani mosque is analogous to the classical Italian Roman Catholic parish, that is, a particular ethnonational expression of a major religion. Likewise, today's Indian regional/linguistic Hindu temples are analogous to German provincial Protestant churches (i.e., Old World parochial variations of a single national religion), while today's Jain temples and Sikh *gurdwārās* are analogous to Polish Roman Catholic churches and Jewish synagogues, respectively (i.e., distinct major religions within a single ethnonational group). A significant departure from such differentiation is found in ecumenically minded congregations such as The Hindu Temple of Greater Chicago and Muslim Community Center, though as we have seen, the ecumenical ideal is not easily realized.

A crucial difference between the experience of the recent immigrant religions and that of the classical period stems from post–World War II urban restructuring. The arrival of the recent immigrants both coincided with and contributed to the new urban context in the latter half of the twentieth century. These immigrants constitute the primary source of the new ethnic, racial, and religious diversity of America's metropolitan regions, and their social bimodalism, patterns of residential settlement, and siting of religious centers have participated in the latest transformation of Chicago and other large American cities. In this sense the recent immigrants share more with their contemporaries in the majority society than did previous immigrant groups.

The evolution of immigrant enclavism is most striking. Classically, Swedes, Italians, Jews, and others formed relatively distinct ethnoreligious neighborhoods within the city of Chicago or in certain suburbs, and when one group moved to a different area, another group occupied its territory and converted its religious centers. It took decades for most classical groups to disperse throughout the metropolitan region; in the Italian case, this did not occur until after World War II.[43] It appears that ethnicity per se no longer constitutes the most salient factor in immigrant enclavism. Rather, socioeconomic status now seems most salient, even though socioeconomic status includes variables of ethnoreligious identity (as seen, for instance, in the geographic distribution of religious centers within the Indo-Pakistani group). Today, well-off groups or subgroups occupy desirable areas while the less well-off cluster in poorer areas of the city of Chicago and in certain suburbs. Classical, neighborhood-type immigrant religious centers can still be found, mostly in the city, but now many exurban commuter-type religious centers serve widely scattered and mobile immigrant congregations. Centers of both types have followed the classical pattern of occupying the facilities of previous religious groups, but only in rare instances, mostly in well-off exurban locations and among certain religious groups, have recent immigrant congregations been able to construct new religious facilities according to Old World architectural models.

An ever-widening gap between America's rich and poor cuts across the entire society, including recent immigrant groups.[44] As Robert Manning and Anita Butera observe, "The old urban centers . . . are becoming increasingly populated by disadvantaged native minorities and recent immigrants who lack the necessary social and human capital for negotiating the more favorable terrain of the suburban economy."[45] Prosperous areas remain few, while many other areas see prosperity receding from sight. America's newest religious immigrants are like their classical predecessors in important ways, yet their experience also differs due to the great "social divide" of the new metropolis where they now live.

NOTES

Some ideas and wording in this chapter previously appeared in Numrich, "Recent Immigrant Religions in a Restructuring Metropolis: New Religious Landscapes in Chicago," *Journal of Cultural Geography* 17, 1.

1. See Park and Miller, *Old World Traits Transplanted;* Handlin, *The Uprooted;* Herberg, *Protestant-Catholic-Jew;* Bodnar, *The Transplanted;* Fenton, *Transplanting Religious Traditions;* Numrich, *Old Wisdom.* Portes and Rumbaut, *Immigrant Americans,* 144, point out the shared etymology of *travel* and *travail.* The term *recent* refers to post–World War II waves of immigrants, particularly those coming since the 1965 Immigration Act. "Classical" immigrants include both the "old" immigrant waves (predominantly northern European and Protestant, up to 1880) and the "new" immigrant waves (largely southern and eastern European, and Roman Catholic, Orthodox Christian, and Jewish, from 1880 to 1924).

2. On the interrelation of recent immigration and urban restructuring, but without consideration of religion, see, e.g., Soja, Morales, and Wolff, "Urban Restructuring"; Waldinger, "Immigration"; Manning and Butera, "From City to Suburbia."

3. The U.S. Immigration and Naturalization Service has counted Indians and Pakistanis separately since 1973, but ethnic studies often conflate them into a single category of "Indo-Pakistanis."

4. Williams, *Religions of Immigrants* and *Sacred Thread*.

5. Rangaswamy, "Asian Indians," 449.

6. Williams, *Religions of Immigrants*, 229.

7. Ibid., 231–33.

8. Rangaswamy, "Asian Indians," 450. Also, on 448, she reports: "Many Indians feel that groupism is far more pronounced in Chicago [than in other U.S. cities] but are at a loss to explain why this is so."

9. Williams, *Religions of Immigrants*, 229.

10. Eck, *Darsan*, 62–63.

11. Some media commentators assumed immediately that the April 1995 bombing of a federal facility in Oklahoma City represented the work of Muslim extremists.

12. Dusenbery, "Introduction."

13. La Brack, *Sikhs of Northern California*, 421.

14. Indian government troops and militant Sikh partisans engaged in a violent confrontation at the Golden Temple in Amritsar. A few months later, Prime Minister Indira Gandhi was assassinated by her Sikh bodyguards.

15. Cf. Williams, *Religions of Immigrants*, 81, 240.

16. Helweg, "Sikh Diaspora," 80.

17. Sikhism's tenth and last historical Guru (Teacher) established the Khalsa (the "Pure"), a status conferred by initiation and characterized by adoption of the surnames Singh (males) or Kaur (females) as well as distinguishing personal marks known as the five Ks: *kesh* (uncut hair, which males cover with a turban), *kanghā* (comb), *karā* (bracelet), *kachhā* (a certain kind of undershorts), and *kirpān* (ceremonial sword).

18. Williams, *Religions of Immigrants*, 240. Our own source pointed out that the congregation gave the architect a free hand in designing the facility because he did so without charge.

19. Reimers offers this useful metaphor in *Still the Golden Door*.

20. Minocha, "South Asian Immigrants," 348–350.

21. Portes and Rumbaut, *Immigrant Americans*, 6–8.

22. Bodnar, *The Transplanted*, 170.

23. Espiritu and Light, "Changing Ethnic Shape," 36, 42; see Rumbaut, "Passages to America," 225, 228.

24. Waldinger, "Immigration and Urban Change," 211.

25. Fuchs, *American Kaleidoscope,* 296–304; Portes and Rumbaut, *Immigrant America,* 36.

26. Portes and Rumbaut, *Immigrant America,* 37.

27. These are 1997 self-estimates reported by the Chicago and Northern Illinois Region of the National Conference for Community and Justice, formerly the National Conference of Christians and Jews.

28. Galloway, "Place to Call Home."

29. Becker, "Ethnicity and Religion," 1477; Conzen et al., "Invention of Ethnicity."

30. E.g., Williams, *Religions of Immigrants,* 290; Haddad, ed., *Muslims of America,* 3.

31. Dart, "Most View Christians."

32. Minocha, "South Asian Immigrants," 363.

33. Takaki, *Strangers;* Xenos, Barringer, and Levin, *Asian Indians.*

34. Espiritu and Light, "Changing Ethnic Shape," 49–50.

35. Williams, *Sacred Thread,* 255.

36. We adopt the generic term *religious center,* i.e., a particular place where a congregation gathers regularly for religious activities, in order to avoid imperialistic use of one group's term (e.g., church) to refer to other groups' sacred places (e.g., temple, mosque, *gurdwārā*). The term *congregation,* defined as "a local, religious association of people" (cf. Wind, *Places of Worship,* xvii), has gained acceptance beyond its initial Judeo-Christian context, though to be sure, temples, mosques, etc., in America do not always function like classical American churches or synagogues. We have not considered size—whether of membership or programming—when including particular religious centers in our tally, but we have excluded special-purpose groups and centers with one-dimensional programming, such as Muslim Student Associations and Friday Islamic prayer places. Note that the eighty-nine total represents the number of *congregations* in our study; the number of *religious centers* is slightly less, due to some congregational sharing of centers.

37. Carlson, "Settling of Asian Immigrant Groups."

38. Ibid.

39. E.g., Pacyga and Skerrett, *Chicago;* Holli and Jones, eds., *Ethnic Chicago,* 3rd and 4th eds.

40. Waldinger, "Immigration and Urban Change"; Espiritu and Light, "Changing Ethnic Shape."

41. Manning and Butera, "From City to Suburbia."

42. Pacyga and Skerrett, *Chicago;* Cutler, *Jews of Chicago.*

43. Candeloro, "Chicago's Italians."

44. Cf. Hirt, "Shifts in Labor Market."

45. Manning and Butera, "From City to Suburbia."

Map 11. The Roman Catholic Archdiocese of Chicago, with more than two million people, is the largest religious body in metropolitan Chicago. Map by Brian Twardosz, BMT Printing and Cartographic Specialists.

Catholic Planning for a Multicultural Metropolis, 1982–1996

Peter R. D'Agostino

A sadness fell over Chicago with the death of Cardinal-Archbishop Joseph Bernardin (1982–1996). Although a principal architect of the postconciliar Catholic Church on the national level, Bernardin also oversaw a host of local (archdiocesan) reforms. These addressed familiar characteristics of late-twentieth-century America such as deindustrialization, multiculturalism, and the shift of power from city neighborhoods to suburbs. The planning processes and institutional changes enacted during Bernardin's episcopacy, although sometimes the source of conflict, became a model for other dioceses. This chapter describes and interprets the normative vision of the local church that drove the reforms enacted during Bernardin's tenure. I construct this vision through a narrative of institutional changes and an analysis of explanations offered to legitimate change. I describe this vision as a process ecclesiology.

This chapter's archdiocesan analysis complements the ethnographic studies of congregations and parishes presented in the rest of this book, at a time when Catholic authorities beyond the reach of congregations are closing parishes and schools. These closings have profound implications for education, politics, and ethnoracial developments in urban America. Church authorities beyond the parish have baptized multiculturalism as the normative ideology of American and Catholic identity, transforming the design of parish programs and shaping interparish dynamics in new ways.

Although not readily apparent to the ethnographer immersed in a rich congregational universe, Catholic parishes increasingly reconstitute archdiocesan organizations and reforms, and they are increasingly forced to work across parish boundaries on terms established by the archdiocese. In other words, the archdiocese both limits and facilitates parochial initiatives. It is what sociologist Anthony Giddens and historian William Sewell call a deep structure.[1] To describe contemporary urban parishes without reference to it is to analyze words without a grammar. We have, of course, learned a great deal about the Archdiocese of Chicago from our ethnographic analysis within parishes. However, the Religion and Urban America Program realized, and this chapter demonstrates, that an understanding of public religion and urban transformation, particularly in Chicago, is greatly illuminated by an analysis of the Archdiocese's process ecclesiology.

By a process ecclesiology I mean the permanent integration of a dynamism of adaptation into the church at all levels of organization. Bernardin's reforms promoted awareness of interdependence among Catholic institutions and people. This consciousness, cultivated through cooperative planning, culminated in institutional reforms made in a dialectic with the larger environment, which itself was always in flux. Bernardin and his coworkers in relevant archdiocesan agencies—planners or "experts"—hoped the church would institutionalize adaptation to the changing realities of modern life, as it simultaneously mobilized its material, social, and spiritual resources to transform society.

Bernardin's reforms diverged from many local traditions. Both the reorganization of the Archdiocese's administration, governance, and ecclesial geography and the theology of structural reforms challenged Chicago's Catholics. To demonstrate the innovative character and limits of Bernardin's fourteen-year episcopacy, I give a brief analysis of the Archdiocese's planning processes, elementary school reforms, and rethinking of the normative relationship between faith and culture.

The Archdiocese of Chicago and the Myth of Chicago Catholicism

The size and history of the Archdiocese of Chicago are daunting. At the end of 1995, the Archdiocese was a geographic space of 1,411 square miles; a political space identical to Lake and Cook Counties in the state of Illinois; an ecclesial space comprising 6 vicariates, 25 deaneries, and 377 parishes; and a complex organization including the Pastoral Center at the hub, 46 cemeteries, 200 operational units of Catholic Charities, 19

Catholic hospitals, 6 Catholic colleges and universities, 377 parishes, 281 elementary schools, 48 high schools, 3 archdiocesan seminaries, and the nation's largest theologate—the Catholic Theological Union. In terms of personnel, the Archdiocese was composed of Bernardin, 7 auxiliary bishops, 988 diocesan priests, 861 religious priests in residence, 457 religious brothers in residence, 3,574 women religious in residence, 587 deacons, 148 pastoral associates (which included some deacons and religious), a total of 6,664 teachers and administrators in the school system, and 4,719 employees of Catholic Charities. There were 18,876 employees of the Catholic archbishop of Chicago, not including those employed at Catholic hospitals and universities. The total population of the Archdiocese was 5,712,000, which included a Catholic population of 2,342,000 of which 62 percent was White (non-Hispanic), 31 percent Hispanic, 4 percent African American, and 3 percent Asian.[2]

These numbers only hint at the pluralism embedded in its many regional, ethnic, clerical, and class subcultures. Thus the Archdiocese has a strong, "thick," multifaceted personality. The shared stories, personalities, movements, and buildings that Chicagoans, American Catholics, and scholars associate with the Archdiocese of Chicago suggest it readily becomes a multivalent symbol. Communities of memory transform the Archdiocese of Chicago into a corporate personality, which I shall call Chicago Catholicism.[3]

The Archdiocese of Chicago transformed by memory and values into Chicago Catholicism functions as a myth. The myth tells the story of tight-knit neighborhoods and struggles of proud ethnic groups for local democracy, land ownership, and political clout. Within the myth, the parish-school plant symbolizes the neighborhood community. It embodies, protects, and dramatizes the values of the neighborhood as it bridges generations of neighborhood residents. The parish-school plant marks urban boundaries, brings order out of chaotic urban space, and gives each neighborhood a distinctive history and name recognizable throughout the metropolitan area. The myth has a normative dimension that preserves the history of the Archdiocese of Chicago in selective ways. Deviations from the myth generate resistance. Thus some Chicagoans assert that every parish once had a school, that every Catholic child attended that school, and therefore, that every parish ought to maintain a school today. Bernardin tried to portray aspects of his reform in continuity with the myth. But pan-parochial planning and alternatives to powerful parochial loyalties met resistance from many

Catholics who were mourning the loss of urban parishes and schools intimately associated with memories of family and community.[4]

Bernardin arrived as an outsider to Chicago Catholicism. Born and raised in Columbia, South Carolina, by immigrants from northeastern Italy, his experiences had been administrative, as auxiliary bishop in Atlanta and as a formative figure in the National Conference of Catholic Bishops. Although he had been the bishop of Cincinnati from 1972 to 1982, a large, deindustrialized, heterogeneous city such as Chicago was new to him. In contrast to his twentieth-century predecessors, Bernardin was not Roman-trained and did not have an authoritarian or autocratic style of leadership. He came to Chicago as a healer to reinvigorate an archdiocese and city that had become disenchanted, with charges of corruption and insensitivity aimed at his predecessor.

Administration, Governance, and Geography

Upon his installation on August 25, 1982, Bernardin oversaw reforms in the administration, governance, and ecclesial geography of the Archdiocese. In December 1982, Bernardin appointed an Administrative Reorganization Advisory Committee to review the organizational structure of the archdiocesan Chancery Office (renamed the Pastoral Center). To delegate authority and promote greater coordination and fiscal efficiency, he consolidated sixty-nine agencies and offices into six departments: Evangelization and Christian Life, Financial Services, Human Services, Ministry Formation, Personnel Services, and Communications and Development.

In March 1985 the Archdiocesan Pastoral Council (APC) held its first regular meeting. Established to receive input from parishes and regions throughout the Archdiocese, the APC had four standing committees with forty-six voting members, 67 percent of whom were laypeople. The APC served as a consultative body to the archbishop. In this way the APC legitimized consolidations and closings of parishes and schools. In 1986, the Presbyteral Senate also formed a task force on consolidations, which the cardinal consulted, as required by canon law. Bernardin oversaw the creation of parish councils, made mandatory by 1990, which were necessary to integrate parishes into archdiocesan long-range planning processes. In January 1988 only 65 percent of the Archdiocese's parishes had a parish council, and only 30 percent of the councils operated according to archdiocesan guidelines. An Office for Parish Councils provided workshops to train parishioners on the theology of parish councils.

By January 1984 the Archdiocese was divided into six territorial vicariates (see map 11), each under an auxiliary bishop acting as an episcopal vicar. Each vicariate included deaneries—whose number rose from twelve to twenty-five by 1995—with a representative pastor serving as dean. Within each deanery, clusters were formed from groups of geographic parishes whose priests or lay representatives met to discuss common concerns. This new ecclesial map encouraged parishes operating in similar urban environments to identify common problems, compare solutions, and form common local strategies. This permitted urban problems to be addressed regionally rather than either parochially—where resources were scarce and knowledge was limited—or on the archdiocesan level, which seemed distant or insensitive to local residents. In this sense, geographic reorganization was both a delegation of authority and decision making from the center to the periphery and a loss of parish autonomy. Furthermore, to the extent that local entities were compelled to meet and plan, one could argue these reforms represented a type of episcopal authority imposed in an indirect bureaucratic manner, rather than through a traditional monarchical personal-command structure.

These ecclesial units—vicariates, deaneries, clusters—were by no means symmetrical in terms of size, resources, or character. They exhibited a variety of levels of cooperation, planning, cohesion, and trust. Ethnicity, race, neighborhood traditions, and leadership qualities conditioned their operation. Many pastors knew little of or actively resisted cooperation and planning within these units. In fact, some pastors generated and maintained parish identity and solidarity by defining themselves against the Pastoral Center as a beleaguered congregation protecting itself against an uncaring "bureaucracy." In contrast, one West Side cluster had a long tradition of lay involvement and activism. Lay representatives from cluster parishes had been meeting for twenty years to discuss common public concerns, and the parishes in that cluster had joint Lenten services. Reforms built on local traditions were more likely to succeed.

These reforms required episcopal reinforcements to man each vicariate. On December 13, 1983, four new bishops were consecrated to Chicago to join the two existing auxiliaries. These appointments reflected sensitivity to the cultural geography of the Archdiocese. The importance of bonds forged between bishops and Catholics of the same race or ethnicity could either weaken or strengthen the territorial identities of the vicariate system. Thus, from 1983 until his reassignment to the Diocese of Belleville, Bishop Wilton Gregory, an African American, was the vicar of the South Side of Chicago (vicariate 6), which included a high proportion of African American residents (69 percent in 1995). Those residents often articulated the idea of a Black Catholic Church on the South Side of Chicago that had its own bishop, in spite of Bishop Gregory's self-proclaimed commitment to be a bishop for all Chicagoans. From 1983 until his reassignment to the Diocese of Lubeck, Bishop Placido Rodriguez was the episcopal vicar of the Near West Side (vicariate 3, 46 percent Hispanic in 1995), which included the overwhelmingly Mexican Pilsen and Little Village neighborhoods. Like the African American Catholics in regard to Bishop Gregory, Hispanics throughout Chicago thought of Bishop Rodriguez as their bishop.

Planning: Modernization and Legitimation

The reforms described above facilitated strategic planning at every level of church organization. Strategic planning, in Bernardin's vision, was the means whereby the corporate reflection of "the people of God" would emerge. While planning embodied the Catholic principle of subsidiarity, it also legitimated change. The reforms of the administration, governance, and geography of the Archdiocese coincided with highly publicized controversial closings and consolidations of schools and parishes. In this conflictual context, the cardinal promoted planning as a type of religious activity, a devotion of the new people of God to discern God's will.

John A. Grindel's work helps us understand how planning linked to institutional change was a religious activity. Grindel describes a pastoral circle with four parts: insertion, social analysis, theological reflection, and pastoral planning, which leads back to insertion to complete the circle. The first moment of the circle, insertion into the individual and corporate Catholic experience, begins with the thoughts and feelings of Catholics, who go on to share and analyze their experiences. Through theological reflection, Catholics understand those experiences in the light of their "faith, Scripture, church teaching and the resources of tradition." Finally, pastoral planning involves designing an effective short- and long-term plan. In a similar way, Bernardin hoped the Archdiocese would internalize this pastoral circle, creating a dynamic organization in a constant process of renewal. Grindel describes the process as a circle because it "must be gone through again and again. Every time a pastoral plan is implemented it gives rise to another set of experiences which once again must be analyzed and reflected on in order to do further pastoral planning." Grindel warns that social analysis enters "into the realm of controversy," and "any analysis is implicitly linked to some ideological tradition." Thus part of the process requires "conversion," the explication of values one brings to social analysis.[5]

In the Archdiocese planning was conceived as a corporate devotion implemented to discover the mission of the church and to transform Catholics. In 1986, archdiocesan Personnel Services director Father J. Cletus Kiley asked:

> What is the mission of this Church? What does it mean to be a Roman Catholic in Cook and Lake County? . . . One of the fears that a lot of us have is we are using management language and we are a Church, not a business. The challenge is to take the best that management has learned and remember to keep our identity as a people of God with a spiritual mission. . . .
>
> We don't know the future. We see trends, we use sociology or whatever. . . . But at the same time there is always room for the Spirit. It's the blending the two, spirituality and science. In management they talk about "organizational transformation." We're using the word "conversion." Business uses the word "good management." We talk about "stewardship."[6]

In 1988, Bernardin published a four-part series in *Chicago Catholic,* the archdiocesan weekly, titled "Why Do We Need to Plan?" in which he linked planning to the core of the church's mission. When "wave upon wave of immigrants" constituted the church, national parishes were "a good and effective approach to pastoral needs," Bernardin noted. He went on to say, however, that they also "tended to go their separate ways, fragmenting the archdiocese. People thought of themselves more as parishioners of a particular parish than as members of the larger church. A certain degree of parochialism or congregationalism set in, and it is still present." Bernardin reasoned that since "we are no longer primarily an immigrant church, . . . the church's mission has changed." In light of demographic changes, "the archdiocese has no choice but to be a careful manager of all its resources—facilities, finances and, especially, personnel. . . . Planning . . . is increasingly becoming a fact of life in the archdiocese."[7] Bernardin believed the situation had reached crisis proportions: "To be candid, the number of parishes in need of archdiocesan assistance, as well as the number of parishes merely breaking even, is somewhat alarming." The financial crisis "make[s] . . . planning essential. Otherwise, there will continue to be an unwise and inequitable allocation and distribution of archdiocesan resources."[8]

Bernardin connected planning with the idea of just, responsible stewardship. "Within the archdiocese in the past, planning has often been somewhat informal, sporadic or local. However, we can no longer afford to proceed with business as usual." Finally, he addressed the larger issue of Catholic identity and its relationship to planning:

> Perhaps the greatest challenge of all is to expand our personal concept of what it means to be a Catholic, to belong to a church that extends beyond our own parish. . . . An authentic theology of the church underlies this concept, however, and it must be reflected in all our pastoral efforts.[9]

His theological reflections on a postconciliar Catholic identity challenged the operative myth of Chicago Catholicism and troubled many Chicago Catholics. Some associated the requirements to participate in planning with a subterfuge to legitimate parish closings. Planning generated suspicion and, in some cases, instigated resistance.

Bernardin had planted the seeds for a permanent process of self-evaluation in his 1985 pastoral letter "In Service of One Another." In November 1986 the cardinal's cabinet distributed *Criteria for Parish Planning and Evaluation,* endorsed by the Presbyteral Senate, which established guidelines for parish self-evaluation. The guidelines included references to distances between parishes (no more than two miles, not less than one-half mile), population (registered families should not exceed three thousand nor dip beneath three hundred in number), ministerial personnel, religious formation and education, and parish finances. Parish planning in the Archdiocese culminated in a program called Tomorrow's Parish, first implemented in 1992 and henceforth required of all parishes. Bernardin's archdiocesan planning process, completed in 1994, culminated in the publication of *Decisions for the Future of our Church.*

Tomorrow's Parish, in theory a nine-month planning process, was implemented in 1992 by twenty-nine parishes and was required of all parishes by 1998. It was designed to create a three- to five-year plan. The materials the Office of Research and Planning provided to implement Tomorrow's Parish offered detailed but flexible criteria that a planning team used to reflect on its parish. These criteria related to ministerial life—spirituality, human concerns, education, parish life—and planning—ministerial personnel, demographics, religious education, finances. Once this assessment was complete, the parish council and pastor implemented changes to realize their vision for the parish. The process allowed for input from parishioners, neighboring parishes, and deanery, vicariate, and archdiocesan representatives. It was meant to be a prayerful as well as a sociological experience, one that promoted greater awareness among active participants of all dimensions of parish life. Archdiocesan planners hoped to see each parish go through this planning process every five years, thus entering a permanent cycle of reflection on identity and mission that would strengthen the parish and perpetually reintegrate it into its ecclesial and social environments.[10]

Before the cardinal's death, the Archdiocese completed the initial stages of an archdiocesan strategic-planning process. In the spring of 1993, Bernardin identified two priorities: (1) evangelization and education and (2) ministerial leadership. With input from two writing teams that consulted with more than eight thousand Catholics, the cardinal put forth *Decisions for the Future of Our Church* in the spring of 1994 and appointed a committee that published a five-year *Decisions Implementation Plan,* with concrete goals based on a financial assessment.[11]

Decisions for the Future of Our Church acknowledged a break with Chicago Catholicism. In *Decisions,* Bernardin emphasized the need to overcome strictly parochial commitments in order to develop cooperation and collaboration across territorial and ethnic and racial boundaries:

> We belong to a universal Church whose teaching and experience we must respect. We are not a "congregational" church. . . . Each of our parishes and institutions is part of the local Church we call the Archdiocese. They do not exist in isolation. Planning for the future requires a greater degree of collaboration and sharing than has been our custom in the past.

The document anticipated further restructuring of deaneries to define them by "natural groupings [which] will make it easier to plan collaboratively for the promotion of the Church's primary mission of evangelization, of which its educational mission is an integral part." While Bernardin promoted collaboration across territorial and ethnic and racial boundaries, he also insisted on the maintenance of traditional structures, particularly schools for all Catholics and the urban poor. Thus, Bernardin asserted the value of regional or consolidated schools—a school for more than one parish—but he agreed that the "*parochial* nature of our elementary schools must be maintained." Thus he broke from Chicago Catholicism's traditional parish-school unit but hoped to harness its spiritual, social, and material capital for his innovation.[12]

Tomorrow's Parish and *Decisions* followed the financial crisis that had culminated in extensive parish and parish school closings. According to Thomas J. Gannon, S.J., and David F. Schwartz, the financial crisis grew out of "a large and continuing increase in grants to parishes; higher costs of labor and employee benefits, specifically medical benefits; and rising operational costs for parish and archdiocesan buildings." In 1989 parish operating revenues fell $26.3 million short of expenses, and the Pastoral Center incurred a $20.8 million deficit. Nearly two-thirds of the Archdiocese's parishes were unable to meet expenses from income. The parochial schools' average collective deficit from 1987 to 1992 was $68 million, a sum historically paid from excess parish income.[13] Bernardin took steps to raise funds and cut budgets, including administrative cutbacks for the Pastoral Center. Since 1986, twenty-seven parishes had already been closed or consolidated. By June 1990 an additional twenty-eight parishes, eighteen elementary schools, two missions, and a minor seminary were closed. Five more parishes and two more elementary schools were closed by June 1991. Many Chicagoans who felt closings were implemented without consultation cried foul. After 1990, they often associated planning with a purely financial response to a financial problem and evinced little interest in the theological framework for planning and for a new postconciliar Catholic identity. This limited the success of planning in the 1990s.

Catholic Elementary Schools

The Archdiocese of Chicago boasts the largest Catholic school system in the United States. Powerful affective bonds to schools constitute a central feature of Chicago Catholicism. But Bernardin inherited a school system in decline. According to the *Official Catholic Directory,* enrollment dropped from 286,670 students in 429 elementary schools in 1965, to 160,129 in 394 schools in 1975, to 125,786 in 361 schools in 1985, to 105,030 in 281 schools in 1995. Of these remaining 281 elementary schools, only 207 (74 percent) were strictly parochial—under the authority of one parish and its pastor—conforming to the parish-school unit that has constituted a principal component of Chicago Catholicism. Seventy-four (26 percent) were not traditional parish-school plants and fell under the authority of two or more parishes or the Archdiocese. These trends represented a break with Chicago Catholicism.[14]

At the Third Plenary Council of Baltimore (1884), the American Catholic bishops had commanded the construction of a school for each parish and required Catholic children to attend. Although these ideals were never realized, the importance of the school in the parish community was considerable. Consequently, many parishioners today have difficulty conceiving of a parish without a school. Furthermore, although some ethnic groups, such as Italians, Puerto Ricans, and Mexicans, never sent a high proportion of their children to Catholic schools, those Chicagoans with stronger familial ties to parochial schools "remember" a time when all Catholic children went to them and learned the Baltimore catechism. Thus, Cardinal Bernardin's efforts to close or consolidate parochial schools, due to a shortage of religious who had formerly administered and taught at Catholic schools for little compensation, came as a challenge to Chicago Catholicism.[15]

In the 1980s, Bernardin reorganized the archdiocesan Offices for Catholic Education and Religious Education to cultivate better communication between the schools, principals, pastors, and archdiocesan offices and to integrate them into the broader planning processes. School planning had become institutionalized in 1976 with the establishment of a Planning Department under the Superintendent of Schools. Between 1977 and 1985, forty-five elementary schools completed a planning process, but in each case it was implemented in isolation from the sponsoring parish or neighboring schools.[16]

From 1985 to 1996, school planning was linked to mandatory parish planning. Each school was required to undergo an evaluation process, developed in response to the 1990 letter from the Catholic Bishops titled "In Support of Catholic Elementary and Secondary Schools." The process entailed a self-evaluation by the principal and teachers, with input from parish staff and board members, followed by a three-day visitation from a team composed of representatives from the Office of Catholic Education, principals, and teachers. The school then became responsible for implementing the recommendations given by the visiting team. In addition, the Office of Catholic Education implemented a "Catholic Identity Process" to help each school reflect on its identity and mission. The Identity Process engaged principal, parents, and faculty in discussion. Although voluntary, by the spring of 1994 more than two hundred Catholic elementary schools had participated. The process cultivated self-awareness of the distinctive identity of each school, which often depended on the character of the neighborhood and its traditions. This process revealed that some schools understood their identity as Catholic because they nurtured students into the life of the church, while others considered themselves Catholic because they had a mission to transform society in line with Catholic social teaching.

The financial strains on the Archdiocese led to a reorganization of the school system. This generated controversy because it usually culminated in closing some parochial schools and consolidating others into regional schools, breaking with the traditions of Chicago Catholicism. Each consolidation required the new regional school to cultivate a new identity not grounded in strictly parochial traditions and conceptions of urban space. Bernardin hoped this new identity would be more inclusive, evincing a greater awareness of cultural and economic diversity.[17]

A Multicultural Church

Ethnic and racial diversity has shaped the Archdiocese. Numerous national parishes were constructed in industrial cities for continental European immigrants. Frequently, religious congregations took the lead in pastoral care over ethnic groups. The Resurrectionists for the Poles, the Scalabrinians for the Italians, the Claretians for the Mexicans, and the Divine Word Fathers for African Americans, served as pastors and representatives to diocesan or Vatican authorities. Italian, Puerto Rican, Mexican, and African American men were rarely found in, or were segregated from, Saint Mary of the Lake, the archdiocesan seminary, and almost never worked in archdiocesan offices before World War II. Chicago's Polonia, in contrast, became a significant Catholic power bloc and still commands considerable leverage.[18]

Before 1965 the metaphor of the "melting pot" symbolized the dominant ideology of the Catholic Church, which sought to facilitate the assimilation of immigrants and their children into a common American Catholic nationality. The segregation of African American Catholics within the church stood out as a contradiction of this ideal, and the pre–World War II separatism of some Poles or Italians, prolonged by their own clergy, lingered, but it did not undermine faith in the process of assimilation. Although divided by language and history, Catholic parishes increasingly resembled one another in most aspects of their liturgical and congregational life.

After 1965 some activists and intellectuals in the Catholic Church advocated cultural pluralism.[19] Within a Catholic context, they sought to recapture or preserve distinctive religious rituals, symbols, and affective experiences associated with European homelands or immigrant neighborhoods. The public affirmation of cultural pluralism, often coupled to a condemnation of the melting pot metaphor, helped legitimate the persistence and even expansion of distinctive archdiocesan offices and cultural centers for ethnic groups whose immigrant populations had dwindled. The investments of some religious congregations, who themselves had become symbols of ethnicity within Catholic culture, also assured an institutional presence. On his arrival in 1982, Bernardin inherited an ethnic apostolate composed of thirteen full-time employees, with eleven offices dedicated to separate ethnic, racial, or language groups. Each office spoke for "its" people, set up programs or events for "its" people, petitioned for resources for "its" people, and worked in relative isolation from other ethnic offices.

With the financial crisis of 1989, Bernardin reorganized these offices into a new Office for Ethnic Ministries, which opened in 1991. I will analyze the significance of this reorganization in regard to theology and multiculturalism after a historical overview of some of the ethnic apostolates that were reorganized. This overview cannot do justice to the tensions among religious congregations, factions of diocesan clergy, archdiocesan institutions, and lay interest groups that spanned the postwar period. Symbolic boundaries based on ethnicity, race, visions of the political and economic order, and conceptions of religious authority make any brief narrative unsatisfactory. My goal is only to provide the background to archdiocesan planning processes that baptized contemporary multiculturalism as an ideology embodied in the Office for Ethnic Ministries in the 1990s.

Hispanic Ministry

Pastoral care for Spanish-speaking immigrants in the 1950s diverged from a pattern in which European immigrant clergy had worked with "their" own, with little archdiocesan oversight. A cohort of progressive

White Chicago diocesan clergy emerged, with an interest in Hispanic urban ministry. No organization of diocesan clergy had ever sought out a specialized ministry among Czech, Italian, African American, or Mexican Catholics before.

In 1956, Cardinal-Archbishop Samuel A. Stritch (1940–1958) formed the Cardinal's Committee for the Spanish Speaking (CCSS) under the direction of diocesan clergy—Fathers Leo Mahon (1956–1963) and Donald Headley (1963–1968).[20] The CCSS grew out of Mahon's initiatives with Puerto Ricans at Holy Cross Church and supplemented the Claretians' work at Mexican parishes. The CCSS, however, integrated Hispanics into parishes where they lived and organized lay Puerto Ricans for leadership roles. In the late 1950s and 1960s, the Hermanos en la Familia de Dios, an organization of lay men founded to organize Puerto Ricans, and El Cursillo de Cristiandad fostered political activism among Hispanics. Eventually the CCSS developed into the Archdiocesan Latin American Committee (ALAC).

In 1963, with the support of Cardinal-Archbishop Albert Meyer (1958–1965), Mahon established a mission at San Miguelito in the Archdiocese of Panama, where he remained until 1975 as vicar of eastern Panama. With Headley after 1968, Mahon cultivated lay leaders through base communities and hoped to expose Chicago seminarians and priests to a lay-led church. Under the tenure of Cardinal-Archbishop John Patrick Cody (1965–1982), however, the Panama mission did not play the role Mahon had envisioned. Although it became an active center for Latin Americans, Cody neither publicized the mission's activities nor tapped its potential to train Chicago clergy.

The change from national parishes of European ethnics under religious clergy into Mexican parishes under diocesan clergy in the Pilsen and Little Village neighborhoods was also significant for Hispanics' pastoral care. In 1968 the ALAC tried a team ministry approach in Pilsen with eleven diocesan priests, eleven sisters, and one layman. This "18th Street Team" coordinated pastoral care of seven area parishes, integrating community organizations and parish resources on behalf of Mexican interests. Not all the parishes in the area participated, however, and by 1971, eight of the sisters and six of the clergy had left the active ministry. The dissolution of the 18th Street Team left priests reluctant to attempt a coordinated approach again.[21]

In 1974 the first Encuentro Hispano held in Chicago recommended the formation of a Center for Hispanic Ministry. Although Cody appointed Bishop Nevin Hayes, O. Carm., as a vicar for Spanish-speaking Catholics in 1978, many clergy believed Cody had ignored their initiatives and was not prepared for the growing Hispanic population. Consequently, in 1978 a committee of thirty-three priests formed the Hispanic Caucus, which soon included a number of women religious. The caucus encouraged better preparation for seminarians, called for improvements to public schools attended by Hispanics, tried to place Hispanic students at Catholic colleges, demanded more priests in Hispanic parishes, and protested against the Immigration Reform and Control Act of 1986.

Soon after his arrival in Chicago, Bernardin created the Office of the Hispanic Apostolate under Claretian priest Father Pedro Rodriguez. The purpose of the office was to promote Hispanic ministry and integrate the concerns of the caucus into archdiocesan organizations. Through the initiatives of the caucus and the Office of the Hispanic Apostolate, programs for Hispanic evangelization, liturgists, and catechists developed. Since 1982, an annual festival to celebrate Hispanic faith and culture has marked the massive Hispanic presence in the Archdiocese. In 1983, Chicago received its first Hispanic bishop, and by 1986 an archdiocesan Spanish-language paper was established. In 1987 the Hispanic Caucus presented a plan to Bernardin for a new mission in Latin America, which opened in July 1989 in Chilapa, Mexico. In 1988, Bernardin established as his advisory body a Hispanic Pastoral Council of fourteen laypeople, with at least two from each vicariate, and the next year the Office of the Hispanic Apostolate was replaced by a Hispanic Pastoral Commission under the direction of Angelina Marquez.

African American Ministry

During the decades before Bernardin's arrival, an active cohort of diocesan clergy worked with African Americans in the struggle for civil rights and to facilitate the difficult racial transition in Chicago parishes. This often pitted progressive clergy advocating interracialism against confreres who maintained segregation. In the years after the civil rights movement, many of the charismatic clergy and sisters who had worked in the Black community left the active ministry. Perhaps this explains in part why no equivalent of the Hispanic Caucus developed among priests and sisters working with African American Catholics in Chicago.

On Bernardin's arrival in Chicago, he conferred with African American Catholics and their priests and affirmed their desire for an African

American auxiliary bishop and an office for Black Catholics. Bishop Gregory was consecrated to Chicago in December 1983. Before the establishment of the Office for Black Catholic Ministries in 1985, the Office for Chicago Catholic Evangelization handled African American affairs. African American Catholics began meeting annually at the "Comfort My People" festival in 1982, which provided a forum to discuss pastoral issues and to plan for evangelization. In 1984 the ten African American bishops in the United States issued their first pastoral letter, "What We Have Seen and Heard." In October 1985, African Americans gathered for the first annual archdiocesan revival, held in Holy Name Cathedral.

In March 1987 the first archdiocesan Black Catholic Congress was held, promoted by the Office for Black Catholic Ministries. The congress developed plans to strengthen lay leadership and to build connections among African American parishes and agencies, and it prepared for Chicago's participation in the National Black Catholic Congress in Washington, D.C., that May. At this first National Black Catholic Congress of the century, fifteen hundred African American delegates from 110 dioceses developed a national pastoral plan. The implementation of the national plan for evangelization revealed the Archdiocese's strengths and weaknesses. While it had both an auxiliary bishop and an Office for Black Catholic Ministries, as of 1990 only one of two hundred pastoral associates and ten of 466 directors of religious education were African Americans. After the national congress, the Archdiocese promoted the training of Ministers of Care, whose parish apostolate stresses African American cultural values, theology, spirituality, and catechetics.

Polonia

The institutional history of Polish pastoral care dates back to the nineteenth century. Chicago quickly became the largest Polish area of settlement outside Europe and has played an important role in the evolution of Polish ethnicity and in Poland–United States relations. The massive network of Polish national parishes and schools, the presence of the Resurrectionists and several Polish orders of women religious, the strife between the Polish Roman Catholic Union and the Polish National Alliance, and the cold war struggle contributed to Polish ethnic consciousness in the Archdiocese.

In May 1984, Bernardin met with four of his bishops and seventy-four priests to begin a study of the Polish apostolate in the Archdiocese, where there were 752,000 Americans of Polish descent. At this heated meeting the cardinal emphasized that he did not want to set up parallel programs for each ethnic group, but he acknowledged the need for better coordination among Polish ministries. Considerable divisions existed between various generations of Polish Americans, Polish immigrants, and Polish and Polish American clergy. Although 282 of 1,232 students in the archdiocesan seminary system were of Polish descent, only ten spoke Polish. In 1988 the Holy Trinity Mission was established to serve post–World War II arrivals, and the archdiocesan Polish Apostolate was reorganized into the Office of Ministry to Polonia. The office worked to integrate Polish immigrants in existing parishes and to promote the teaching of Polish language and liturgy at Saint Mary of the Lake Seminary.

Chicago auxiliary bishop Alfred Abramowicz served as the national executive director of the Catholic League for Religious Assistance to Poland, established in 1943. Its annual collection instigated division between those who believed Polish American resources ought to support Polish American concerns and those who wanted the resources to support Poles in Poland. Nevertheless, in 1991, Bishop Abramowicz provided the Polish church with $270,000 for the training of priests; $143,000 for churches, convents, monasteries, and soup kitchens; and $25,000 for radio broadcasting and Vatican communications. The collection also supported the Polish Pontifical College in Rome and the Polish Seminary in Paris.

Centers and Missions

Other groups in the Archdiocese established ethnic ministry centers and missions that hosted social and sacramental services to Latin- and non-Latin-rite Catholics. Furthermore, cultural centers with a Catholic affiliation, such as the Lithuanian Cultural Center in Lemont and the Italian Cultural Center in Stone Park, institutionalized ethnic identity in the Archdiocese. Centers and missions are of particular importance to Asian Catholics. By 1990, Chicago hosted the Holy Trinity Polish Mission, the Blessed George Matulaitis Lithuanian Mission, the Angel Guardian Croatian Catholic Mission, the Saint Therese Chinese Catholic Mission, the Syro-Malabar Catholic Mission, the Knanite Syro-Malabar Catholic Mission, the Kananaya Catholic Mission, the Syro-Malankara Catholic Mission, the Haitian Catholic Center, the Indo-Chinese Catholic

Center, the Korean North Suburban Catholic Center, and the Korean Catholic Center at Queen of Angels Parish.

Office for Ethnic Ministries

From Bernardin's arrival until the financial crisis of 1989, the ethnic apostolates were reorganized to express solidarity between the archbishop and his people. The new archdiocesan offices were meant to be receptive to input from ethnic and racial groups, input many felt had not been welcomed by Bernardin's predecessor. Still, the institutional organization of ethnic and racial apostolates reflected a cultural pluralist model in which each group with enough "clout" had an autonomous office. The distinctive history of African Americans in comparison with European ethnic groups and the enormous Hispanic presence had not been institutionally affirmed in any clear manner. Furthermore, the diverse groups of Asian Catholics, who lacked the institutional history that provided patrons and power, required greater attention. The new Office for Ethnic Ministries, created in 1991, emerged both from downsizing the Pastoral Center during the financial crisis of 1989 and from reconceptualizing pastoral care. Its organizational structure embodied a Catholic baptism of the ideology of multiculturalism, and its mission of evangelization was linked to a Catholic theology of inculturation.

In the new office, four consultants were hired to direct four "desks"— for European Americans, Hispanic Americans, Asian Americans, and African Americans. A full-time director assisted by two secretaries coordinated the office. There was also a part-time Polish liaison, a Resurrectionist appointed to coordinate the transfer of clergy and seminarians from Poland to the Archdiocese.

Each consultant oversaw an advisory board that represented either ethnic groups within each desk or regions of the Archdiocese. For example, the European consultant had an advisory board that met bimonthly and included eleven representatives (Slovak, German, Latvian, Italian, Croatian, Polish, Lithuanian, Hungarian, Czech, Irish, and Slovenian). This advisory board kept the office aware of festivals, conflicts, and other concerns in its respective ethnic communities. Similarly, the Asian American and Hispanic American consultants had advisory boards that represented the variety of ethnic groups within their desks. Because the African American desk housed less ethnic diversity (although it included Haitians), its representatives where chosen from geographical regions of the Archdiocese. The Hispanic American desk, unlike the others, had vicariate Hispanic coordinators in each of the six vicariates, who served as regional representatives of the office. The office was reorganized along the lines of the National Conference of Catholic Bishops and the United States Catholic Conference, which in 1990 had four similar desks, thus anticipating coordinated national and international networks and initiatives.

The Office for Ethnic Ministries served as a consultant to parishes and archdiocesan agencies with regard to intercultural relations. Sharing a common space with the other desks in the Pastoral Center, each consultant had responsibilities beyond advocacy for one group. Put another way, the organization of the office acknowledged a need not only to represent distinct constituencies but also to cultivate sensitivity to minority issues among all groups and to promote the recognition and celebration of diverse Catholic identities. This task included educating Catholics about the theological significance of diversity, and encouraging residents to welcome newcomers in their parishes. The office institutionalized a commitment to interaction and understanding among groups, in contrast to isolated ethnic factions bickering for resources.

Organized in a manner sensitive to changes in immigration patterns, American cultural self-understanding, and Catholic theology, the office institutionalized the ideology of multiculturalism. Multiculturalism divides the American population into what David Hollinger has called an "ethno-racial pentagon" of European Americans, African Americans, Hispanic Americans, Asian Americans, and Native Americans.[22] The office's alignment with national and international Catholic institutional networks signaled how a multiculturalism conceptualized within a global framework had become normative for the church in Chicago. The ethic of mutual recognition among all Catholics across racial or ethnic boundaries, along with the emphasis on intercultural interaction and celebration, was a break from the separatist ethnic boosterism of the past. This ethic, described by Charles Taylor in his commentary on multiculturalism as the "politics of recognition," shapes the activities of the consultants.[23]

"Inculturation," a concept used to understand the proper relationship between faith and culture in the process of evangelization, provided the theological underpinnings for the Office for Ethnic Ministries. Conciliar and postconciliar documents have emphasized the need for local churches to embrace the plurality of cultures the church meets. The church has endorsed the idea that it must evangelize cultures, not merely individuals within cultures. A. A. Roest Crollius states:

> Inculturation of the Church is the integration of the Christian experience of a local Church into the culture of its people, in such a way that this experience not only expresses itself in elements of this culture, but becomes a force that animates, orients and innovates this culture so as to create a new unity and communion, not only within the culture in question but also as an enrichment of the Church universal.[24]

The dialogical relationship between church and culture implied in the concept of inculturation has served to legitimate multiculturalism among Catholics engaged in evangelization.

Conclusion

Planning and institutional reorganization marked Bernardin's fourteen years as the archbishop of Chicago. He envisioned what I have called a process ecclesiology: an integrated institutional structure, in a dialectical relationship with a changing environment, animated by an ethic of responsibility and stewardship among members. He tried to harness the resources of Chicago Catholicism, although he acknowledged that many changes were a break from that tradition.

Bernardin's tenure spanned a period of economic scarcity for significant sectors of the city of Chicago, while the Archdiocese's edge cities and suburbs grew in numbers and power. Most urban neighborhoods did not have resources to build new institutions. Before 1960, the Archdiocese had been built upon a century of remarkable industrial growth. What has been called "the immigrant church" might also be called "the industrial church." Many Chicago Catholics were industrial workers, civil servants, and small-scale entrepreneurs who lived in urban industrial neighborhoods. The relatively unregulated economy, notwithstanding unpredictable booms and depressions, allowed European immigrants and their children to attain high levels of property ownership and to build parish-school plants.

Postconciliar Catholicism is largely a "post-industrial church." Deindustrialization, out-migration of middle-class Catholics, weakened labor unions, and diminished urban social services and neighborhood political power have drastically restricted the possibilities for the Catholic Church in urban America. Sadly, many Catholic discussions about the closing of institutions do not fully take into account this transformation. These discussions tend to evaluate the moral intentions of fellow Catholics and can become highly accusational. Bernardin did not initiate a massive reallocation of resources from suburbs to the city. Through voluntarism, such as the Big Shoulders program or parish sharing efforts, some suburban resources were directed toward city parishes and schools. But like all American bishops reigning over midwestern and eastern urban dioceses in the 1980s, Bernardin presided over the dismantling of the industrial church in urban neighborhoods. In that context, Bernardin tried to give institutional reorganization theological meaning linked to a new Catholic identity.

Bernardin claimed that this identity was more genuinely Catholic than an exclusively parish-centered consciousness of Chicago Catholicism. Nothing Bernardin said, however, indicated a hostility toward the territorial or national parish, the parish school, or the preconciliar devotional ethos that had passed away among middle-class Catholics. He tried to mobilize the symbolic and social capital of Chicago Catholicism to support his reforms. But the parish, according to Bernardin, while fundamental to Catholic formation and identity, could no longer be the only commitment, particularly because parishes were competing with one another for scarce resources.

One generous interpretation of the reorganization of institutions would be that postconciliar Catholicism is analogous to the immigrant church. Between 1880 and 1940 the church promoted assimilation through "Americanization," generating confusion and conflict as a new American Catholic identity was forged from the children of European immigrants. Today, new forms of Catholic consciousness that require higher levels of activity, planning, and sharing across parish and racial boundaries will also take a generation to become normative in the imagination of a new generation of Catholics.

Two factors limit the realization of Bernardin's vision. First, in some cases collaborative planning and decision making do not work smoothly because lay Catholics harbor ambivalence about taking responsibilities, setting agendas, and forming visions. Many Catholics do not participate in their parishes with enough regularity or at a level of sufficient intensity to experience the corporate reality of the church. Unlike those whom James Castelli and Joseph Gremillion have defined as "core" Catholics, they prefer to have clerical authorities lead, and they remain unaware of or indifferent to planning processes or church governance.[25]

The ambiguity of authority in postconciliar Catholicism also hampers the realization of Bernardin's vision. Tension exists between democratic and hierarchical church structures. The laity, or in some cases the clergy, are not certain that their decisions will be followed even after they participate in an intensive planning process.

This ambiguity of authority is systemic. Since Vatican Council II, Catholic bureaucracies, agencies, councils, and conferences have proliferated. Many are canonically required consultative and advisory bodies that give Catholics a voice, but not power, in the church. The collaborative participatory model of the church, which some contend is normative for postconciliar Catholicism and which Bernardin's career symbolized, exists in tension with the juridical-canonical definition of the church. On the one hand, local organizations sensitive to local needs suggest a church with empowered laity, in which the Pastoral Center functions as a resource to help Catholics develop innovative approaches to solve their own problems. This is a church not explicitly hierarchical. It uses social-scientific research to implement decisions in a pragmatic, responsive manner. On the other hand, a hierarchical structure remains. Canonically, bishops remain the monarchs of dioceses and pastors remain the princes of their parishes and schools. In sum, consultative and advisory bodies have no formal authority.

Observers have noted the ambiguity of authority in the postconciliar church. John Grindel states, "Gradually, the bishops have been opting for a participative style of life in the Church. This participative style has its roots in the American principle of 'self-governing association' that is at the basis of all other aspects of life in the United States." But he adds a caveat. The church's "ecclesial structure has remained quite Roman and hierarchical, a structure that is creating tensions with a membership much more attuned to equality, due process, and participation in decision making."[26]

NOTES

The data for this essay are derived from the archdiocesan weekly *Chicago Catholic* (renamed the *New World*), 1982–1996; more than fifty structured interviews with Catholic administrators, priests, and laypeople; many more informal conversations with Catholics throughout Chicago; and numerous observations of liturgical services and religious group activities. Thanks to Religion in Urban America Program colleagues and to John McGreevy for comments on earlier drafts.

1. Giddens, *Constitution of Society;* and Sewell, "Theory of Structure."

2. *Data on the Organization, Resources and Activities of the Archdiocese of Chicago* (1996).

3. On the history of Catholicism in Chicago, see Shanabruch, *Chicago's Catholics;* Kantowicz, *Corporation Sole;* Avella, *This Confident Church;* Dahm, *Power and Authority;* Sanders, *Education of an Urban Minority.*

4. For works that question the notion that the parish-school unit was the central marker of the neighborhood, see Zorbaugh, *Gold Coast and Slum;* Suttles, *Social Order of the Slum;* Hunter, *Symbolic Communities.*

5. Grindel, *Whither the U.S. Church?* 10, 11, 12.

6. *Chicago Catholic,* September 12, 1986, 1, 14.

7. Ibid. June 3, 1988, 2.

8. Ibid. June 10, 1988, 2.

9. Ibid. June 24 and July 1, 1988, 2.

10. *Tomorrow's Parish: Guide for Planning; Tomorrow's Parish: Criteria for Planning.*

11. Bernardin, *Decisions for the Future of Our Church* (Spring 1994); *Decisions for the Future of Our Church: Implementation Plan* (Fall 1994).

12. Bernardin, *Decisions* (Spring 1994), 2 n. 1, 6, 10.

13. Gannon and Schwartz, "Church Finances in Crisis," 112.

14. *Data,* 81, 99. For similar trends in high schools, see Fornero, "Expansion and Decline."

15. Buetow, *Of Singular Benefit;* Hunt and Kunkel, "Catholic Schools."

16. Schuster, "Study of the Local School Long-Range Planning Process."

17. On schools and controversies, see Beaudoin, "Elementary Schools"; Harris, "Is the American Catholic Church Getting Out?"; O'Brien, *Mixed Messages;* Kealey, "Collision Course"; McCready, "Catholic Schools and Catholic Identity."

18. Parot, *Polish Catholics in Chicago;* Davis, *History of Black Catholics;* D'Agostino, "Missionaries in Babylon."

19. Gleason, *Keeping the Faith.*

20. The next several paragraphs draw on an unpublished working paper by Charles Dahm, O.P., "A Brief Analysis of Some Historical Developments in Hispanic Ministry in the Archdiocese of Chicago."

21. Kelliher, "Mexican Catholics and Chicago's Parishes."

22. Hollinger, *Postethnic America.*

23. Taylor, *Multiculturalism.*

24. Schreiter, "Faith and Cultures," quotes Crollius, "What Is So New about Inculturation? A Concept and Its Implications"; quote on p. 735.

25. Castelli and Gremillion, *Emerging Parish.*

26. Grindel, *Whither the U.S. Church?* 92, 96, 97.

Part IV

Epilogue

Epilogue

Building Religious Communities at the Turn of the Century

R. Stephen Warner

When I met Lowell Livezey late in 1991, he had received a planning grant for this project from the Lilly Endowment, and as I recall Lilly wanted him to investigate what "urban ministry"—an ideal that had flourished in Chicago from the 1920s through the 1950s—could mean in the context of radically changed American cities at the end of the twentieth century. In the years surrounding World War II, urban ministry had come to center on the responsibility that privileged white Protestant denominations assumed for cities that were increasingly alien to their own once rural, now increasingly suburban, constituencies, as the cities of the nation's industrial heartland became more Catholic, more colored, and more poor. At the end of the century, it was time for another look at the place of religion in such cities. Their industrial base had eroded into a "Rust Belt" that their white inhabitants, Protestant and Catholic alike, continued to flee in the face of newer and yet more alien people—new immigrants from the third world—even as white Protestant religious institutions had lost much of the vigor that had sustained urban ministry ideals. Such, as I understood it, was the agenda with which Livezey was presented.

During the planning process, Livezey made three fateful decisions that decisively shaped the research that he and his associates report in this book—locating the project at the University of Illinois at Chicago (UIC), defining the city as a place of ongoing religious activity, and conducting the field research from the neighborhood up.

First, Livezey knew that the project would have to engage non-Christian religious communities, and, as he told me, he thought that entrée to such communities would be facilitated if the project were to be housed at a secular university. For many reasons, McCormick Theological Seminary, the distinguished Presbyterian institution where his wife, Lois Gehr Livezey, teaches theology and ethics, would have been a suitable home, not least for its having housed Carl Dudley's Church and Community Ministry Project in the late 1980s.[1] But Livezey wanted to allay any suspicion on the part of Muslims and Jews, among others, that the project had a particularly Christian agenda, and so he shopped around for a more neutral venue. John Gardiner, of UIC's Office of Social Science Research, whose significant contributions to the project are acknowledged in the Preface, opened doors for the project at UIC, promising office space and administrative savvy and introducing Livezey to me and other potential collaborators. Settling in at UIC, not previously known as a home for research in contemporary American religion and oblivious to urban ministry, Livezey's Religion in Urban America Program (RUAP) was enmeshed in a matrix of urban-oriented social science departments, including a sociology department that enshrined the tradition of Chicago school field research. Elfriede Wedam, who had been trained in that tradition and was soon to finish her Ph.D., became central to the RUAP team. UIC was also home to a large and diverse student body of undergraduate and graduate students, for many of whom Chicago was home, from whose number RUAP was able to recruit many capable research assistants.

The second decision, bound up with the first, was a far-ranging conceptual one: to define the city for religious purposes not in terms of its needs or deficits but in terms of the religious communities already on the ground. Instead of assuming that the city was the religious responsibility of the white Protestant elite who had dominated its early years,[2] RUAP would approach the city expecting to find a diverse array of religious institutions—fledgling, struggling, and flourishing—who understood one or another part of the city's territory or population to be their special bailiwick.[3] It makes a huge difference whether one's approach toward urban populations is foremost concerned with what they lack (good jobs, decent housing, effective schools, anchor institutions, and so forth) or one instead assumes that the point of departure must be their religious activities and self-understandings. Foreign missionaries face an analogous conceptual choice, but for them the challenge is to respect the indigenous, usually non-Christian, religious tradition. In the case of contemporary American cities, the indigenous population is very likely to be Christian but followers of Christian traditions that practitioners of urban ministry often find alien and suspect, such as fundamentalism, evangelicalism, and Pentecostalism. Defining "religion in urban America" from the ground up and having at hand potential research assistants stemming from some of these indigenous urban religious communities, Christian and otherwise, RUAP avoided the deficit perspective.

Finally, as Livezey organized his RUAP research team, they decided to follow the Chicago school tradition of urban research (including the *Local Community Fact Book,* which since 1985 has been produced at UIC)[4] and to conduct the research primarily from the perspective of neighborhoods. Thus, for the most part the field sites of the research were local religious communities—congregations, parishes, Islamic centers, temples, and *gurdwārās*—that were found, prominently or obscurely, by surveying the neighborhoods. The exceptions are mostly represented in part 3, where we read about one Roman Catholic congregation (or "magnet parish") that serves a population drawn from the entire metropolitan area (chapter 9), congregations of new immigrants, many of which draw their members from similarly dispersed residential communities (chapter 10), and the most important supracongregational judicatory in Chicago, the Roman Catholic archdiocese (chapter 11).

The neighborhood-based method is a decisive alternative to focusing the study on those religious institutions identified with Chicago's ecumenical and interfaith movement, as represented for example in the local chapter of the National Conference for Community and Justice (NCCJ) and the Council for a Parliament of the World's Religions (CPWR). Had RUAP sampled religious institutions for the study through the NCCJ or the CPWR, it no doubt would have encountered a higher proportion of religious energies directed toward social activism and external ministry, but it would have missed the smaller, less ecumenically inclined but arguably no less effective churches, synagogues, mosques, and other nascent institutions that turned up in RUAP's exhaustive, on-the-ground inventory of local congregations.[5] The neighborhood-based method may thus underrepresent what metropolitanwide activism exists. Yet the particular neighborhoods chosen for the study also underrepresent other religious communities that are similar to those sampled, including those of Korean Protestants, Chinese Evangelicals, and Puerto Rican Pentecostals, as well as the nation's most prominent megachurch, Willow Creek

Community Church, located in one of the edge cities of the metropolitan region. Inclusion of such communities would, as I shall argue below, only have strengthened the findings of the study.

On the basis of these three practical, conceptual, and methodological commitments, RUAP was poised to discover the actual ways that religious institutions in Chicago engage their urban (and metropolitan) context. RUAP's findings will likely disappoint those who expect urban churches to be activist cadres dedicated to social change.[6] Indeed, the picture of American religion that emerges in these pages is, although far more varied in confessional terms, not unlike one that could be drawn about other American times and places characterized by rapid population movement and economic change, whether in the early republican period, on the frontier in the 1830s, in the cities between the wars, suburbia in the 1950s, or exurbia in the 1970s: Americans are inclined to use their religious institutions to build community in the face of social change.[7]

Throughout this book, we read of religious institutions made up of people of every color and creed that invite their members to get acquainted with one another, provide safe havens for members' (and neighbors') children, promote family values, facilitate homeownership, attempt to channel behavior in constructive directions and discourage indulgence in temptations, promote concern for others who themselves are expected to hew to the standards of the group, nurture positive identifications when negative ones are so near at hand, offer moral support and a psychological shield against a perceivedly hostile society, and promote spiritual growth where pressures of the job are experienced as soul-deadening.

Adapting for our purposes Penny Becker's typology of congregations,[8] we can say that religious institutions tend to specialize in one of four callings, being primarily (1) places of worship, where the religious ideals of the group are inculcated and expressed, (2) networks of relationships, where quasi-kinship bonds and interpersonal networks of caring are nurtured, (3) communities of discourse, where members' values are expressed and implications debated, or (4) activist organizations, where members' values and leaders' initiatives are devoted to changing the surrounding society. In terms conventional around Protestant seminaries, activities of the first two types tend to be classified as focusing on "private" religion while the fourth type, and lately the third, are lifted up as "public" involvements.[9] From this point of view, it is remarkable how much religion of the second type, where members work at building internal solidarity, shows up in RUAP's Chicago. Shall we follow the conventional wisdom and call this a pattern of "privatization"?

It was perhaps easier to do that in the 1950s, when the nascent communities tended to be suburban and their constituents so heavily white and middle class and disproportionately Protestant.[10] Under such circumstances, for white middle-class Protestant social critics to call their own people to moral account, demanding that they subordinate their "private" interests to their "public" obligations, was seen as prophecy, not prejudice. The new suburbanites were affluent, they appeared to have good jobs and stable families, and public policies like federally guaranteed mortgages and federally subsidized highways were stacked in their favor. They seemed to have no moral right to be collectively involuted, and to the extent that they were so, they were perceived as socially conformist, politically quiescent, and religiously effeminate.[11]

But when the inhabitants of urban America themselves, the people that self-centered suburbanites were cajoled to care about, show up in research like that reported in this book as dedicated to the social construction and moral self-improvement of their own communities (alongside the development of their material infrastructure), what are the erstwhile critics to say? Stepping out of the mode of conventional thought, Livezey boldly asserts (chapter 1), that their efforts at cultural production (which one might classify under Becker's first type) are one form of public religious action.

The fact is that community, which was to be the necessary infrastructure for religious social action and urban ministry, cannot be taken for granted at the end of the twentieth century, whether we are speaking of the formation of noninstrumental social bonds in a suburban development, an urban ethnic neighborhood, a church congregation, or even a family. It is not that community has been eclipsed or that it is only a relic of the past. In America, communities have been and must still be regularly created anew, particularly in times, like our own, of rapid social change. Robert Putnam has recently raised the specter of "bowling alone," leisure activity without social bonds, in his concern for the erosion of social capital.[12] Although his portrait has been criticized for its exaggeration (and although his concentration on the decline of service clubs and sports leagues ignores the greater vitality of local religious congregations), it is not absurd to worry with him about individualistic fragmentation in American society, where each person can feel so free to go his or her own way and so lonely in the going.[13] Much of modern art and drama is built around such themes, where even the joining of one person to one other has to count as a triumph.

But the precariousness of social capital is not only a problem for our time, nor—and this is a major theme in this book—are the worries about fragmentation only those of white Americans feeling displaced by multiculturalism. Those new to America recognize what many of the natives ignore, that American culture is thoroughly steeped in individualism.[14] Long before the supposedly unprecedented 1960s, Americans had been urged to follow Jesus regardless of mother and father, to go west and leave family behind, to sample the charms of Kansas City and not to be fenced in. Individualism was, and likely still is, a functional ethic for a society so devoted to economic growth and mastery of the natural environment, where the lessons a father learned about making a living were likely to be obsolete by the time his son was old enough to have to earn his own keep. Surely the value of individualism—practical as well as moral—was accentuated by the 1960s, when with postwar prosperity and the baby boom more and more Americans became heir to the culture's promises. Adapting older aspirations, some of them replaced Jesus with Buddha, others went north instead of west, and the lure of Kansas City was eclipsed by that of San Francisco's Castro district for gay men.[15] The economic devaluation of parents' learning, which young men had long been led to expect, became something many young women experienced; to the father-son disjunction was added one between mothers and daughters.[16] These individualizing currents were new but distinctly American; our culture has always been one that values mobility and individual opportunity.

The American middle class—the old WASP establishment now firmly upper middle class—has long lived with the tension between individualistic ideals and sociological realities. In the middle third of the century the nuclear family ideal—where the unit of mobility was the "two-person career"—was an apparent temporary resolution to the tension between individual and community, and parents had the expectation, backed by their resources, that prodigal children would return to the fold after their experiment with youth culture.[17] Not only did this ideal eventually reveal its bias against the aspirations of women,[18] but it also was vulnerable at the less privileged end of the white social scale to employers who had no interest in supporting more than the one person who could be induced to work for wages offered. For the lower middle class and the working class who in the 1960s finally became heirs to its promises, the nuclear-family ideal was undermined by the economic system to which it had seemed so exquisitely adapted.[19] One response of the white middle class was to lay even more stress on small-scale interpersonal responsibilities, women to men, men to women, parents to children and children to parents, an appeal to family values.

For white Appalachians, African Americans and other people of color, and Hispanics, as well as new immigrants, the American system offered both promise and threat, as barriers to mobility were lowered along with guarantees against disaster and where ethics of mutual help and deference that had helped sustain these communities in older times and other places seemed to be in jeopardy. In the post-1960s world, a family could hope for fame and fortune for a child but had good reason also to fear disgrace and poverty. Hear how often the religious communities portrayed in this book express their distrust of "the culture": the Hispanic families of Emmanuel Presbyterian and *Iglesia de Cristo,* who worry about gang recruitment of their children; the struggling African American families of the Revival Center Church of God in Christ on the West Side, who call by the name of Satan the many threats to their members; the Muslim families repulsed by the "cesspool" of un-Islamic influences to be found in American culture; the black middle-class families of New Covenant Missionary Baptist Church who are told not to trust the culture of the surrounding society; even the affluent edge-city families who think "Naperville is scary."

Largely missing, except among the volunteer tutors at Fourth Presbyterian, is the confident conviction that young people of all backgrounds need to learn the tools that would allow them full participation in the society, both its economy and its culture. Also heard little in these chapters is the idea that the wider culture should be changed. (This lacuna may be an artifact of the concentration of chapters 2 and 11 on organizational aspects of the tall-steeple Protestant churches and the archdiocesan office to the relative neglect of the sermons preached in their respective cathedrals, and of the absence altogether of megachurches in the conservative Calvinist mold.) Instead one reads that each community in question typically finds the culture lacking in religiocultural and moral guidelines for them and their children to live by; providing these guidelines for their own people they take to be their responsibility.[20]

"The culture" that is so distrusted seems for the most part nameless, except for the label "American." It seems clear enough implicitly that what one group disdains (e.g., sexual permissiveness for Muslims) may not be the same as another's anathema (e.g., violence, drugs, or even stress). It is doubtful than any single package of reforms would mend the culture to the satisfaction of all the groups; they have different complaints. Yet it also seems that the threat perceived from the culture is to a large extent an internal one, where the culture is seen as posing moral temptations to members of the group itself, particularly its young people, rather than physical threats to their possessions. What threatens most of the groups here is not other groups or other persons but less tangible cultural and ideological currents that are thought to undermine the group's intergenerational and interpersonal solidarity. Thus, moral boundaries are often drawn within the group (as they are by the Revival Center) rather than between groups. Backsliders and the nonobservant are harshly or lovingly corrected and admonished, but few of the groups portrayed here enjoy the kind of unambiguous group solidarity that would be capable of identifying the threat as coming solely from outside.[21]

Within-group moral boundaries are what we might expect to find, at least on the surface, in a culture so heavily influenced by evangelical Protestantism and its ideology of individual responsibility, including the ideal of the self-made man. In such a culture, it is incumbent on the individual to maintain his or her respectability, and dereliction weighs more heavily on the miscreant and reflects less on the reputation of the family or community than is the case in more communal cultures. Protestant churches can surely foster interreligious prejudice, especially anti-Semitism, and, in their guise as social clubs, they offer breeding grounds for narrow intergroup sympathies. Yet evangelical Protestantism is universalistic—salvation is open to all—and gives no ideological support for ethnic particularism between groups of evangelicals (a communion that includes most African Americans and increasingly Asian Americans). Evangelical churches are *supposed to* welcome everyone regardless of race or nationality; that is their value system. With spiritualized conceptions of virtue (where lust in the heart is seen as equivalent to adultery), there is no way other than vigilant self-control to keep the enemy at bay.

Similarly, perhaps because American Jews have come to recognize intermarriage and assimilationism as a greater threat to their future than pogroms,[22] the Jewish enclave of West Rogers Park that Livezey writes about is "defined by the concentration of the Jewish population and institutions, not by exclusion of or hostility toward others." For Rogers Parks in general "Far from having negative attitudes toward outsiders, these groups are primarily concerned with themselves. . . . [The] boundaries [are] within ethnoracial groups, not between them" (chapter 6).

Many religious communities whose stories are missing from these pages because of RUAP's sampling method manifest similar within-group boundaries, as Korean American churches are increasingly differentiated by generation, the first generation oriented to Korean culture and the Korean language and the second to American-style evangelicalism and the English language.[23] Korean immigrant parents have learned not to scorn "Americans," for that category now includes their own children. Community building in the form of intergenerational solidarity is a problem and a priority for most new immigrant communities; they cannot easily build fences to protect themselves because who they are is precisely what is at issue.[24]

Similarly, it is not only conservatives who seek to build community in the face of socially destructive forces, to bolster internal solidarity as much as to keep enemies at bay. Gays and lesbians, who owe to a culture of individualism their greater freedom to "come out" and express their sexual identities, nonetheless have to exert themselves to reconstruct relationships that were strained by their disclosures and to build new ones in place of the old.[25] The social centrifuge of the 1960s and 1970s both freed them from roles and expectations to which they were not suited and sorted them into new enclaves where they could begin to build their own cities on a hill.[26] Had RUAP sampled religious institutions in other Chicago neighborhoods—particularly Lakeview—this book would have featured more, and more diverse, instances of internally directed community building.

In sum, the religious institutions portrayed in this book devote considerable energies to community construction; they attempt to counteract the demoralizing effects of American culture on their members' lives by strengthening the group's subculture and promoting awareness of mutual accountability. Yet their enhancement of subcultural particularity is not tantamount to the promotion of divisiveness in American society. Religious communities in our country do not simply mirror preexisting social divisions.

The organizational repertoires of American religion offer two contrasting modes of building local communities, the congregational model prevalent in the reformed branch of American Protestantism (especially the Baptist churches) and among American Jews, and the parish model most thoroughly institutionalized until recently in the U.S. Roman Catholic Church.[27] As the word etymologically implies, the congregational model defines the local community socially as a gathering of like-minded people, people brought together by virtue of their ideals. By contrast, the parish model (from a Greek word indicating propinquity) defines the community geographically, as the territory under the authority of the local representative of the broader church. Within Janise Hurtig's Pilsen we see both models, in Emmanuel Presbyterian and Saint Pius, respectively. More broadly, we see the congregational model across the entire religious spectrum of Livezey's Rogers Park and Paul Numrich's Naperville, whereas the parish model still seems to dominate the public culture of Wedam's Southwest Side.

Both parishes and congregations can be moral communities and networks of concern, and those who are struggling to rebuild communities can operate on either set of paradigms, building a new neighborhood community within the frame of the Catholic parish (as in the Southwest Side) or a series of congregational enclaves (as in Rogers Park). We see in the case of Pilsen's Saint Pius and the churches of the Southwest Side that the parish is oriented to taking care of people, feeling responsible for them whether or not they participate. They do not really have to participate in religious activities to fall under the care of the parish, because the parish is responsible for the territory. But precisely that expectation makes for conflict with newcomer "others," because they are not "us," they are not "my neighbor." The congregation, by contrast, looks after itself and demands a lot of its members in terms of both participation and behavior. In order for care to be given, congregations tend to demand that the recipient be morally accountable to the group, not merely a resident of the neighborhood, and they therefore tend to discriminate, in terms discussed by Matthew Price, between the deserving and undeserving poor. Congregations tend to promote moral crusades, whereas parishes lend themselves to turf wars.

But that demand for moral accountability means that the congregation has a stronger impact on changing people; it gets under their skin. Livezey proposes that under conditions of a restructured metropolis, the social network of the congregation can conceivably provide social bridges to the outside, thus alleviating the social isolation that is the most serious problem of the urban underclass. But Wedam gives us reason to think that the parish model is better than the congregation at providing a potential forum for intergroup contact and dialog.

Because of its comprehensiveness as a local community, the parish model requires explicit negotiation among groups and invites the question, "Whose place is this?" and the demand, "You have to speak my language to come in." Congregations, however, are built on cultural, especially religiomoral, consensus, instead of place. Coexistence among different congregations may require only mutual toleration and civil inattention. The Jews of West Rogers Park, who are congregational, seem to understand how to deal with religious diversity at both the community and the enclave levels. As we have seen, Protestants may not always welcome cultural diversity, but unlike Catholics, they are not used to owning urban turf.

The racial history of Chicago offers mixed lessons about these two models and no clear verdict on the superiority of one over the other. As Chicago neighborhoods have undergone racial change, it is relatively easy for congregationally based institutions to move with their constituents to new city neighborhoods or the suburbs, depriving the old neighborhood of some of its social capital, whereas parish-based institutions are far more likely to stay as anchors in old neighborhoods and to be ready to minister to their new residents. On the other hand, the physical capital of fleeing congregations, their often substantial buildings, can be made available by sale to the congregations that actually represent the newcomer population. Moreover, the carefully inculcated loyalty to parish territory has tragically fueled fierce resistance to neighborhood racial change.[28] It is not clear that one model is superior to another in building community relations.

As much as they cannot be dismissed as "privatized," the efforts at community construction and restructuring portrayed in these pages still leave much to be desired. Too few of them seem to address issues of concern across the entire metropolitan area, let alone the nation as a whole, an important matter given the decreasing capacity of the city, even of its elites, to govern its own destiny. Those who might have the resources to do so—the churches of affluent, growing Naperville—seem not to address tractable issues that their members appear to be aware of, their hard-driven, materialistic lifestyles. Another church of the affluent, Old Saint Pat's, seems to offer little challenge to its parishioners to employ humanely what power they enjoy in their workplaces. The downtown churches seem on the verge of losing much of the raison d'être of their urban ministry, as the Cabrini Green housing project, whose children they tutor, seems doomed before the rising tide of real estate values. None of these congregations seems to have much to say about extreme and rising economic inequality in the United States. In these chapters, only the Catholic archdiocese seems even remotely capable of a policy of modest redistribution, in which affluent suburban churches might subsidize the efforts of poor urban ones. Perhaps more along such lines is going on in these churches than appears in this book, as well as in the many religious institutions RUAP could not cover.

Yet the achievement of the book—and the efforts of the religious institutions we read of in it—should not be slighted. These churches, synagogues, mosques, temples, and *gurdwārās* devote themselves to building cultural coherence and social bonds in the face of powerful individualizing currents. Those who attempt to improve the material lot of their constituents do so using methods that are both material and spiritual, both structural and cultural. State-centered attempts to further economic equality should take seriously the methods found in at least some of these churches, where effective material aid in the form of the Earned Income Tax Credit (to cite one example of an effective tool of social policy) would be insufficient without a continuing rhetorical attack on drug and alcohol abuse. Although none of these religious communities may have the right answer for improving the condition of the truly disadvantaged, thoughtful outsiders who would like to call themselves progressives should respectfully consider as models of policy the religious schooling some provide and the moral strings others attach to charitable aid. The stalemate of left/right politics and the dichotomy of "structural" versus "moral" approaches to policy should end, and this book makes an important contribution to that goal.

NOTES

1. Dudley, *Basic Steps toward Community Ministry.*

2. Stockwell, "A Better Class of People."

3. A similar shift in perspective can be seen in comparing the chapter on context in Carroll, Dudley, and McKinney, eds., *Handbook,* with the chapter on ecology in Ammerman et al., eds., *Studying Congregations.*

4. Chicago Fact Book Consortium, *Local Community Fact Book,* 1980 and 1990.

5. There is a paradox to interfaith efforts, which, sampling on the dependent variable of willingness to engage in cross-boundary dialog, misrepresent the range of American religious diversity, typically excluding those who do not wish

to be included among the ecumenically inclined—Pentecostal Christians, Orthodox Jews, and conservative Muslims, among others.

6. See Ducey, *Sunday Morning.*

7. See Mathews, "Second Great Awakening as an Organizing Process";
Miyakawa, *Protestants and Pioneers;* McGreevy, *Parish Boundaries;* Winter, *Suburban Captivity of the Churches;* and Warner, *New Wine in Old Wineskins.*

8. Becker, *Congregations in Conflict.*

9. Marty, "Public and Private."

10. W. H. Whyte, in *The Organization Man,* and Bennett M. Berger, in *Working-Class Suburb,* wrote of Jewish and working-class suburbs, respectively.

11. Warner, "Changes in the Civic Role of Religion," 238.

12. Putnam, "Bowling Alone."

13. Wuthnow, *Restructuring of American Religion.*

14. Bellah et al., *Habits of the Heart.*

15. See Tipton, *Getting Saved from the Sixties;* Lemann, *Promised Land;* and
FitzGerald, *Cities on a Hill.*

16. Stacey, *Brave New Families.*

17. Parsons, "Age and Sex in Social Structure."

18. Friedan, *Feminine Mystique.*

19. Stacey, *Brave New Families.*

20. Warner, "Changes in the Civic Role of Religion."

21. See also Pattillo, "Sweet Mothers and Gangbangers."

22. Notwithstanding the racism and anti-Semitism that Benjamin Smith and
the World Wide Church of the Creator brutally visited upon this community on
July 2, 1999.

23. Kwon, Kim, and Warner, eds., *Korean Americans and Their Religions.*

24. Warner and Wittner, eds., *Gatherings in Diaspora.*

25. Wilson, *Our Tribe.*

26. FitzGerald, *Cities on a Hill;* Warner, "Metropolitan Community Churches
and the Gay Agenda."

27. Warner, "The Place of the Congregation."

28. McGreevy, *Parish Boundaries.*

Appendix

Religious Organizations Studied and Names of Principal Contact Persons

Chapter 2. Pilsen

Iglesia Presbiteriana Emanuel
1850 S. Racine Avenue
Chicago, IL 60608
Rev. Rolando Cuellar, pastor

Pilsen Resurrection Project
1818 S. Paulina Street
Chicago, IL 60608
Raoul Raymundo, executive director

St. Paul Roman Catholic Church
2127 W. 22nd Place
Chicago, IL 60608
Rev. George Ruffolo, pastor

St. Pius V Roman Catholic Church
1919 S. Ashland Avenue
Chicago, IL 60608
Rev. Charles W. Dahm, O.P., pastor

Temple Bethel Church of God
1924 S. Leavitt Street
Chicago, IL 60608
Rev. Jose Vasquez, pastor

Chapter 3. Loop and Near North Side

First United Methodist Church, Chicago Temple
77 W. Washington Street
Chicago, IL 60602
Rev. Eugene Winkler, pastor

Fourth Presbyterian Church
126 E. Chestnut Street
Chicago, IL 60611
Rev. John M. Buchanan, pastor

LaSalle Street Church
1136 N. LaSalle Street
Chicago, IL 60610
Rev. Bruce Otto, associate pastor

The Moody Church
1609 North LaSalle
Chicago, IL 60614
Rev. Erwin Lutzer, pastor
Rev. Daryl Worley, associate pastor

Old St. Patrick's Roman Catholic Church
122 S. Des Plaines Street
Chicago, IL 60661
Rev. John J. Wall, pastor

Park Community Church
108 W. Germania Place
Chicago, IL 60610
Jim Sharkey

Episcopal Cathedral of St. James
65 E. Huron Street
Chicago, IL 60611
Rev. Todd Smelser, dean

St. Joseph's Roman Catholic Church and School
1065 N. Orleans Street
Chicago, IL 60610
Sr. Stephanie Schmidt

Temple Sholom
3480 N. Lake Shore Drive
Chicago, IL 60657
Rabbi Frederick Schwartz

Chapter 4. Near West Side

First Baptist Congregational Church
1613 W. Washington Boulevard
Chicago, IL 60612
Rev. Arthur D. Griffin, pastor

Greater Pleasant Valley Missionary Baptist Church
1709 W. Washington Boulevard
Chicago, IL 60612
Rev. Robert Skinner, pastor

People's Church of God in Christ
4244 W. Madison Street
Chicago, IL 60624
Rev. William M. Elder, pastor

Presentation Roman Catholic Church
734 S. Springfield Avenue
Chicago, IL 60624
Rev. Thomas P. Walsh, pastor

Revival Center Church of God in Christ
1956 W. Washington Boulevard
Chicago, IL 60612
Rev. Benjamin Bowman, pastor

St. Malachy Roman Catholic Church
2248 W. Washington Boulevard
Chicago, IL 60612
Rev. Ralph E. Starus, pastor

St. Stephen AME Church
2000 W. Washington Boulevard
Chicago, IL 60612
Rev. Albert D. Tyson III, pastor

Spirit of Joy Lutheran Church
1345 N. Karlov Avenue
Chicago, IL 60651
Rev. Maxine Washington, pastor

Chapter 5. Southwest Side

Almuhajireen Mosque and School
Pulaski Avenue at 63rd Street
Chicago, IL 60629
Khawla Razeq, lay member

Congregation Lawn Manor Beth Jacob
6601 S. Kedzie Avenue
Chicago, IL 60629
Janice Kay, lay member

Covenant Group of Churches
6012 S. Laflin Street
Chicago, IL 60636
Mary Foley, coordinator

Greater Southwest Development Corporation
2601 W. 63rd Street
Chicago, IL 60629
Jim Capraro, director

St. Adrian Roman Catholic Church
7000 S. Fairfield Avenue
Chicago, IL 60629
Rev. Theodore Ostrowski, pastor

St. Bruno Roman Catholic Church
4751 S. Harding Avenue
Chicago, IL 60632
Rev. Joseph P. Grembla, pastor

St. Clare de Montefalco Roman Catholic Church
5443 S. Washtenaw Avenue
Chicago, IL 60632
Rev. Anthony Pizzo, pastor

St. Gall Roman Catholic Church
5511 S. Sawyer Avenue
Chicago, IL 60629
Rev. David Dowdle, pastor

Nativity BVM Roman Catholic Church
6812 S. Washtenaw Avenue
Chicago, IL 60629

St. Nicholas of Tolentine Roman Catholic Church
3721 W. 62nd Street
Chicago, IL 60629
Rev. Stanley G. Rataj, pastor

St. Rita of Cascia Roman Catholic Church
6243 S. Fairfield Avenue
Chicago, IL 60629
Rev. William E. Lego, O.S.A., pastor

Southwest Organizing Project
(formerly Southwest Catholic Cluster Project)
2601 W. 63rd Street
Chicago, IL 60629
Jay Caponigro, executive director

Southwest Youth Collaborative
3154 W. 63rd Street
Chicago, IL 60629
Camille Odeh, director

New Life Community Church
1700 W. 44th Street
Chicago, IL 60609
Rev. Mark Jobe, pastor

First Christian Church
3600 W. 79th Street
Chicago, IL 60652
Rev. Alan White, pastor

Ashburn Lutheran Church
3345 W. 83rd Street
Chicago, IL 60652

Chapter 6. Rogers Park and West Rogers Park

Al-Madina Islamic Center
(also Wallen Community Center)
1701 W. Wallen Avenue
Chicago, IL 60626

The Ark
6450 N. California Avenue
Chicago, IL 60645
Renee Lepp, executive director

Congregation Ezra Habonim
2620 W. Touhy Avenue
(now 2800 W. Sherwin)
Chicago, IL 60645
Rabbi Robert Rhodes
Fred Sinay, president
Ralph Reubner, chair, Pulpit Committee

First Telugu Methodist Church
1545 W. Morse Avenue
Chicago, IL 60626
Rev. Jacob Agepog, pastor

Good News Church/Iglesia Buenas Nuevas
7649 N. Paulina Street
Chicago, IL 60626
Rev. Karen Mosby-Avery, pastor
Rev. Haracio Sedio-Peralta, pastor

Iglesia de Cristo–Misión Cristiana Elim
1615 W. Morse Avenue
Chicago, IL 60626
Rev. Hector Nufio, pastor

International Society for Krishna Consciousness (ISKCON)
(Hare Krishna Temple)
1716 W. Lunt Avenue
Chicago, IL 60626
Prithusrava Dasa, president
Shankara Pandit, vice president

St. Jerome Roman Catholic Church
1709 W. Lunt Avenue
Chicago, IL 60626
Rev. Harold A. Bonin, pastor

Sephardic Congregation
1819 W. Howard Street
Evanston, IL 60202
Rabbi Michael Azose
Yehoshua Ben Avraham, president

United Church of Rogers Park
1545 W. Morse Avenue
Chicago, IL 60626
Rev. Kermit Krueger, pastor
Anita Alcantara, minister of community life

Unity Church
1925 W. Thome Avenue
Chicago, IL 60660

Chapter 7. Chatham and Greater Grand Crossing

Carter Temple CME Church
7841 S. Wabash Avenue
Chicago, IL 60619
Rev. Henry M. Williamson Sr., pastor

Ingleside-Whitfield United Methodist Church
929 E. 76th Street
Chicago, IL 60619
Rev. Danita Anderson, pastor

Israel Methodist Community Church
7620 S. Cottage Grove Avenue
Chicago, IL 60619
Rev. Hiram Crawford, pastor

New Covenant Missionary Baptist Church
740 E. 77th Street
Chicago, IL 60619
Rev. Stephen J. Thurston, pastor

St. Columbanus Roman Catholic Church
331 E. 71st Street
Chicago, IL 60619
Rev. Phillip Cyscon, pastor

Vernon Park Church of God
9011 S. Stony Island Avenue
Chicago, IL 60617
Rev. Claude Wyatt and Rev. Addie Wyatt, pastors

Chapter 8. Naperville, Illinois

Calvary Church
9S200 Route 59
Naperville, IL 60564
Rev. Robert Schmidgall, pastor (deceased)
Rev. Keith Boucher, assistant pastor
Mark Strohm, principal, Calvary Christian School

Congregation Beth Shalom
1433 N. Main Street
Naperville, IL 60563
Rabbi Michael M. Remson

First Congregational Church
25 E. Benton Avenue
Naperville, IL 60540
Harold Gosselink, lay member and historian

Islamic Center of Naperville
450 S. Olsen Drive
Naperville, IL 60540
Faisel Hamoudeh, president

Lotus Sangha
1520 Canyon Run Road
Naperville, IL 60565
Amelia Nguyen, lay member

St. James Lutheran Church
2844 W. Ogden Avenue (Route 34)
Naperville, IL 60567
Rev. Roger Timm, pastor

Wheatland Salem Church
Route 59 and 95th Street
Naperville, IL 60564
Rev. Scott Field, pastor

Chapter 9. Old Saint Patrick's Roman Catholic Church

Old St. Patrick's Roman Catholic Church
122 S. Des Plaines Street
Chicago, IL 60661
Rev. John J. Wall, pastor
Rev. John C. Cusick, associate pastor
Eileen Smith, lay member

Chapter 10. Recent Immigrant Congregations

Chinmaya Mission
11 S. 80, Route 83
Hinsdale, IL 60521
Brother Sharan Chaitanya

The Hindu Temple of Greater Chicago
10915 Lemont Road
Lemont, IL 60439
Marella L. Hanumadass, president

International Society of Krishna Consciousness (ISKCON)
1716 W. Lunt Avenue
Chicago, IL 60626
Prithusrava Dasa

Jain Society of Metropolitan Chicago
435 N. Route 59
Bartlett, IL 60103

Mosque Foundation
Harlem Avenue and 93rd Street
Bridgeview, IL 60455
Rafeeq A. Jaber, president

Muslim Community Center
4380 N. Elston Avenue
Chicago, IL 60641
NeQuiniso Abdulla, president

Sikh Religious Society of Chicago
P.O. Box 864
Palatine, IL 60067
Granthi Mohinder Singh

Sri Venkateswara (Balaji) Temple of Greater Chicago
1145 Sullivan Road
P.O. Box 1536
Aurora, IL 60507-1536

The Thai Buddhist Temple (Wat Dhammaram)
7059 W. 75th Street
Chicago, IL 60638-5934
Ven. Chuen Phangcham

Wat Phrasriratanamahadhatu
4735 N. Magnolia
Chicago, IL 60640
Phra Ratana Thongkrajai

Chapter 11. Archdiocese of Chicago

The Pastoral Center
155 E. Superior Street
Chicago, IL 60611
Joseph Cardinal Bernardin, archbishop of Chicago (deceased)
Rev. David E. Baldwin, director of the research and planning
Elaine Schuster, superintendent of Catholic schools

Bibliography

Adelman, William J. *Pilsen and the West Side*. Chicago: Illinois Labor History Society, 1977.

Ammerman, Nancy T. *Congregation and Community*. New Brunswick, NJ: Rutgers University Press, 1997.

Ammerman, Nancy T., Jackson W. Carroll, Carol S. Dudley, and William McKinney, eds. *Studying Congregations: A New Handbook*. Nashville, TN: Abingdon, 1998.

Anderson, Alan B., and George W. Pickering. *Confronting the Color Line: The Broken Promise of the Civil Rights Movement in Chicago*. Athens: University of Georgia Press, 1986.

Anderson, Elijah. "The Code of the Streets." *Atlantic Monthly,* May 1994, 81–94.

———. *Streetwise: Race, Class, and Change in an Urban Community*. Chicago: University of Chicago Press, 1990.

Anderson, Nels. *The Hobo*. Chicago: University of Chicago Press, 1923.

Anzaldúa, Gloria. *Borderlands/La Frontera: The New Mestiza*. San Francisco: Spinsters/Aunt Lute, 1987.

The Archdiocese of Chicago: Antecedents and Developments. Des Plaines, IL: St. Mary's Training School, 1920.

Asante, Molefi Kete. *Afrocentricity*. Trenton, NJ: Africa World, 1988.

Asian American Handbook. Chicago: National Conference of Christians and Jews, Asian American Journalists Association, and Association of Asian Pacific American Artists, 1991.

Avella, Steven. *This Confident Church: Catholic Leadership and Life in Chicago, 1940–1965*. Notre Dame, IN: University of Notre Dame Press, 1992.

Badillo, David. "The Catholic Church and the Making of Mexican-American Parish Communities in the Midwest." In *Mexican Americans and the Catholic Church, 1900–1965*, edited by Jay P. Dolan and Gilberto M. Hinojosa, 254–256. Notre Dame, IN: University of Notre Dame Press, 1994.

Bakke, Raymond J. *The Expanded Mission of "Old First" Churches*. Valley Forge, PA: Judson, 1986.

———. *A Theology as Big as the City*. Downers Grove, IL: InterVarsity, 1997.

Banner-Haley, Charles. *The Fruits of Integration: Black Middle Class Ideology 1960–1990*. Jackson: University Press of Mississippi, 1994.

Barton, Timothy. "Celtic Revived: The Artistry of Thomas O'Shaughnessy." In *At the Crossroads: Old Saint Patrick's and the Chicago Irish*, edited by Ellen Skerrett, 85–101. Chicago: Wild Onion, 1997.

Bass, Dorothy C. "Congregations and the Bearing of Traditions." In *American Congregations*, vol. 2: *New Perspectives in the Study of Congregations*, edited by James P. Wind and James W. Lewis. Chicago: University of Chicago Press, 1994.

———, ed. *Practicing Our Faith: A Way of Life for a Searching People*. San Francisco: Jossey-Bass, 1996.

Beaudoin, David M. "Elementary Schools in the United States: Catholic and American." *Chicago Studies* 28 (November 1989): 303–319.

———. "Evangelization, Christian Initiation and Catholic Schools." *Catechumenate* 14 (July 1992): 12–20.

Becker, Laura L. "Ethnicity and Religion." In *Encyclopedia of the American Religious Experience: Studies of Traditions and Movements*, edited by Charles H. Lippy and Peter W. Williams, 1477–1491. New York: Scribner's, 1988.

Becker, Penny E. *Congregations in Conflict: Cultural Models of Local Religious Life*. Cambridge: Cambridge University Press, 1999.

Becker, Penny E., and Nancy L. Eiesland, eds. *Contemporary American Religion: An Ethnographic Reader*. Walnut Creek, CA: AltaMira, 1997.

Bellah, Robert N., Richard Madsen, William M. Sullivan, Ann Swidler, and Steven M. Tipton. *Habits of the Heart: Individualism and Commitment in American Life*. Berkeley: University of California Press, 1985.

Berger, Bennett M. *Working-Class Suburb*. Berkeley: University of California Press, 1960.

Bernardin, Joseph Cardinal. *Decisions for the Future of Our Church*. Archdiocese of Chicago, Chicago, Spring 1994.

———. *Decisions for the Future of Our Church: Implementation Plan, Evangelization and Education, Ministerial Leadership*. Archdiocese of Chicago, Chicago, Fall 1994.

———. *The Gift of Peace: Personal Reflections*. Chicago: Loyola University Press, 1997.

Billingsley, Andrew. *Climbing Jacob's Ladder: The Enduring Legacy of African-American Families*. New York: Simon & Schuster, 1992.

Blank, Rebecca M. *It Takes a Nation: A New Agenda for Fighting Poverty*. Princeton, NJ: Princeton University Press, 1997.

Bluestone, Daniel. *Constructing Chicago*. New Haven, CT: Yale University Press, 1991.

Bodnar, John. *The Transplanted: A History of Immigrants in Urban America*. Bloomington: Indiana University Press, 1985.

Bole, William. "Closing the Doors." *Catholic World Report* 4, no. 5 (May 1994): 30–33.

Boyer, Horace Clarence. *How Sweet the Sound: The Golden Age of Gospel.* Washington, DC: Elliott & Clark, 1995.

Braden, William. "Chatham: An African-American Success Story." In *Ethnic Chicago: A Multicultural Portrait,* edited by Melvin G. Holli and Peter d'A. Jones, 4th ed., 341–345. Grand Rapids, MI: William B. Eerdmans, 1995.

Branch, Taylor. *Parting the Waters: America in the King Years, 1954–1963.* New York: Simon & Schuster, 1988.

Browning, Don S. *A Fundamental Practical Theology: Descriptive and Strategic Proposals.* Minneapolis: Fortress, 1991.

Buchanan, John M. *Being Church, Becoming Community.* 1st ed. Louisville, KY: Westminster John Knox, 1996.

Buetow, Harold A. *Of Singular Benefit: The Story of U.S. Catholic Education.* New York: Macmillan, 1970.

Burgess, Ernest W. "The Growth of the City: An Introduction to a Research Project." In *The City,* by Robert E. Park and Ernest W. Burgess. Chicago: University of Chicago Press, 1925.

Butler, Francis J., ed. *American Catholic Identity: Essays in an Age of Change.* Kansas City, MO: Sheed & Ward, 1994.

"Cabrini Youths Take Shot at Film Making." *Chicago Defender,* 28 September 1994.

Candeloro, Dominic. "Chicago's Italians: A Survey of the Ethnic Factor, 1850–1990." In *Ethnic Chicago: A Multicultural Portrait,* edited by Melvin G. Holli and Peter d'A. Jones, 4th ed., 229–259. Grand Rapids, MI: William B. Eerdmans, 1995.

Carlson, Alvar W. "The Settling of Asian Immigrant Groups in the Chicago Metropolitan Area, 1965–76." *Philippine Geographical Journal* 28 (1984): 22–40.

Carroll, Jackson W., Carl S. Dudley, and William McKinney, eds. *Handbook for Congregational Studies.* Nashville, TN: Abingdon, 1986.

Caruso, Jorge, and Eduardo Camacho. "Latino Chicago." In *Ethnic Chicago,* edited by Melvin G. Holli and Peter d'A. Jones, 4th ed. Grand Rapids, MI: William B. Eerdmans, 1995.

Casanova, José. *Public Religions in the Modern World.* Chicago: University of Chicago Press, 1994.

Castelli, James, and Joseph Gremillion. *The Emerging Parish: The Notre Dame Study of Catholic Life since Vatican II.* San Francisco: Harper & Row, 1987.

Cateura, Linda Brandi, ed. *Growing Up Italian: How Being Brought Up as an Italian-American Helped Shape the Characters, Lives, and Fortunes of Twenty-four Celebrated Americans.* New York: William Morrow, 1987.

Cenkner, William. *The Multicultural Church: A New Landscape in U.S. Theologies.* New York: Paulist, 1995.

Chapman, Mark L. *Christianity on Trial: African American Religious Thought before and after Black Power.* Maryknoll, NY: Orbis Books, 1996.

Chaves, Mark. "Secularization as Declining Religious Authority." *Social Forces* 72, no. 3 (March 1994): 749–774.

Chicago Fact Book Consortium. *Local Community Fact Book, Chicago Metropolitan Area: Based on the 1980 Census.* Chicago: The Chicago Review, 1985.

———. *Local Community Fact Book Chicago Metropolitan Area 1990.* Chicago: Academy Chicago, 1995.

Chicago Housing Authority. *Statistical Profile: The Chicago Housing Authority, 1991–1992.* Chicago: Chicago Housing Authority, 1992.

Chicago Regional Report. National Growth Management Leadership Project, October 1996.

Cohen, Anthony. *The Symbolic Construction of Community.* London: Routledge, 1985.

Cohen, Martin A., and Abraham J. Peck, eds. *Sephardim in the Americas: Studies in Culture and History.* Tuscaloosa: University of Alabama Press, 1993.

Coleman, James. "Families and Schools." *Educational Researcher* 32 (August 1987): 32–38.

———. *Foundations of Social Theory.* Cambridge, MA: Belknap Press of Harvard University Press, 1990.

———. "Social Capital in the Creation of Human Capital." *American Journal of Sociology* 94 (1988): S95–121.

Coleman, John, S.J. "True and False Multi-Culturalism." Address to National Catholic Charities Convention, Washington, DC, 1 October 1994.

Condit, Celeste Michelle, and John Louis Lucaites. *Crafting Equality: America's Anglo-African Word.* Chicago: University of Chicago Press, 1993.

Conzen, Kathleen Neils. "Forum: The Place of Religion in Urban and Community Studies." *Religion and American Culture* 6, no. 2 (1996): 112.

Conzen, Kathleen Neils, David A. Gerber, Ewa Morawska, George E. Pozetta, and Rudolph Vecoli. "The Invention of Ethnicity: A Perspective from the U.S.A." *Journal of American Ethnic History* 12, no. 1 (1992): 3–41.

Copeland, Warren R. *And the Poor Get Welfare: The Ethics of Poverty in the United States.* Nashville, TN: Abingdon, 1994.

Coriden, James A. *The Parish in Catholic Tradition: History, Theology and Canon Law.* New York: Paulist, 1997.

Coriden, James A., Thomas J. Green, and Donald E. Heintschel, eds. *The Code of Canon Law: A Text and Commentary.* New York: Paulist, 1985.

Cose, Ellis. *The Rage of a Privileged Class: Why Are Middle-Class Blacks Angry? Why Should America Care?* New York: HarperCollins, 1993.

"Criteria for a Good Parish." *Origins* 24, no. 3 (2 June 1994): 1, 35.

Cruse, Harold. *Plural but Equal: A Critical Study of Blacks and Minorities and America's Plural Society.* New York: William Morrow, 1987.

Cutler, Irving. *The Jews of Chicago: From Shtetl to Suburb.* Chicago: University of Illinois Press, 1996.

D'Agostino, Peter R. "The Crisis of Authority in American Catholicism: Urban Schools and Cultural Conflict." *Records of the American Catholic Historical Society of Philadelphia* 108 (Fall–Winter 1997–1998): 87–122.

———. "Missionaries in Babylon: The Adaptation of Italian Priests to Chicago's Church, 1870–1940." Ph.D. diss., University of Chicago, 1993.

———. "Recent Research." *American Catholic Studies Newsletter, Cushwa Center for the Study of American Catholicism* 21, no. 2 (September 1994): 16–18.

Dahm, Charles, O.P. "A Brief Analysis of Some Historical Developments in Hispanic Ministry in the Archdiocese of Chicago." Unpublished paper, October 1990.

———. *Power and Authority in the Catholic Church: Cardinal Cody in Chicago.* Notre Dame, IN: University of Notre Dame Press, 1981.

Daniel, Vattel Elbert. "Ritual Stratification in Chicago Negro Churches." *American Sociological Review* 7 (June 1942): 73.

Daniels, David D., III. "The Cultural Renewal of Slave Religion: Charles Price Jones and the Emergence of the Holiness Movement in Mississippi." Ph.D. diss., Union Theological Seminary, 1992.

Danzger, M. Herbert. *Returning to Tradition: The Contemporary Revival of Orthodox Judaism.* New Haven, CT: Yale University Press, 1989.

Dart, John. "Most View Christians, Jews as Good Influences, Survey Finds." *Los Angeles Times,* 17 February 1996, B1.

Data on the Organization, Resources and Activities of the Archdiocese of Chicago: Facts and Figures for Year Ending 1995. Chicago: Archdiocese of Chicago Office of Research and Planning, 1996.

Davis, Cyprian. *The History of Black Catholics in the United States.* New York: Crossroad, 1993.

"Declaration on Religious Freedom." In *The Documents of Vatican II: In a New and Definitive Translation,* edited by Walter M. Abbott, S.J., 675–696. New York: Herder & Herder, 1966.

Demerath, N. J., III, and Rhys H. Williams. *A Bridging of Faiths: Religion and Politics in a New England City.* Princeton, NJ: Princeton University Press, 1992.

———. "Secularization in a Community Context: Tensions of Religion and Politics in a New England City." *Journal for the Scientific Study of Religion* 31, no. 2 (1992): 189–206.

"Developer Building a Dream at Cabrini." *Chicago Tribune,* 20 June 1998.

Díaz-Stevens, Ana María, and Anthony M. Stevens-Arroyo. *Recognizing the Latino Resurgence in U.S. Religion.* Boulder, CO: Westview, 1998.

"Diocesan Offices: Organization and Reorganization." *Center Papers* 6 (1994): 1–12.

"Diocesan Reorganization." *Center Papers* 2 (December 1985): 1–12.

Dolan, Jay P. *The American Catholic Experience: A History from Colonial Times to the Present.* Garden City, NY: Doubleday, 1985.

Dolan, Jay P., and Gilberto M. Hinojosa, eds. *Mexican Americans and the Catholic Church, 1900–1965*. Notre Dame, IN: University of Notre Dame Press, 1994.

Drake, St. Clair, and Horace R. Cayton. *Black Metropolis: A Study of Negro Life in a Northern City*. New York: Harper & Row, 1962.

Drucker, Peter F. "The Age of Social Transformation." *Atlantic Monthly,* November 1994, 53–80.

Ducey, Michael. *Sunday Morning: Aspects of Urban Ritual*. New York: Free Press, 1977.

Dudley, Carl S. *Basic Steps toward Community Ministry: Guidelines and Models in Action*. Washington, DC: Alban Institute, 1991.

Dudley, Carl S., and Sally A. Johnson. "Congregational Self-Images for Social Ministry." In *Carriers of Faith: Lessons from Congregational Studies,* edited by Carl S. Dudley, Jackson W. Carroll, and James P. Wind, 104–124. Louisville, KY: Westminster John Knox, 1991.

Dudley, Carl S., Jackson W. Carroll, and James P. Wind, eds. *Carriers of Faith: Lessons from Congregational Studies*. Louisville, KY: Westminster John Knox, 1991.

DuPage County Development Department, Planning Division. *Profile: DuPage County Statistical Handbook*. 1992.

DuPage County Regional Planning Commission. *DuPage County Jobs/Housing Study*. February 1991.

Dusenbery, Verne A. "Introduction: A Century of Sikhs beyond Punjab." In *The Sikh Diaspora: Migration and the Experience Beyond Punjab,* edited by N. Gerald Barrier and Verne A. Dusenbery, 1–28. Delhi: Chanakya, 1989.

Dyson, Michael E. *Reflecting Black: African-American Cultural Criticism*. Minneapolis: University of Minnesota Press, 1993.

Ebner, Michael H. "Technoburb." *Inland Architect* 37, no. 1 (January 1993): 54–59.

Eck, Diana L. *Darsan: Seeing the Divine Image in India*. 2d ed. Chambersburg, PA: Anima, 1985.

———. *World Religions in Boston: A Guide to Communities and Resources*. Cambridge, MA: Pluralism Project, Harvard University, 1995.

Edington, Howard. *Downtown Church: The Heart of the City*. Nashville, TN: Abingdon, 1996.

Ehrenhalt, Alan. *The Lost City: Discovering the Forgotten Virtues of Community in the Chicago of the 1950s*. New York: Basic Books, 1995.

Eiesland, Nancy L. *A Particular Place: Urban Restructuring and Religious Ecology in a Southern Exurb*. New Brunswick, NJ: Rutgers University Press, 2000.

Elshtain, Jean Bethke. *Democracy on Trial*. New York: Basic Books, 1995.

Engel, Ronald J. *Sacred Sands: The Struggle for Community in the Indiana Dunes*. Middletown, CT: Wesleyan University Press, 1983.

Espiritu, Yen Le, and Ivan Light. "The Changing Ethnic Shape of Contemporary

Urban America." In *Urban Life in Transition,* edited by Mark Gottdiener and Chris G. Pickvance, 35–54. Newbury Park, CA: Sage, 1991.

Etzioni, Amitai. "The Responsive Community: A Communitarian Perspective— 1995 Presidential Address." *American Sociological Review* 61, no. 1 (February 1996): 1–11.

Faith and Culture: A Multicultural Catechetical Resource. Washington, DC: United States Catholic Conference, 1987.

Faramelli, Norman, Edward Rodman, and Anne Scheibner. "Seeking to Hear and Heed in the Cities: Urban Ministry in the Postwar Episcopal Church." In *Churches, Cities, and Human Community: Urban Ministry in the United States 1945–1985,* edited by Clifford J. Green, 97–122. Grand Rapids, MI: William B. Eerdmans, 1996.

Farr, Marcia. "Language, Culture, and Literacy in a Transnational Community: Old Traditions in New Settings." Unpublished manuscript, 1997.

Fenton, John Y. *Transplanting Religious Traditions: Asian Indians in America.* New York: Praeger, 1988.

Ferguson, Margaret Geneva. *The History of St. Paul C.M.E. Church, Chicago, Illinois 1907–1988.* Chicago: Margaret G. Ferguson, 1988.

Ferman, Barbara. *Challenging the Growth Machine: Neighborhood Politics in Chicago and Pittsburgh.* Lawrence: University Press of Kansas, 1996.

Fichter, Joseph H. *Social Relations in the Urban Parish.* Chicago: University of Chicago Press, 1954.

Field, Scott N. "'Let My People Go!' Breaking the Two Hundred Barrier at Wheatland Salem United Methodist Church through Lay Ministries." Ph.D. diss., Asbury Theological Seminary, 1991.

Fischer, Claude S. "The Subcultural Theory of Urbanism: A Twentieth-Year Assessment." *American Journal of Sociology* 101, no. 3 (November 1995): 543–577.

———. *To Dwell among Friends: Personal Networks in Town and City.* Chicago: University of Chicago Press, 1982.

Fish, John, Gordon Nelson, Walter Stuhr, and Lawrence Witmer. *The Edge of the Ghetto: A Study of Church Involvement in Community Organization.* New York: Seabury, 1968.

Fishman, Robert. *Bourgeois Utopias: The Rise and Fall of Suburbia.* New York: Basic Books, 1987.

FitzGerald, Frances. *Cities on a Hill: A Journey through Contemporary American Cultures.* New York: Simon and Schuster, 1986.

Fitzpatrick, Joseph P., S.J. *One Church, Many Cultures: The Challenge of Diversity.* Kansas City, MO: Sheed & Ward, 1987.

Fontana, John. "A Religious Entrepreneur in the World of Work." *Catholic World* 237 (July 1994): 1420.

Fornero, George V. "The Expansion and Decline of Enrollment and Facilities of

Secondary Schools in the Archdiocese of Chicago, 1955–1980: A Historical Study." Ph.D. diss., Loyola University of Chicago, 1990.

Fox Valley Genealogical Society. *Copenhagen Cemetery.* Naperville, IL, 1997.

Franklin, Robert M. *Another Day's Journey: Black Churches Confronting the American Crisis.* Minneapolis: Fortress, 1997.

———. "My Soul Says Yes: The Urban Ministry of the Church of God in Christ." In *Churches, Cities, and Human Community: Urban Ministry in the United States 1945–1985,* edited by Clifford J. Green, 77–96. Grand Rapids, MI: William B. Eerdmans, 1996.

———. "The Safest Place on Earth: The Culture of Black Congregations." In *American Congregations,* vol. 2: *New Perspectives in the Study of Congregations,* edited by James P. Wind and James W. Lewis, 257–284. Chicago: University of Chicago Press, 1994.

Frazier, E. Franklin. *Black Bourgeoisie.* New York: Collier Books, 1962.

———. *The Negro Church in America.* New York: Schocken Books, 1974.

———. *The Negro Family in Chicago.* Chicago: University of Chicago Press, 1932.

———. *The Negro Family in the United States.* Chicago: University of Chicago Press, 1939.

Friedan, Betty. *The Feminine Mystique.* New York: Norton, 1963.

Fuchs, Lawrence H. *The American Kaleidoscope: Race, Ethnicity, and the Civic Culture.* Hanover, NH: Wesleyan University Press, 1990.

Galloway, Paul. "A Place to Call Home: Assyrian Church Brings Headquarters to Chicago." *Chicago Tribune,* 8 September 1995, sec. 2, p. 9.

Gannon, Thomas. "Religious Tradition and Urban Community." *Sociological Analysis* (1979): 283–302.

Gannon, Thomas, and David F. Schwartz. "Church Finances in Crisis." *Social Compass* 39, no. 1 (March 1992): 111–120.

Garraghan, Gilbert J. *The Catholic Church in Chicago, 1673–1871: An Historical Sketch.* Chicago: Loyola University Press, 1921.

Garreau, J. *Edge City: Life on the New Frontier.* New York: Doubleday, 1991.

Geertz, Clifford. *The Interpretation of Cultures.* New York: Basic Books, 1973.

———. *Local Knowledge: Further Essays in Interpretive Anthropology.* New York: Basic Books, 1983.

Giddens, Anthony. *The Constitution of Society: Outline of a Theory of Structuration.* Berkeley: University of California Press, 1984.

Gilkes, Cheryl Townsend. "The Storm and the Light: Church, Family, Work, and Social Crisis in the African-American Experience." In *Work, Family, and Religion in Contemporary Society,* edited by Nancy T. Ammerman and Wade C. Roof, 177–198. New York: Routledge, 1995.

Gilkey, Langdon. "The Christian Congregation as Religious Community." In *American Congregations,* vol. 2: *New Perspectives in the Study of Congregations,* edited by James P. Wind and James W. Lewis, 100–132. Chicago: University of Chicago Press, 1994.

Gilligan, Carol. *In a Different Voice: Psychological Theory and Women's Development*. Cambridge, MA: Harvard University Press, 1982.

Gitlin, Todd. *The Twilight of Common Dreams: Why America Is Wracked by Culture Wars*. New York: Metropolitan Books–Henry Holt, 1995.

Glazer, Nathan. *American Judaism*. 2d rev. ed. The Chicago History of American Civilization, edited by Daniel J. Boorstin. Chicago: University of Chicago Press, 1989.

———. *We Are All Multiculturalists Now*. Cambridge, MA: Harvard University Press, 1997.

Gleason, Philip. *Keeping the Faith: American Catholicism Past and Present*. Notre Dame, IN: University of Notre Dame Press, 1987.

———. "What Made Catholic Identity a Problem?" In *The Challenge and Promise of a Catholic University,* edited by Theodore M. Hesburgh, C.S.C., 91–102. Notre Dame, IN: University of Notre Dame Press, 1994.

Goozner, Merrill. "What Ails Post-Industrial Chicago." In *Chicago's Future in a Time of Change,* edited by Dick Simpson, 77–87. Champaign, IL: Stipes, 1993.

Gottdiener, Mark. *The Social Production of Urban Space*. 2nd ed. Austin: University of Texas Press, 1994.

Gottdiener, Mark, and Joe R. Feagin. "The Paradigm Shift in Urban Sociology." *Urban Affairs Quarterly* 24 (1988): 163–187.

Gottdiener, Mark, and Chris G. Pickvance, eds. *Urban Life in Transition*. Newbury Park, CA: Sage, 1991.

Greeley, Andrew M. *The American Catholic: A Social Portrait*. New York: Basic Books, 1977.

———. *The Catholic Myth: The Behavior and Belief of American Catholics*. New York: Scribner's, 1990.

——. "Catholic Schools: A Golden Twilight?" *America* (11 February 1989): 106–118.

Green, Cathy, and Monique Irvin. "The National Black Catholic Congress." *In a Word* 5 (July–August 1987): 2.

Green, Clifford J. "History in the Service of the Future: Studying Urban Ministry." In *Churches, Cities, and Human Community: Urban Ministry in the United States 1945–1985,* edited by Clifford J. Green, 1–22. Grand Rapids, MI: William B. Eerdmans, 1996.

———, ed. *Churches, Cities, and Human Community: Urban Ministry in the United States 1945–1985.* Grand Rapids, MI: William B. Eerdmans, 1995.

Green, Paul M., and Melvin G. Holli, eds. *Restoration 1989: Chicago Elects a New Daley,* Chicago: Lyceum Books, 1991.

Grimshaw, William J. *Bitter Fruit: Black Politics and the Chicago Machine, 1931–1991*. Chicago: University of Chicago Press, 1992.

Grindel, John A., C.M. *Whither the U.S. Church? Context, Gospel, Planning.* Maryknoll, NY: Orbis Books, 1991.

Griswold, Wendy. *Cultures and Societies in a Changing World.* Thousand Oaks, CA: Pine Forge, 1994.

Gronbjerg, Kirsten A., Katy Crossley, Lorri Platek, Natalya Zhezmer, and Toni Migliore. *Rogers Park: A Tradition of Diversity—Laying the Foundation for Economic Development.* Loyola University, Chicago, November 1993.

"Growth Is at the Root of Cabrini Youth Garden." *Chicago Tribune,* 30 June 1993.

Guidelines for Development Strategy for Metropolitan Mission. New York: Division of Church Strategy and Development, Board of National Missions, United Presbyterian Church U.S.A., 1967.

Hacker, Andrew. *Two Nations: Black and White, Separate, Hostile, Unequal.* New York: Macmillan, 1992.

Haddad, Yvonne Yazbeck, ed. *The Muslims of America.* New York: Oxford University Press, 1991.

Haider, Donald. "Chicagoland 2005." In *Chicago's Future in a Time of Change,* edited by Dick Simpson, 114–132. Champaign, IL: Stipes, 1993.

Hall, John R., and Mary Jo Neitz. *Culture: Sociological Perspectives.* Englewood Cliffs, NJ: Prentice-Hall, 1993.

Hall, Suzanne E. *A Catholic Response to the Asian Presence.* Washington, DC: National Catholic Educational Association, 1990.

Hammond, Phillip E. *Religion and Personal Autonomy: The Third Disestablishment in America.* Columbia: University of South Carolina Press, 1992.

Handlin, Oscar. *The Uprooted: The Epic Story of the Great Migrations That Made the American People.* Boston: Little, Brown, 1951.

Handy, Robert T. "The Voluntary Principle in Religion and Religious Freedom in America." In *Voluntary Associations,* edited by D. B. Robertson. Richmond, VA: John Knox, 1966.

Harding, Vincent. "Toward a Darkly Radiant Vision of America's Truth: A Letter of Concern, an Invitation to Re-Creation." In *Community in America: The Challenge of Habits of the Heart,* edited by Charles H. Reynolds and Ralph V. Norman, 67–83. Berkeley: University of California Press, 1988.

Harkins, William. *Introducing the Catholic Elementary School Principal: What Principals Say about Themselves, Their Values, Their Schools.* Washington, DC: National Catholic Educational Association, 1993.

Harris, Joseph C. "Is the American Catholic Church Getting Out of the Elementary School Business?" *Chicago Studies* 31, no. 1 (April 1992): 81–92.

Harris, Michael W. *The Rise of Gospel Blues: The Music of Thomas Andrew Dorsey in the Urban Church.* New York: Oxford University Press, 1992.

Hefley, James C. *The Church That Takes on Trouble.* Elgin, IL: D. C. Cook, 1976.

Helgesen, Sally. *Everyday Revolutionaries: Working Women and the Transformation of American Life.* New York: Doubleday, 1998.

Helweg, Arthur W. "The Sikh Diaspora and Sikh Studies." In *Studying the Sikhs: Issues for North America,* edited by John Stratton Hawley and Gurinder Singh Mann, 69–93. Albany: State University of New York Press, 1993.

Herberg, Will. *Protestant-Catholic-Jew: An Essay in American Religious Sociology.* Garden City, NY: Doubleday, 1956.

Higginbotham, Evelyn B. *Righteous Discontent: The Women's Movement in the Black Baptist Church, 1880–1920.* Cambridge, MA: Harvard University Press, 1993.

Hirsch, Arnold. *Making the Second Ghetto: Race and Housing in Chicago, 1940–1960.* New York and Cambridge: Cambridge University Press, 1983.

Hirt, Jane. "Shifts in Labor Market Increase Wage Gap between Rich and Poor." *Chicago Tribune,* 20 June 1996, sec. 1, p. 6.

Hochschild, Jennifer L. *Facing Up to the American Dream: Race, Class, and the Soul of the Nation.* Princeton, NJ: Princeton University Press, 1995.

Holli, Melvin G., and Peter d'A. Jones, eds. *Ethnic Chicago: A Multicultural Portrait.* 3rd ed. Grand Rapids, MI: William B. Eerdmans, 1984.

———. *Ethnic Chicago: A Multicultural Portrait.* 4th ed. Grand Rapids, MI: William B. Eerdmans, 1995.

Hollinger, David A. *Postethnic America: Beyond Multiculturalism.* New York: Basic Books, 1995.

Hopewell, James F. *Congregation: Stories and Structures.* Edited by Barbara G. Wheeler. Philadelphia: Fortress, 1987.

Hovda, Robert W., ed. *This Far by Faith: American Black Worship and Its African Roots.* Washington, DC: National Office for Black Catholics, 1977.

Hunt, Thomas C., and Norlene M. Kunkel. "Catholic Schools: The Nation's Largest Alternative School System." In *Religious Schooling in America,* edited by James C. Carper and Thomas C. Hunt, 1–34. Birmingham, AL: Religious Education, 1984.

Hunter, Albert. "The Gold Coast and the Slum Revisited: Paradoxes in Replication Research and the Study of Social Change." *Urban Life* 11, no. 4 (1983): 461–476.

———. *Symbolic Communities: The Persistence and Change of Chicago's Local Communities.* Chicago: University of Chicago Press, 1974.

Hunter, James Davison. *Culture Wars: The Struggle to Define America.* New York: Basic Books, 1991.

Interfaith Organizing Project. *The New "West Side Story": The Story of the Interfaith Organizing Project.* Chicago: Interfaith Organizing Project, 1992.

Irvin, Dona L. *The Unsung Heart of Black America: A Middle-Class Church at Midcentury.* Columbia: University of Missouri Press, 1992.

Jackson, Joseph H. *A Story of Christian Activism.* Nashville, TN: Townsend, 1980.

Jackson, Kenneth T. *Crabgrass Frontier: The Suburbanization of the United States.* New York: Oxford University Press, 1985.

Janowitz, Morris. *The Community Press in an Urban Setting*. Chicago: University of Chicago Press, 1967.

Jones, Ezra Earl, and Robert L. Wilson. *What's Ahead for Old First Church*. 1st ed. New York: Harper & Row, 1974.

Kantowicz, Edward R. *Corporation Sole: Cardinal Mundelein and Chicago Catholicism*. Notre Dame, IN: University of Notre Dame Press, 1983.

Kasarda, John D. "Urban Industrial Transition and the Underclass." In *The Ghetto Underclass: Social Science Perspectives,* edited by William J. Wilson, 26–47. Newbury Park, CA: Sage, 1993.

Kealey, Robert J. "Collision Course: Clergy and Laity on Catholic Schools." *Chicago Studies* 28 (November 1989): 277–291.

Keating, Ann Durkin, and Pierre Lebeau. *North Central College and Naperville: A Shared History, 1870–1995*. Naperville, IL: North Central College, 1995.

Kelliher, Thomas G. "Mexican Catholics and Chicago's Parishes." *Working Paper Series, Cushwa Center for the Study of American Catholicism* 25, no. 2 (March 1993).

Kennedy, Eugene C. *Cardinal Bernardin: Easing Conflicts and Battling for the Soul of American Catholicism*. Chicago: Bonus Books, 1989.

———. *My Brother Joseph: The Spirit of a Cardinal and the Story of a Friendship*. New York: St. Martin's, 1997.

Kerr, Louise Año Nuevo. "Mexican Chicago." In *Ethnic Chicago: A Multicultural Portrait,* edited by Melvin G. Holli and Peter d'A. Jones, 3rd ed. Grand Rapids, MI: William B. Eerdmans, 1984.

Kincheloe, Samuel C. "The Behavior Sequence of a Dying Church." In *The Church in the City,* edited by Yoshio Fukuyama, 31–50. Chicago: Exploration, 1989.

Kniss, Fred. "Culture Wars: Remapping the Battleground." In *Cultural Wars in American Politics: Critical Reviews of a Popular Myth,* edited by Rhys H. Williams, 259–282. New York: Aldine de Gruyter, 1997.

Koenig, Harry C., ed. *A History of the Parishes of the Archdiocese of Chicago*. 2 vols. Chicago: Archdiocese of Chicago, 1980.

Kostarelos, Frances. *Feeling the Spirit: Faith and Hope in an Evangelical Black Storefront Church*. Columbia: University of South Carolina Press, 1995.

Kotlowitz, Alex. *There Are No Children Here: The Story of Two Boys Growing Up in the Other America*. New York: Anchor Books, 1992.

Kunjufu, Jawanza. *Countering the Conspiracy to Destroy Blacks Boys*. 2 vols. Chicago: African-American Images, 1985–86.

Kwon, Ho-Youn, Kwang Chung Kim, and R. Stephen Warner, eds. *Korean Americans and Their Religions*. University Park: Pennsylvania State University Press, 2000.

La Brack, Bruce. *The Sikhs of Northern California 1904–1975*. New York: AMS, 1988.

Laderman, Gary, ed. *Religions of Atlanta: Religious Diversity in the Centennial Olympic City.* Atlanta: Scholars, 1996.

Lamont, Michele, and Marcel Fournier, eds. *Cultivating Differences: Symbolic Boundaries and the Making of Inequality.* Chicago: University of Chicago Press, 1992.

Landry, Bart. *The New Black Middle Class.* Berkeley: University of California Press, 1987.

Lasch, Christopher. *The Culture of Narcissism.* New York: W. W. Norton, 1978.

Lawrence, Beverly H. *Reviving the Spirit: A Generation of African Americans Goes Home to the Church.* New York: Grove, 1996.

Lemann, Nicholas. "Stressed Out in Suburbia." *Atlantic Monthly,* November 1989, 34–48.

———. *The Promised Land: The Great Black Migration and How It Changed America.* New York: Knopf, 1991.

Lerner, Michael. *The Politics of Meaning: Restoring Hope and Possibility in an Age of Cynicism.* Reading, MA: Addison-Wesley, 1996.

Levitt, Peggy. "Local-Level Global Religion: The Case of U.S. Dominican Migration." *Journal for the Scientific Study of Religion* 37, no. 1 (1988): 74–89.

Lewis, James W. *The Protestant Experience in Gary, Indiana, 1906–1975: At Home in the City.* Knoxville: University of Tennessee Press, 1992.

Lincoln, C. Eric. *The Black Church since Frazier.* New York: Schocken Books, 1974.

———. "Black Methodists and the Middle-Class Mentality." In *Experiences, Struggles, and Hopes of the Black Church,* edited by James S. Gadsen, 58–68. Nashville, TN: Tidings, 1975.

Lincoln, C. Eric, and Lawrence H. Mamiya. *The Black Church in the African American Experience.* Durham, NC: Duke University Press, 1990.

Linnan, John, C.S.V. "Re-thinking the Urban Parish." Unpublished manuscript, 1995.

Liptak, Dolores. *Immigrants and Their Church.* New York: Macmillan, 1989.

Livezey, Lois Gehr. "The Fourth Presbyterian Church of Chicago: One Congregation's Response to the Challenges of Family Life in Urban America." In *Tending the Flock: Congregations and Family Ministry,* edited by K. Brynolf Lyon and Archie Smith Jr., 119–144. Louisville, KY: Westminster John Knox, 1998.

Livezey, Lowell W., ed. *Religious Organizations and Structural Change in Metropolitan Chicago: The Research Report of the Religion in Urban America Program.* Chicago: Office of Social Science Research, University of Illinois at Chicago, 1996.

Lydersen, Kari. "Lawsuits Claim Realtors Pander to Racial Fears." *Streetwise,* 22 December 1998, 5.

Mamiya, Lawrence H. "A Social History of the Bethel African Methodist Episcopal Church in Baltimore: The House of God and the Struggle for Freedom." In

American Congregations, vol. 1: The Portraits of Twelve Religious Communities, edited by James P. Wind and James W. Lewis, 221–293. Chicago: University of Chicago Press, 1994.

Manning, Robert D., and Anita C. Butera. "From City to Suburbia: The 'New' Immigration, Native Minorities, and the Post-Industrial Metropolis." American Sociological Association Meeting, New York, 19 August 1996.

Marciniak, Edward, and William Droel. "The Future of Catholic Churches in the Inner City." *Chicago Studies* 34 (2 August 1995): 172–186.

Marty, Martin E. *The Public Church: Mainline-Evangelical-Catholic.* New York: Crossroad, 1981.

———. "Public and Private: Congregation as Meeting Place." In *American Congregations, vol. 2: New Perspectives in the Study of Congregations,* edited by James P. Wind and James W. Lewis, 133–166. Chicago: University of Chicago Press, 1994.

Massey, Douglas, Rafael Alarcón, Jorge Durand, and Humberto Gonzalez. *Return to Aztlan: The Social Process of International Migration from Western Mexico.* Berkeley: University of California Press, 1987.

Mathews, Donald G. "The Second Great Awakening as an Organizing Process, 1780–1830: An Hypothesis." *American Quarterly* 21 (Spring 1969): 23–43.

Mays, Benjamin E., and Joseph W. Nicholson. *The Negro's Church.* New York: Arno, 1969.

McAlister, Elizabeth. "The Madonna of 115th Street Revisited: Vodou and Haitian Catholicism in the Age of Transnationalism." In *Gatherings in Diaspora: Religious Communities and the New Immigration,* edited by R. Stephen Warner and Judith G. Wittner, 123–160. Philadelphia: Temple University Press, 1998.

McClain, William B. "What Is Authentic Black Worship?" In *Experiences, Struggles, and Hopes of the Black Church,* edited by James S. Gadsen, 69–84. Nashville, TN: Tidings, 1975.

McCready, William C. "Catholic Schools and Catholic Identity: Stretching the Vital Connection." *Chicago Studies* 28 (November 1989): 217–231.

McGreevy, John. "Faith and Morals in the U.S., 1865–Present." *Reviews in American History* 26 (1998): 239–254.

———. *Parish Boundaries: The Catholic Encounter with Race in the Twentieth-Century Urban North.* Chicago: University of Chicago Press, 1996.

McRoberts, Omar M. "Understanding the 'New' Black Pentecostal Activism: Lessons from Ecumenical Urban Ministries in Boston." *Sociology of Religion* 60, no. 1 (March 1999): 47–70.

Meyers, Eleanor Scott, ed. *Envisioning the New City: A Reader on Urban Ministry.* Louisville, KY: Westminster John Knox, 1992.

Minocha, Urmil. "South Asian Immigrants: Trends and Impacts on the Sending and Receiving Societies." In *Pacific Bridges: The New Immigration from Asia and the Pacific Islands,* edited by James T. Fawcett and Benjamin V. Carino, 347–373. New York: Center for Migration Studies, 1987.

Mitchell, Henry H. "Black Power and the Christian Church." *Foundations* 11 (April–June 1968): 99–109.

Miyakawa, T. Scott. *Protestants and Pioneers: Individualism and Conformity on the American Frontier.* Chicago: University of Chicago Press, 1964.

Moore, Joan. "'Hispanic/Latino': Imposed Label or Real Identity?" *Latino Studies Journal* 1, no. 2 (1990): 33–47.

Mukenge, Ida Rousseau. *The Black Church in Urban America: A Case Study in Political Economy.* Lanham, MD: University Press of America, 1983.

Murnion, Philip J. "Parish: Covenant Community." *Church* 12, no. 1 (March 1996): 7.

———. Review of *The Parish in Catholic Tradition: History, Theology, and Canon Law. Church* 14, no. 4 (Winter 1998): 50.

"The National Black Catholic Congress." *In a Word* 10 (August–September 1992): 2.

Nelson, Ellis. *Where Faith Begins.* Richmond, VA: John Knox, 1967.

Niebuhr, H. Richard. *The Social Sources of Denominationalism.* New York: Henry Holt, 1957.

Novak, Michael. *The Catholic Ethic and the Spirit of Capitalism.* New York: Free Press, 1993.

———. *The Rise of the Unmeltable Ethnic: Politics and Culture in the Seventies.* New York: Macmillan, 1972.

Numrich, Paul D. "Facing Northeast in a Midwestern Metropolis: The Growth of Islam and the Challenge of the Ummatic Ideal in Chicago." In book forthcoming from the Auburn Project on the History of Religion and Urban America, 1875–present. Auburn Theological Seminary, NY.

———. *Old Wisdom in the New World: Americanization in Two Immigrant Theravada Buddhist Temples.* Knoxville: University of Tennessee Press, 1996.

———. "A Pentecostal Megachurch on the Edge: Calvary Church, Naperville, Illinois." In *Tending the Flock: Congregations and Family Ministry,* edited by K. Brynolf Lyon and Archie Smith Jr., 78–97. Louisville, KY: Westminster John Knox, 1998.

———. "Recent Immigrant Religions in a Restructuring Metropolis: New Religious Landscapes in Chicago." *Journal of Cultural Geography* 17, no. 1 (Fall/Winter 1997): 55–76.

Oboler, Suzanne. *Ethnic Labels, Latino Lives: Identity and the Politics of (Re)Presentation in the United States.* Minneapolis: University of Minnesota Press, 1995.

O'Brien, J. Stephen. *Mixed Messages: What Bishops and Priests Say about Catholic Schools.* Washington, DC: National Catholic Education Association, 1987.

Omi, Michael, and Howard Winant. *Racial Formation in the United States: From the 1960's to the 1990's.* New York: Routledge, 1994.

Orellana, Marjorie Faulstich, and Barrie Thorne. "Year-Round Schools and the Politics of Time." *Anthropology and Education Quarterly* 29, no. 4 (1998): 446–471.

O'Rourke, Lawrence M. *Geno: The Life and Mission of Geno Baroni.* New York: Paulist, 1991.

Orr, John B., Donald E. Miller, Wade Clark Roof, and J. Gordon Melton. *Politics of the Spirit—Religion and Multiethnicity in Los Angeles.* Los Angeles: University of Southern California Press, 1994.

Orsi, Robert A. *The Madonna of 115th Street: Faith and Community in Italian Harlem, 1880–1950.* New Haven, CT: Yale University Press, 1985.

———. *Thank You, St. Jude: Women's Devotion to the Patron Saint of Hopeless Causes.* New Haven, CT: Yale University Press, 1996.

Orum, Anthony M. *City-Building in America.* Boulder, CO: Westview, 1995.

Pacyga, Dominic A. "Chicago's Ethnic Neighborhoods: The Myth of Stability and the Reality of Change." In *Ethnic Chicago: A Multicultural Portrait,* edited by Melvin G. Holli and Peter d'A. Jones, 4th ed., 604–617. Grand Rapids, MI: William B. Eerdmans, 1995.

Pacyga, Dominic A., and Ellen Skerrett. *Chicago: City of Neighborhoods.* Chicago: Loyola University Press, 1986.

Padilla, Felix M. *Latino Ethnic Consciousness: The Case of Mexican Americans and Puerto Ricans in Chicago.* Notre Dame, IN: University of Notre Dame Press, 1985.

Paris, Arthur E. *Black Pentecostalism: Southern Religion in an Urban World.* Amherst: University of Massachusetts Press, 1982.

Paris, Peter J. *Black Religious Leaders: Conflict in Unity.* Louisville, KY: Westminster John Knox, 1991.

———. *The Social Teaching of the Black Churches.* Philadelphia: Fortress, 1985.

Park, Robert E. "The City as a Social Laboratory." In *Chicago: An Experiment in Social Science Research,* edited by T. V. Smith and Leonard D. White. Chicago: University of Chicago Press, 1968.

Park, Robert E., and Ernest W. Burgess. *The City.* Chicago: University of Chicago Press, 1925.

Park, Robert E., and Herbert A. Miller. *Old World Traits Transplanted.* Salem, NH: Ayer, 1921.

Parot, John Joseph. *Polish Catholics in Chicago, 1850–1920: A Religious History.* De Kalb: Northern Illinois University Press, 1981.

Parsons, Talcott. "Age and Sex in the Social Structure of the United States." *American Sociological Review* 7 (October 1942): 604–616.

"Pastoral Constitution on the Church in the Modern World." In *Catholic Social Thought: The Documentary Heritage,* edited by David J. O'Brien and Thomas A. Shannon, 166–237. Maryknoll, NY: Orbis Books, 1992.

Pattillo, Mary E. "Sweet Mothers and Gangbangers: Managing Crime in a Black Middle-Class Neighborhood." *Social Forces* 76 (March 1998):747–774.

Philpott, Thomas Lee. *The Slum and the Ghetto*. New York: Oxford University Press, 1978.

Policy Research Action Group. *The Black Churches of West Humboldt Park*. Chicago: DePaul University, January 1999.

Portes, Alejandro, and Rubén G. Rumbaut. *Immigrant America: A Portrait*. Berkeley: University of California Press, 1990.

Provost, James, and Knut Walf, eds. *Catholic Identity*. Concilium 5. New York: Orbis Books, 1994.

Putnam, Robert D. "Bowling Alone: America's Declining Social Capital." *Journal of Democracy* 6, no. 1 (January 1995): 65–78.

———. "The Prosperous Community." *American Prospect* (March 1993): 5–19.

Racially and Ethnically Diverse Urban Neighborhoods. Cityscape: A Journal of Policy and Research 4, no. 2 (1998): 1–269. Special issue.

Rangaswamy, Padma. "Asian Indians in Chicago: Growth and Change in a Model Minority." In *Ethnic Chicago: A Multicultural Portrait,* edited by Melvin G. Holli, and Peter d'A. Jones, 4th ed., 438–462. Grand Rapids, MI: William B. Eerdmans, 1995.

Ranney, David C. "Transnational Investment and Job Loss in Chicago." In *Chicago's Future in a Time of Change,* edited by Dick Simpson, 88–98. Champaign, IL: Stipes, 1993.

Reardon, Patrick T. "The New Geography." *Chicago Tribune Magazine* 10, 5 November 1995: 15–28.

Reese, Thomas J. *Archbishop: Inside the Power Structure of the American Catholic Church*. New York: Harper & Row, 1989.

Reimers, David M. *Still the Golden Door: The Third World Comes to America*. New York: Columbia University Press, 1992.

Reynolds, Charles H., and Ralph V. Norman, eds. *Community in America: The Challenge of Habits of the Heart*. Berkeley: University of California Press, 1988.

Richesin, L. Dale. "Eighty Years of Ministry 1907–1987." In *1988–1990 Greater Chicago Religions Directory and Buyers Guide,* edited by L. Dale Richesin, 153–170. Chicago: Church Federation of Greater Chicago, 1988.

Rieder, Jonathan. *Canarsie: The Jews and Italians of Brooklyn against Liberalism*. Cambridge, MA: Harvard University Press, 1985.

Rieff, Philip. *The Triumph of the Therapeutic*. New York: Harper & Row, 1966.

Rivers, Clarence Joseph. *Soulful Worship*. Washington, DC: National Office for Black Catholics, 1974.

Roeser, Thomas R. "A Letter from Chicago: Is America's Greatest Archdiocese Really in Decline?" *Crisis: A Journal of Catholic Lay Opinion* 12 (July 1994): 43–47.

Roozen, David A., William McKinney, and Jackson W. Carroll. *Varieties of Religious Presence: Mission in Public Life.* New York: Pilgrim, 1984.

Rouse, Roger. "Mexican Migration and the Social Space of Postmodernism." *Diaspora* 1, no. 1 (1991): 8–23.

———. "Questions of Identity: Personhood and Collectivity in Transnational Migration to the United States." *Critique of Anthropology* 15, no. 4 (1995): 351–380.

Rumbaut, Rubén G. "Passages to America: Perspectives on the New Immigration." In *America at Century's End,* edited by Alan Wolfe, 208–244. Berkeley: University of California Press, 1991.

Sánchez, George J. *Becoming Mexican American: Ethnicity, Culture, and Identity in Chicano Los Angeles, 1900–1945.* New York: Oxford University Press, 1993.

Sandel, Michael J. *Democracy's Discontent: America in Search of a Public Philosophy.* Cambridge, MA: Belknap Press of Harvard University Press, 1996.

Sanders, Cheryl J. *Saints in Exile: The Holiness-Pentecostal Experience in African American Religion and Culture.* New York: Oxford University Press, 1996.

Sanders, James W. *The Education of an Urban Minority: Catholic in Chicago, 1822–1965.* New York: Oxford University Press, 1977.

Sandoval, Moises. *On the Move: A History of the Hispanic Church in the United States.* Maryknoll, NY: Orbis Books, 1990.

Schaller, Lyle E. "Foreword." In *Downtown Church: The Heart of the City,* by Howard Edington. Nashville, TN: Abingdon, 1996.

Schiller, Nina Glick, Linda Basch, and Cristina Blanc-Szanton. "From Immigrant to Transmigrant: Theorizing Transnational Migration." *Anthropology Quarterly* 68, no. 1 (January 1995): 48–63.

———. "Transnationalism: A New Analytic Framework for Understanding Migration." In *Towards a Transnational Perspective on Migration: Race, Class, Ethnicity, and Nationalism Reconsidered,* edited by Nina Glick Schiller, Linda Basch, and Cristina Blanc-Szantin, 1–24. Annals of the New York Academy of Sciences, vol. 645. New York: New York Academy of Sciences, 1992.

Schlesinger, Arthur M., Jr. *The Disuniting of America: Reflections on a Multicultural Society.* New York: W. W. Norton, 1992.

Schreiter, Robert J. "Faith and Cultures: Challenges to a World Church." *Theological Studies* 50 (1989): 744–760.

Schroeder, W. Widick, and Victor Obenhaus. *Religion in American Culture: Unity and Diversity in a Midwestern County.* New York: Free Press of Glencoe, 1964.

Schuster, Elaine. "A Study of the Local School Long-Range Planning Process in the Archdiocese of Chicago." Ph.D. diss., University of Illinois at Chicago, 1987.

Scott, Daryl Michael. *Contempt and Pity: Social Policy and the Image of the Damaged Black Psyche, 1880–1996.* Chapel Hill: University of North Carolina Press, 1997.

Scroggs, Marilee Munger. "Making a Difference: Fourth Presbyterian Church of Chicago." In *American Congregations*, vol. 1: *Portraits of Twelve Religious Communities*, edited by James P. Wind and James W. Lewis, 464–519. Chicago: University of Chicago Press, 1994.

Sennett, Richard, ed. *Classic Essays on the Culture of Cities*. Englewood Cliffs, NJ: Prentice-Hall, 1969.

Sewell, William H., Jr. "A Theory of Structure: Duality, Agency, and Transformation." *American Journal of Sociology* 98, no. 1 (July 1992): 1–29.

Shanabruch, Charles. *Chicago's Catholics: The Evolution of an American Identity*. Notre Dame Studies in American Catholicism 4. Notre Dame, IN: University of Notre Dame Press, 1981.

Shaw, Stephen J. *The Catholic Parish as a Way-Station of Ethnicity and Americanization: Chicago's Germans and Italians, 1903–1939*. New York: Carlson, 1991.

Simpson, Dick, ed. *Chicago's Future in a Time of Change*, Champaign, IL: Stipes, 1993.

Skerrett, Ellen, ed. *At the Crossroads: Old Saint Patrick's and the Chicago Irish*. Chicago: Wild Onion, 1997.

Skerrett, Ellen, Edward R. Kantowicz, and Steven M. Avella. *Catholicism: Chicago Style*. Chicago: Loyola University Press, 1993.

Sklare, Marshall. "The Conservative Movement: Achievements and Problems." In *The Jewish Community in America*, edited by Marshall Sklare, 175–192. New York: Behrman House, 1974.

Slater, Philip E. *The Pursuit of Loneliness: American Culture at the Breaking Point*. Boston: Beacon, 1970.

Slayton, Robert A. *Back of the Yards: The Making of a Local Democracy*. Chicago: University of Chicago Press, 1986.

Smith, Carl S. *Urban Disorder and the Shape of Belief: The Great Chicago Fire, the Haymarket Bomb, and the Model Town of Pullman*. Chicago: University of Chicago Press, 1995.

Smith, Gary Scott. "When Stead Came to Chicago: The 'Social Gospel Novel' and the Chicago Civic Federation." *American Presbyterian* 68 (1990): 193–205.

Soja, Edward W. *Postmodern Geographies: The Reassertion of Space in Critical Social Theory*. New York: Verso, 1989.

Soja, Edward, Rebecca Morales, and Goetz Wolff. "Urban Restructuring: An Analysis of Social and Spatial Change in Los Angeles." *Economic Geography* 59 (1983): 195–230.

Sollors, Werner, ed. *The Invention of Ethnicity*. New York: Oxford University Press, 1989.

Soot, Siim, Ashish Sen, Kevin Curtin, and Paul Metaxatos. "Analysis of Employment Hubs and Work Trip Patterns in the Chicago Metropolitan Region." Urban Transportation Center, University of Illinois at Chicago, Chicago, 12 October 1994.

Spalding, David. "The Negro Catholic Congresses, 1889–1894." *Catholic Historical Review* 55 (1969): 337–357.

Squires, Gregory D. *Capital and Communities in Black and White: The Intersections of Race, Class, and Uneven Development.* Albany: State University of New York Press, 1994.

Squires, Gregory D., Larry Bennett, Kathleen McCourt, and Philip Nyden. *Chicago: Race, Class, and the Response to Urban Decline.* Comparative American Cities series, edited by Joe T. Darden. Philadelphia: Temple University Press, 1987.

Stacey, Judith. *Brave New Families: Stories of Domestic Upheaval in Late Twentieth Century America.* New York: Basic Books, 1990.

Stark, Robert. "Religious Ritual and Class Formation: The Story of Pilsen, St. Vitus Parish and the 1977 Via Crucis." Ph.D. diss., University of Chicago Divinity School, 1981.

Stead, William T. *If Christ Came to Chicago! A Plea for the Union of All Who Love in the Service of All Who Suffer.* Chicago: Laird & Lee, 1894.

Stockwell, Clinton E. "A Better Class of People: Protestants in the Making of Early Chicago." Ph.D. diss., University of Illinois at Chicago, 1992.

———. "Graham Taylor—Urban Pioneer." *Chicago Theological Seminary Register* 86, no. 1 (December 1996): 1–23.

Stout, Harry S. "The Place of Religion in Urban and Community Studies." *Religion and American Culture: A Journal of Interpretation* 6, no. 2 (June 1996): 110–122.

Sugrue, Thomas J. *The Origins of the Urban Crisis.* Princeton, NJ: Princeton University Press, 1996.

Suttles, Gerald D. *The Social Construction of Communities.* Chicago: University of Chicago Press, 1972.

———. *The Social Order of the Slum: Ethnicity and Territory in the Inner City.* Chicago: University of Chicago Press, 1968.

Swidler, Ann. "Culture in Action: Symbols and Strategies." *American Sociological Review* 51 (1986): 273–286.

Takaki, Ronald. *Strangers from a Different Shore: A History of Asian Americans.* Boston: Little, Brown, 1989.

Taub, Richard P., D. Garth Taylor, and Jan D. Dunham. *Paths of Neighborhood Change: Race and Crime in Urban America.* Chicago: University of Chicago Press, 1984.

Taylor, Charles. *Multiculturalism: Examining the Politics of Recognition.* Princeton, NJ: Princeton University Press, 1992.

Thompson, Richard H. *Theories of Ethnicity: A Critical Appraisal.* New York: Greenwood, 1989.

Tipton, Steven M. *Getting Saved from the Sixties: Moral Meaning in Conversion and Cultural Change.* Berkeley: University of California Press, 1982.

Todd, George C. "Presbyterian Ministry in Urban America, 1945–1980." In *Churches, Cities, and Human Community: Urban Ministry in the United States 1945–1985*, edited by Clifford J. Green, 151–178. Grand Rapids, MI: William B. Eerdmans, 1996.

Tomasi, Silvano M., C.S. "A Lesson from History: The Integration of Immigrants in the Pastoral Practice of the Church in the United States." *CMS: Occasional Papers: Pastoral Series* 7 (1987).

———. *Piety and Power: The Role of the Italian Parishes in the New York Metropolitan Area, 1880–1930*. New York: Center for Migration Studies, 1975.

———. "The Response of the Catholic Church in the United States to Immigrants and Refugees." *CMS: Occasional Papers: Pastoral Series* 3 (August 1984).

Tomorrow's Parish: Criteria for Planning. Chicago: Office of Research and Planning, Archdiocese of Chicago, 1993.

Tomorrow's Parish: Guide for Planning. Chicago: Office of Research and Planning, Archdiocese of Chicago, 1993.

Towsley, Genevieve. "A View of Historic Naperville from the Sky-Lines: A Collection of Articles of Historic Significance." *Naperville Sun*, 1975.

Travis, Dempsey J. *An Autobiography of Black Politics*. Volume 1. Chicago: Urban Research Press, 1987.

———. *"Harold" the People's Mayor: An Authorized Biography of Mayor Harold Washington*. Chicago: Urban Research Press, 1989.

Troy, Leander, O. Carm. *The Dandelion Bishop: Nevin Hayes of Chicago*. Chicago: Croatian Franciscan Press, 1994.

Tutor/Mentor Connection 2 (September 1994).

U.S. Bureau of the Census. *1990 Census of Population and Housing*. Summary tape file 3. September 1992.

Van Engen, Charles. "Constructing a Theology of Mission for the City." In *God So Loves the City: Seeking a Theology for Urban Mission*, edited by Charles Van Engen and Jude Tiersma, 241–269. Monrovia, CA: Mission Advanced Research and Communication Center, 1994.

Van Engen, Charles, and Jude Tiersma, eds. *God So Loves the City: Seeking a Theology for Urban Mission*. Monrovia, CA: Mission Advanced Research and Communication Center, 1994.

Vecoli, Rudolph J. "Prelates and Peasants: Italian Immigrants and the Catholic Church." *Journal of Social History* 2 (March 1969): 217–268.

Verba, Sidney, Kay Lehman Schlozman, and Henry E. Brady. *Voice and Equality: Civic Voluntarism in American Politics*. Cambridge, MA: Harvard University Press, 1995.

Villafañe, Eldin. *The Liberating Spirit: Toward an Hispanic American Pentecostal Social Ethic*. Lanham, MD: University Press of America, 1992.

———. *Seek the Peace of the City: Reflections on Urban Ministry*. Grand Rapids, MI: William B. Eerdmans, 1995.

Walch, Timothy. *The Diverse Origins of American Catholic Education: Chicago, Milwaukee and the Nation.* New York: Garland, 1988.

Waldinger, Roger. "Immigration and Urban Change." *Annual Review of Sociology* 15 (1989): 211–232.

Wall, A. E. P. *The Spirit of Cardinal Bernardin.* Chicago: Thomas Moore, 1983.

Wallwork, Ernest. "A Constructive Freudian Alternative to Psychotherapeutic Egoism." In *Community in America: The Challenge of Habits of the Heart,* edited by Charles H. Reynolds and Ralph V. Norman, 202–216. Berkeley: University of California Press, 1988.

Warner, R. Stephen. "Changes in the Civic Role of Religion." In *Diversity and Its Discontents: Cultural Conflict and Common Ground in Contemporary American Society,* edited by Neil J. Smelser and Jeffrey C. Alexander, 229–243. Princeton, NJ: Princeton University Press, 1999.

————. "The Metropolitan Community Churches and the Gay Agenda: The Power of Pentecostalism and Essentialism." In *Sex, Lies, and Sanctity: Religion and Deviance in Contemporary North America,* edited by Mary Jo Neitz and Marion S. Goldman, 81–108. Greenwich, CT: JAI Press, 1995.

————. *New Wine in Old Wineskins: Evangelicals and Liberals in a Small-Town Church.* Berkeley: University of California Press, 1988.

————. "The Place of the Congregation in the Contemporary American Religious Configuration." In *American Congregations,* vol. 2: *New Perspectives in the Study of Congregations,* edited by James P. Wind and James W. Lewis, 54–99. Chicago: University of Chicago Press, 1994.

————. "Work in Progress toward a New Paradigm for the Sociological Study of Religion in the United States." *American Journal of Sociology* 98, no. 5 (March 1993): 1044.

Warner, R. Stephen, and Judith G. Wittner, eds. *Gatherings in Diaspora: Religious Communities and the New Immigration.* Philadelphia: Temple University Press, 1998.

Warner, Sam Bass, Jr. *The Urban Wilderness: A History of the American City.* New York: Harper & Row, 1972.

Washington, Joseph R. *Black Sects and Cults.* Garden City, NY: Doubleday Anchor Books, 1973.

Wedam, Elfriede, and Stephen R. Warner. "Sacred Space on Tuesday: A Study of the Institutionalization of Charisma." In *"I Come Away Stronger": How Small Groups Are Shaping American Religion,* edited by Robert Wuthnow, 148–178. Grand Rapids, MI: William B. Eerdmans, 1994.

Wellman, James K. Jr. "Boundaries of Taste: A Gold Coast Church and Cabrini Green." Unpublished manuscript, 19 February 1994.

————. "A Counter-Example of Liberal Protestant Decline: A Case-Study of an Elite Downtown Protestant Church." Paper presented at the Association for the Sociology of Religion, Los Angeles, CA, August, 1994.

West, Cornel. *Race Matters*. Boston: Beacon, 1993.

Whyte, William H. *The Organization Man*. New York: Simon and Schuster, 1956.

Williams, Melvin D. *Community in a Black Pentecostal Church: An Anthropological Study*. Pittsburgh: University of Pittsburgh Press, 1974.

Williams, Raymond Brady. *Religions of Immigrants from India and Pakistan: New Threads in the American Tapestry*. New York and Cambridge: Cambridge University Press, 1988.

——. *A Sacred Thread: Modern Transmissions of Hindu Traditions in India and Abroad*. Chambersburg, PA: Anima, 1992.

Williams, Rhys H. "Religion as Political Resource: Culture or Ideology?" *Journal for the Scientific Study of Religion* 35, no. 4 (1996): 368–378.

Williams, Rhys, and Fred Kniss. "Approaching Religion as Culture." *Newsletter of the Sociology of Culture* 8, no. 1 (December 1994): 1, 5–8.

Wilson, Nancy L. *Our Tribe: Queer Folks, God, Jesus, and the Bible*. San Francisco: Harper Collins, 1995.

Wilson, William Julius. *The Truly Disadvantaged: The Inner City, the Underclass, and Public Policy*. Chicago: University of Chicago Press, 1987.

——. *When Work Disappears: The World of the New Urban Poor*. New York: Alfred A. Knopf, 1996.

——, ed. *The Ghetto Underclass: Social Science Perspectives*, Newbury Park, CA: Sage, 1993.

Wind, James P. *Places of Worship: Exploring Their History*. Nashville, TN: American Association for State and Local History, 1990.

Wind, James P., and James W. Lewis. "Memory, Amnesia, and History." In *Carriers of Faith: Lessons from Congregational Studies*, edited by Carl S. Dudley, Jackson W. Carroll, and James P. Wind, 15–39. Louisville, KY: Westminster John Knox, 1991.

——, eds. *American Congregations*. vol. 1, *Portraits of Twelve Religious Communities*. vol. 2, *New Perspectives in the Study of Congregations*. Chicago: University of Chicago Press, 1994.

Winter, Gibson. *The Suburban Captivity of the Churches: An Analysis of Protestant Responsibility in the Expanding Metropolis*. New York: Macmillan, 1962.

Wirth, Louis. *The Ghetto*. Chicago: University of Chicago Press, 1928.

——. "Urbanism as a Way of Life." In *Classic Essays on the Culture of Cities*, edited by Richard Sennett, 143–164. Englewood Cliffs, NJ: Prentice-Hall, 1969.

"Without Sweeps, CHA Crime Might Be Worse." *Chicago Tribune*, 26 October 1992, sec. 1, p. 9.

Wolfe, Alan, ed. *America at Century's End*. Berkeley: University of California Press, 1991.

Wuthnow, Robert. *Loose Connections: Joining Together in America's Fragmented Communities*. Cambridge, MA: Harvard University Press, 1998.

Wuthnow, Robert. *Meaning and Moral Order: Explorations in Cultural Analysis.* Berkeley: University of California Press, 1987.

———. *Producing the Sacred.* Chicago: University of Illinois Press, 1994.

———. *Restructuring of American Religion,* Princeton, NJ: Princeton University Press, 1988.

———, ed. *"I Come Away Stronger": How Small Groups Are Shaping American Religion.* Grand Rapids, MI: William B. Eerdmans, 1994.

Xenos, Peter, Herbert Barringer, and Michael J. Levin, *Asian Indians in the United States: A 1980 Census Profile.* Honolulu: East-West Population Institute, 1989.

Young, Iris Marion. *Justice and the Politics of Difference.* Princeton, NJ: Princeton University Press, 1990.

Younger, George D. *The Church and Urban Power Structure: Christian Perspectives on Social Problems.* Philadelphia: Westminster, 1952.

Zenner, Walter P. "Chicago's Sephardim: A Historical Exploration." *Chicago Jewish History* 12, no. 3 (March 1989).

Zorbaugh, Harvey Warren. *The Gold Coast and the Slum: A Sociological Study of Chicago's Near North Side.* Chicago: University of Chicago Press, 1929.

Zukin, Sharon. *The Cultures of Cities.* Cambridge, MA: Blackwell, 1995.

———. "The Hollow Center." In *America at Century's End,* edited by Alan Wolfe, 245–261. Berkeley: University of California Press, 1991.

———. *Landscapes of Power: From Detroit to Disney World.* Berkeley: University of California Press, 1991.

Contributors

Peter R. D'Agostino
Assistant Professor of History and Religious Studies, Stonehill College

David D. Daniels III
Associate Professor of Church History, McCormick Theological Seminary

Janise D. Hurtig
Postdoctoral Research Associate, Center for Research on Women and Gender, University of Illinois at Chicago

Isaac B. Laudarji
Pastor, Evangelical Church of West Africa

Lowell W. Livezey
Director, Religion in Urban America Program, University of Illinois at Chicago

Paul D. Numrich
Research Associate, The Park Ridge Center for the Study of Health, Faith, and Ethics

Matthew J. Price
Postdoctoral Fellow, J. M. Ormond Center, Duke University Divinity School

R. Stephen Warner
Professor of Sociology, University of Illinois at Chicago

Elfriede Wedam
Senior Research Associate, The Polis Center, and Adjunct Assistant Professor of Sociology, Indiana University–Purdue University at Indianapolis

Index

Page numbers followed by f refer to figures; page numbers followed by t refer to tables.